Cultural Responsiveness in Assisted Reproductive Technology

Danielle A. Kaplan
Editor

Cultural Responsiveness in Assisted Reproductive Technology

Best Practices for Clinics and Affiliated Providers

Springer

Editor
Danielle A. Kaplan
Department of Psychiatry
NYU Langone Medical Center
New York, NY, USA

ISBN 978-3-031-76203-1 ISBN 978-3-031-76204-8 (eBook)
https://doi.org/10.1007/978-3-031-76204-8

This Springer imprint is published by the registered company Springer Nature Switzerland AG
The registered company address is: Gewerbestrasse 11, 6330 Cham, Switzerland

It is not enough to be compassionate. You must act. There are two aspects to action. One is to overcome the distortions and afflictions of your own mind... This is action out of compassion. The other is more social, more public. When something needs to be done in the world to rectify the wrongs, if one is really concerned with benefitting others, one needs to be engaged, involved.

—Dalai Lama, XIV

Preface

This book speaks in many voices. Some are data-heavy, replete with information about the neurological correlates of behavior or research-driven findings on pregnancy outcomes after ART. Some are deeply personal, speaking from the experience of giving birth in a Black body, being labeled with new descriptors and identities after emigrating, or celebrating holidays and passing on traditions to the next generation.

Some of these voices agree, amplifying each other in the call to diversify representation in reproductive healthcare and challenge our assumptions about the patients we serve. Sometimes they argue. In some chapters, you will read about the need to recognize and challenge our implicit biases. Others question whether these biases are so implicit after all, and whether our time and energy wouldn't be better spent on advocacy, increasing access to care, and establishing procedural safeguards and protocols to increase the odds that all patients have an equitable experience of reproductive healthcare. As the young people say, it's complicated.

That's because race, ethnicity, and culture are complicated. Although I am honored to have had the participation of international contributors, this book is primarily written by authors who live and practice in the United States. The United States isn't the most diverse country in the world. By measures of fractionalization—the odds that any two randomly selected people in a country will differ by ethnicity, religion, or language—that's Uganda. The United States isn't even in the top ten, coming in well behind most of Africa and comfortably behind Mexico, Tajikistan, and Malaysia.

However, the United States is perhaps unique in being both a country of ever-increasing diversity and one whose structures and systems confer enduring advantages for a small subset of its population—primarily those who are cisgender, heterosexual, able-bodied, and White. In many ways, reproductive and infertility care mirror this contradiction. The population seeking infertility care is changing; ART clinics now routinely see patients who hold a multiplicity of identities, all of whom desire parenthood. However, there is a gap between the demographics of the patients in need of treatment and our understanding of how to meet their cultural, linguistic, and medical needs to improve their outcomes in care.

The process of researching and editing this volume has made several points clear. First, the experiences of diverse patients in reproductive care cannot be discussed in isolation. Rather, patients come to infertility treatment with the full weight of history—both their own and those of the groups with which they identify—behind them. Intergenerational experiences of inequitable health care practices impact the overall health and fertility of marginalized populations. Relatedly, they impact providers' learned biases about patients and patients' expectations of their providers. These factors collude to lead to inequitable access and worse outcomes in infertility care for patients from many marginalized groups. Even among patients whose outcomes in ART care are more favorable, providers' lack of cultural responsiveness can still leave them feeling unheard or poorly understood.

It is therefore clear that ameliorating healthcare disparities for patients in infertility care requires coordinated efforts. Throughout this book, you will read about proposed interventions at the level of the individual practitioner, the clinic, and the larger systems with which patients interface. These include schools, insurers, and the overall system of healthcare. Chapter authors exhort providers to engage in self-reflection and individual behavioral change, and clinics and training programs to reexamine their intake procedures and criteria for admission. All of us are asked to serve as advocates and allies for patients whose voices are less likely to be heard by systems that were not designed to serve them. All these interventions are necessary. None of them alone is sufficient.

The information presented in this book is not comprehensive. Much work remains to capture the experiences and needs of the increasingly diverse patient populations that hope to grow their families through ART. Underscored throughout this volume is the need for researchers in reproductive endocrinology and infertility (REI) to recruit study participants who mirror the diversity of the US population (and those of other nations). In particular, the reader will note the absence of a chapter reviewing research on infertility care for Asian American patients. Comprising just over seven percent of the US population, the category of Asian American encompasses a wide variety of countries of heritage, socioeconomic circumstances, and cultural values. It is not uncommon for anyone who shares this census designation, however, to be subjected to the myth of the "model minority" and, consequently, to have their experiences of racism and discrimination overlooked. I regret any similar consequences of the absence of a chapter on Asian Americans in infertility care in this volume, which is due solely to the complexity of capturing the experiences of such a diverse set of patients in a single chapter.

Incorporating diverse populations in research is generally considered in terms of race and ethnicity; however, truly purposive sampling would also require the participation of sexual and gender minorities, members of diverse religious groups, neurodivergent individuals, and patients who hold intersectional marginalized identities. It is my hope that researchers will take up the call to diversify their samples and that the next iteration of this work will be informed by more comprehensive data on infertility care for patients with additional diverse identities. I am grateful to the researchers and healthcare professionals who began the dialogue about cultural responsiveness in ART care. I invite you, the reader, to continue the conversation.

New York, NY, USA Danielle A. Kaplan

Acknowledgments

I am deeply indebted to the chapter authors, who gave freely of their knowledge and time to contribute to this volume. The authors are anthropologists, educators, medical residents and fellows, nurse educators, psychologists, reproductive endocrinologists, and social workers. People from these specialties, along with attorneys, embryologists, office staff, and representatives of numerous other professions, play critical roles in determining the experiences of diverse patients in reproductive care. I am grateful for their voices here and their dedication to the patients they serve.

I am also grateful to those who worked behind the scenes to provide input and feedback on the writing that appears in this book. Thank you to Bill Petok, Eleanor Stevenson, and Jennifer Matta Wood, herself a contributor to this volume, for helping to secure the participation of some key contributors to this endeavor, and to Drs. Marcia Inhorn and Soraya Tremayne for graciously giving me permission to reprint their seminal work on Muslims in ART. Joelle Ehre, Karima Clayton Forbes, Sarah Katz, Raoul Meyer, and my husband, Alan Wolpert, were instrumental in insuring that the information you are about to read is both factually accurate and emotionally honest about the complexity of providing equitable care to marginalized patients. Thanks are especially due to Kristopher Spring, Lillie Mae Gaurano, and Swathiga Karthikeyan at Springer Nature for their patience and collaboration in bringing this volume into existence. Any remaining errors are my responsibility.

The inspiration for this work comes from two sources. The first is the lived experiences of the many patients whose journey through reproductive and infertility care I have supported in my role as a clinical psychologist. I am grateful to them for their vulnerability in sharing their journeys with me, their courage in pursuing treatment in systems that do not always recognize their experiences, and their willingness to let me hold their babies in session. The second is the work I have done through the Mental Health Professionals Group (MHPG) of the American Society for Reproductive Medicine. My participation as a member of MHPG, and especially its Anti-Racism and Inclusion Task Force, has given me far more than I have given in return. Many thanks to my colleagues and dear friends in MHPG for giving me an intellectual home and so much more.

This book is dedicated to all our patients and the families they hope to have, and to my own ART babies, Jonathan and Annalise. It is also dedicated to my grandmother, Norma Fox Odintz, age 97 3/4 at the time of this writing. Grandma, you told me that if I wrote this, you'd buy it. I did it as fast as I could. I love you.

Contents

Part I
Understanding the Issue

Chapter 1
Understanding the Issue: Race, Ethnicity, Culture, and the Structural Determinants of Health

Danielle A. Kaplan

Introduction

The first successful recorded pregnancy achieved via intrauterine insemination (IUI) occurred in 1793, when London physician John Hunter inseminated a woman with the sperm of her husband, who had been diagnosed with hypospadias [1]. Almost 200 years later and about 200 miles further north, Louise Brown became the first baby born via in vitro fertilization (IVF) in 1978 [2]. The intervening years have brought both refinements in assisted reproductive technology techniques and procedures and a dramatic increase in their use. As of 2023, over ten million children have been born through IVF, with the total number of ART cycles exceeding three million per year. Current estimates suggest that between 2 and 4% of children born worldwide are conceived with the help of IVF [3, 4].

For individuals and couples experiencing medical or social infertility, these numbers represent a hopeful trend. However, they also obscure a persistent reality. Across all ages, geographic locations, and socioeconomic statuses, non-Hispanic White and Asian American/Pacific Islander patients are overwhelmingly more likely to access infertility treatment and less likely to discontinue treatment prematurely than are Black, Hispanic, and Native American/Indigenous patients. Among patients of all races and ethnicities who do access care, treatment is also overwhelmingly more likely to result in a live birth among White and AAPI patients [5–8]. Other minoritized groups, such as LGBTQ+ patients and those with disabilities, face similar disparities [9, 10]. These disparities are the result of a confluence of factors that disproportionately impact minoritized and racialized patients irrespective of their other sociodemographic characteristics such as level of education and socioeconomic status.

D. A. Kaplan (✉)
Department of Psychiatry, NYU Langone Medical Center, New York, NY, USA

D. A. Kaplan (ed.), *Cultural Responsiveness in Assisted Reproductive Technology*, https://doi.org/10.1007/978-3-031-76204-8_1

To understand why these disparities exist, it is helpful to begin by considering the myriad internal and external resources required to access ART services at all. Initially, the potential ART patient must recognize that they are struggling to conceive or have a medical or social characteristic that makes it likely that they will have difficulty conceiving. The patient must then know what services to access and, in many cases, receive a referral for specialized care. That care and associated expenses such as medication must be affordable, whether through insurance coverage, fertility grants, or the ability to pay out of pocket. Care must also be accessible, both geographically and linguistically, and the patient must be able to secure an appointment within a reasonable time frame [11, 12]. The potential ART patient must also be able to manage the demands of treatment. This includes being able to arrange their work schedule to accommodate monitoring and procedures, managing the associated stress of treatment, and balancing time spent on treatment with competing psychosocial needs such as caring for aging parents or already-existing children [13].

In all these spheres, there is evidence to suggest that members of marginalized groups face disproportionate challenges when accessing ART services [14–16]. These challenges can result in critical delays in accessing care, leading to worse outcomes for patients who are Black, Indigenous, or People of Color (BIPOC) [17]. Even among patients who can access care in a timely fashion, however, BIPOC and other minoritized patients face additional challenges. Minoritized patients requiring the assistance of gamete donors may be faced with a scarcity of donors who share their heritage, compounding the loss of a genetic connection to their child with the loss of resemblance to the child they conceive. They might struggle to find a medical or mental healthcare provider who understands their experiences with the healthcare system, provides them with treatment options that are consistent with their values, and partners with them in decision making [12, 18, 19]. Some of these patients may ultimately be lost to care entirely, while others find themselves educating the providers whose job it is to care for them.

Across the continuum of infertility care, providers enter the field with the best of intentions and a commitment to providing high-quality care to the patients who seek their services. The remainder of this book focuses on strategies for narrowing the gap between these intentions and the experiences of an increasingly diverse population of patients seeking infertility care. Understanding why the gap exists at all requires us to understand how categories of race, ethnicity and culture were invented and how their use as meaningful identifiers changes the lived experiences and health outcomes of people who are assigned to these categories.

A Brief History of Race and Ethnicity

The concept of race, now used incorrectly as a distinguishing marker of identity, rarely appeared in speech or writing before the 1500s. When it did, it referred to a group of people who were descendants of a common ancestor or held membership in a common group.[1] When referenced at all during this time, "whiteness" was a characteristic held by elite English women, whose pale skin was seen as a reflection of the high social status that exempted them from outdoor labor. Describing a man of the time as "white" would have been seen as an insult, suggesting that he was too lazy or physically infirm to leave his home to work [20].

It was only in the 1600s that conceptions of race began to comprise assumptions about biology, genetics, and phenotypic markers. Historians of race attribute this phenomenon in part to the dawn of the Enlightenment in the late seventeenth century, when it was believed that humans could be classified along with the rest of the natural world according to distinct physical and biological characteristics [21–23]. In the United States, however, the development of racial categories was tied directly to the desire to justify the permanent enslavement and physical and economic exploitation of Africans and their descendants [24, 25]. By categorizing enslaved people as biologically distinct from their enslavers, for example, through spurious claims that people of African descent required less sleep and felt less pain than people of European descent [26, 27], those who benefited politically and economically from the system of slavery could continue to justify its abusive and exploitative practices.

The use of racial categories to justify hierarchy, power, and exclusion was not limited to the system of slavery. As successive waves of immigrants and refugees entered the United States, changes in racial categorizations were used as justification for excluding groups whose presence was believed to represent a threat to the "good order" of the United States. Laws such as the Chinese Exclusion Act of 1882 and restrictions on Italian immigration in the late 19th and early 20th centuries were justified through pseudoscientific claims about the inherent criminality and intellectual and moral inferiority of the groups seeking legal entry [28–30].

Attempts to divide people into distinct categories by race obscure the overwhelming biological and genetic similarity that exists among groups and the significant genetic and phenotypic heterogeneity that exists within any single putative racial or ethnic category [31]. Racial classifications also fail to recognize the fluidity of these categories across geographic, linguistic, and socioeconomic boundaries. For example, among Latin Americans with the same light brown skin color, nearly 70% of Argentines and Uruguayans identified as white, as compared to less than 10% of Bolivians, Dominicans, Ecuadorians, and Peruvians [32]. Similarly, subjects in Brazil presented with photographs of two people with the same skin color describe the person depicted in business attire as being "whiter" than the person depicted in a janitor's uniform [33].

Like race, ethnicity is a concept with fluid and socially constructed boundaries. For example, some estimates suggest that there are over fifty distinct ethnic groups

[1] Thus, the children, grandchildren, and great-grandchildren of John Farmer (occupation, farmer) might have been considered a race unto themselves in medieval Scotland. So might the 3861 people who lived in Canterbury, England in 1377.

in China, each with its own language, culture, religious observance, and geographic origins. In China, a member of one of these groups might identify as Han, Zhuang, Uyghur, or Mongolian. Should they immigrate to the United States, they would likely be identified as either "Chinese" or "Asian"—a category which would also include people whose geographic origins are in Japan, the Philippines, Vietnam, Thailand, or Indonesia [34, 35]. People who identify as Puerto Rican, Mexican, Peruvian, or Argentine may find that their differences in language, diet, religious observance, and traditions are obscured by their shared United States Census designation as "Hispanic/Latino" [36].

Although links have been made in the medical literature between ethnicity and health outcomes (for example, the increased prevalence of sickle cell disease in patients with sub-Saharan and Mediterranean ancestry, or cystic fibrosis in people of Northern European descent), current wisdom suggests that shared geography is a better predictor of genetic differentiation than other shared characteristics of putative race or ethnicity [37–40]. Any contemporary definition of race or ethnicity in medicine, therefore, more accurately refers to the experience of being *minoritized*—that is, the experience of being designated by the larger society in which a person lives as a member of a specific racial or ethnic group subject to differential treatment. As Flanagin and colleagues remind us,

> Race and ethnicity are social constructs, without scientific or biological meaning. The indistinct construct of racial and ethnic categories has been increasingly acknowledged, and concerns about use of these terms in medical and health research, education, and practice have been progressively recognized...The reporting of race and ethnicity should not be considered in isolation but should be accompanied by reporting of other sociodemographic factors and social determinants, including concerns about racism, disparities, and inequities, and the intersectionality of race and ethnicity with these other factors. ([41], p. 621).

Culture

Like many terms that are commonly used but poorly defined, *culture* is at times used as a near synonym for ethnicity or race. Race and ethnicity, however, are categories used primarily to place people in a hierarchy of privilege and access. In contrast, *culture* comprises the values, behaviors, and beliefs chosen through degrees of self-identification with a particular group [42]. Thus, a person can simultaneously celebrate Jewish holidays and embrace Jewish cultural values of education, social justice, *and tikkun olam* (repair of the world) and eschew ritualized religious practice [43]. Similarly, any number of people who share an ethnic designation of "Asian" can differ in their dietary practices, mourning rituals, and help-seeking practices depending on the specific cultures with which they identify [44, 45].

Not all cultural identities are formed through shared familial, ethnic, or geographic origins. For example, many people who are born deaf are exposed to Deaf culture, which values the use of sign language and involves specific communication norms and etiquette, only once they enter a social or educational community of Deaf people [46, 47]. Similarly, not all people who identify as LGBTQIA+ are exposed to the history of the gay rights movement or given a vocabulary with which to describe their identities and experiences unless they have the opportunity for contact with other LGBTQIA+-identified peers and chosen families [48–50].

Culturally responsive infertility care practitioners should be cognizant of the fact that a patient's racial or ethnic designation provides limited information on the factors that may inform their treatment preferences. Like all patient-centered care, culturally responsive care involves a dialogue [51] in which patients' beliefs, preferences, and histories are inquired about rather than assumed.

Intersectionality

Patients presenting for reproductive health and infertility care can hold many identities simultaneously. Law professor and civil rights activist Kimberlé Crenshaw coined the term *intersectionality* to refer to the cumulative effects of holding multiple marginalized identities. Scholars of intersectionality posit that people's experiences of oppression or privilege are shaped by the multiple identities they hold and the ways that people with these identities are viewed by the systems with which they interact. First used to describe the interaction of race and gender as they impact Black women's experiences of employment discrimination and interpersonal violence [52–54], intersectional identities can impact patients' experience of infertility care. For example, a Black patient in a wheelchair may require different physical accommodations than one who can independently transfer to an exam table for an ultrasound. Similarly, a provider working with a transfeminine Latinx patient might use different language when referring to the process of obtaining a semen sample than one working with a cisgender Latino man. For both of these patients, however, race or ethnicity can factor into access to and experiences of infertility care. Although many of the chapters in this book discuss the treatment of patients who hold one minoritized identity, it is important to recognize that many infertility patients belong to more than one marginalized group simultaneously. For these patients, access to infertility care, much less equitable and culturally responsive care, may be particularly limited.

Racism and Bias

Though race and ethnicity hold no essential meaning, living in a racialized or minoritized body has significant implications for the patients we serve. Racialized and minoritized patients can experience bias at the individual, internalized, institutional, and structural levels. Each of these has implications for patients' well-being; in the aggregate, they can compromise patients' mental and physical health and limit their access to timely and high-quality infertility care. Although the majority of the discussion that follows pertains to racism, it applies equally to discriminatory beliefs and practices that result from bias and discrimination against sexual minorities, people with disabilities, or anyone who holds a marginalized identity and is located in a position of relative disadvantage on the hierarchy of power and privilege.

In the popular imagination, racism and bias exist primarily at the *individual* level. When well-intentioned people assert that they "aren't racist," they are likely envisioning acts of exclusion, or verbal or physical aggression directed from one person to another [55, 56]. A White infertility patient who refuses care from a Black nurse is demonstrating individual racism. So, too, is the classmate described by Nicole Chung, a Korean-American adoptee raised in an almost exclusively White town, who writes the following about an interaction she experienced as a child: "I couldn't lie to myself about why I struggled to feel I belonged in my own life; not since the day I'd finally asked a classmate why she didn't like me, and she pulled her eyes back and said, "The same reason no one else likes you." ([57], p. 35).

Racialized and minoritized individuals exist in a larger cultural context in which they are exposed to repeated negative messaging about people who share their characteristics. *Internalized racism* occurs when that messaging is accepted as true by members of the minoritized group, who may then act in a manner consistent with inferior self-definition. High levels of internalized racism are associated with poor mental health outcomes and lower levels of self-esteem among people of color [58, 59] and may be associated with poorer physical health outcomes, higher levels of substance abuse, and lower levels of help seeking [60, 61].

Healthcare practitioners may aspire to be free of racism and bias on an individual level. Whether this is an accurate self-perception or an achievable goal is the subject of significant discussion in the chapters in this volume that deal with provider bias. Regardless of providers' individual intentions, however, the policies and structures within which they practice may deny equitable access to marginalized patients, leading to avoidable differences in outcomes. *Institutional racism* has been defined as "the collective failure of an organization to provide an appropriate and professional service to people because of their colour, culture or ethnic origin" ([62], p. 47). This might comprise such seemingly disparate practices as failing to provide interpreters for infertility patients with Limited English Proficiency and locating ART clinics far from neighborhoods with high concentrations of minoritized residents, making them functionally inaccessible to particular groups of patients.

An organization can be complicit in institutional racism without the intention of discriminating against specific individuals or groups; any policies and procedures that result in inequitable access and service delivery can perpetuate institutional racism regardless of the reasons that they were instituted. Institutional bias in reproductive medicine can also manifest outside the context of race. For example, patients with physical disabilities can be functionally denied equitable access to fertility treatment if practices lack the adaptive equipment necessary to conduct a diagnostic workup [63].

Racism and bias can exist at the level of a single institution. However, institutional racism occurs in a context in which multiple structures and systems interact to reinforce discrimination through inequitable access to basic resources. *Structural racism* impacts the access of racialized or minoritized people to health-promoting resources including education, credit and employment, fair treatment in the criminal justice system, and healthcare [64, 65]. According to the American Medical Association [66], "structural racism results in systemic variation in opportunity according to race or ethnic background," providing multiple enduring advantages to White people and perpetuating harmful narratives and stereotypes about racialized populations that are used to justify ongoing discrimination and withholding of resources. Structural racism pervades the daily experiences of minoritized populations; increasingly, it is also recognized to have a direct impact on patients' physical and psychological health.

Structural Racism and the Social Determinants of Health

Disparities in reproductive health experiences and outcomes are the major focus of this volume and will be covered at length throughout. However, health disparities exist for many patients long before they seek out reproductive healthcare. Differences in health outcomes for minoritized and racialized people are well documented across the spectrum of disease and wellness, with people from marginalized groups at greater risk for a wide variety of adverse health outcomes including cardiovascular disease, Alzheimer's disease, asthma, and a variety of psychiatric conditions [67–70]. Explicating the reasons for these health disparities requires a complex exploration of the social, educational, employment, and economic realities of living as a racialized or minoritized person in the United States and other nations where categories of race and ethnicity are salient.

The Office of Disease Prevention and Health Promotion groups the social determinants of health into five categories: economic stability, education access and quality, health care access and quality, neighborhood and built environment (for example, access to grocery stores and opportunities for physical activity, and safe air and water quality), and social and community context [71]. In the COVID-19 pandemic, some scholars advocated for the inclusion of broadband internet access as a sixth determinant [72, 73], citing the ability to access work, education, and medical care remotely as a key protective factor in the ability to decrease risk of exposure. For each of these factors, living as a racialized or minoritized person decreases the likelihood of being able to access health-promoting systems and resources. For example, the historical practice of redlining, which involved the withholding of low-interest mortgages for the purchase of homes in neighborhoods graded as "declining" or "hazardous," resulted in decreased property ownership among the predominantly Black residents of these neighborhoods. Today residents of these same neighborhoods remain significantly more likely to experience food insecurity due to the limited availability of nearby supermarkets and decreased rates of car ownership [74]. Similarly, low-income Latinx mothers are more likely than low-income White mothers to lack a traditional checking account and to use predatory lending services such as high-interest payday loans and high-fee check-cashing services, further compromising their economic stability and decreasing access to safe housing and healthy food [75].

The social determinants of health also play a critical role in the fertility and ART outcomes of racialized and minoritized patients. For example, residents of areas with higher-than-average concentrations of Black, Asian, and Hispanic populations are more likely to be exposed to air quality that is compromised by high levels of particulate matter [76]. Such exposure is a documented risk factor for male-factor infertility; air pollution has been associated with an increase in compromised semen quality and an increase in DNA fragmentation [77]. Similarly, environmental exposures, living in food deserts, and having inconsistent access to reproductive healthcare have been linked to an increased prevalence of uterine fibroids among Black women [78, 79], reducing the odds of successful implantation and gestation among those trying to conceive [80].

Even absent direct physiological effects, social determinants play a critical role in the timely assessment and diagnosis of infertility. As will be discussed at length in the chapter on bias in reproductive healthcare, limited access to consistent and high-quality reproductive healthcare can delay the diagnosis of infertility for patients who hold a variety of minoritized identities. Similarly, decreased access to comprehensive sexual health education may result in compromised fertility literacy for many marginalized groups, including LGBTQIA+ patients and those with disabilities [81]. Both factors can result in a critical delay in referral to infertility care, decreasing the likelihood of successful treatment. Notably, this finding is replicated internationally; for example, higher levels of educational attainment among Taiwanese patients are associated with decreased time to a diagnosis of infertility [82].

Structural Competency and the Provision of Culturally-Responsive Care

Race, ethnicity, and other cultural factors impact patient experiences and outcomes in care. In recognition of this truth, scholars interested in the equitable provision of healthcare have exhorted providers to examine their biases and practice cultural humility in the treatment of a diverse patient population. Indeed, much of this volume centers on patient and provider-level variables that can influence the experiences of diverse patients in infertility care. However, the provision of truly equitable care requires providers to look beyond individual patient–provider interactions to examine the structures and systems that lead to disparities in care and health outcomes for oppressed groups.

Structural competency requires us to recognize that the structural and social determinants of health and health inequities impact the wellness of minoritized patients [83]. Structurally competent care involves not just understanding the cultural expression of illness and health, but recognizing the often-invisible systems that perpetuate adverse health outcomes for minoritized populations. Patients who are advised to follow a low-sodium diet are better able to do so when they have easy access to healthy food; those who are advised to exercise to promote cardiovascular health are better able to do so when they live in safe neighborhoods with parks and green space [84]. Similarly, infertility patients who require surgical procedures to aid in conception are more likely to access required care when they have jobs that provide paid sick leave to aid in their recovery [13], and those who would benefit from IUI or IVF are more likely to initiate treatment when they live within reasonable travel distance of an IVF clinic [85].

For REIs and affiliated providers, moving toward structural competency involves being aware of the upstream factors that may compromise the fertility of marginalized patients. In a large multicenter clinical trial comparing methods of ovarian stimulation, for example, patient income was the third most important predictor of treatment outcomes, with patients with higher income experiencing higher pregnancy and live birth rates [86]. Similarly, patients with higher incomes, higher levels of education, and access to private insurance report better mental health outcomes during infertility treatment than do poorer, less educated patients, who experience higher rates of depression and anxiety [87].

Thus, structural competency in infertility care requires more than an awareness of the cultural factors that influence patients' uptake of and preferences for infertility services. It requires us to consider the factors that facilitate access to care for some populations while simultaneously creating barriers to care for others [88]. It requires us to consider our hiring practices, our paperwork, and our cultural collaborators to increase the chances that diverse patients will be treated in a system that recognizes their needs and the ways that they can best access treatment. Finally, practicing infertility care with an eye towards structural competency requires us to examine the root causes of healthcare disparities. True equity in infertility care is impossible to achieve without larger systemic changes aimed at creating health-promoting environments, providing preventative care, improving fertility education, and advocating for insurance coverage that will enable the greatest number of patients to access and benefit from ART.

Interventions

Throughout this book, you will be asked to consider how individual-level provider bias and lack of cultural awareness, institutional policies and procedures, and larger political and economic systems interact to influence the experiences of minoritized patients in ART. In some chapters, the intention is to provide information about the cultural beliefs and experiences of specific groups so clinicians can be aware of treatment issues that may arise in the provision of reproductive healthcare. Other sections focus on bias at the level of the provider and the clinic. These chapters include individual and structural suggestions for reducing the impact of provider bias on minoritized patients. Finally, some chapters are focused on proposed interventions to make ART accessible to a wider variety of patients and third-party collaborators. Though each of these chapters can be used as a stand-alone resource, they can also be considered pieces of a whole, each of which plays a role in increasing equity and improving the experiences of marginalized patients in infertility care. The chart below may serve as a useful guide for understanding the ways that inequities operate at the level of the provider, the clinic, and the larger system, along with the ways that interventions at each of these levels can work in conjunction to improve patient outcomes.

Issue	Examples	Proposed interventions
Provider bias	Use of negative language about minoritized patients in EHR; not leaving time for patient questions; not suggesting costly treatment options to minoritized patients	Standardize documentation; collaborate with diverse colleagues; increase patient talk time; practice self-reflection and cultural humility
Institutional bias	Forms and signage written in English only; forms use heteronormative language; exam rooms and equipment inaccessible to people with disabilities	Diversify REI pipeline and affiliated workforce; review forms, policies, and procedures for bias; provide interpreter services; ensure that exam rooms and equipment are physically accessible
Structural bias	Health disparities; differences in insurance coverage; poor fertility literacy; income disparities; limited information about ART outcomes for BIPOC and other marginalized patients	Include diverse populations in ART research; advocate for broader insurance coverage of IVF; implement affordable IVF protocols; address upstream determinants of health inequities

Summary and Conclusions

The factors that influence the experiences and outcomes of marginalized patients in infertility care begin long before these patients enter the REI clinic or seek mental health support for their fertility journey. Holding one or more minoritized identities, whether they feel consistent with one's own experience or are externally imposed by the majority culture, has implications for the treatment that patients are likely to receive by both individuals and systems. When a minoritized patient presents for infertility care, they may have already experienced bias and discrimination at the individual, institutional, and structural level. These intersecting systems of bias impact patients' willingness and ability to use ART and may ultimately decrease their likelihood of treatment success. Patients' racial and cultural identities can also influence their preferences for treatment, the ways that they prefer to receive information, and the reproductive technologies that they find acceptable. Membership in any given cultural group is only one among a host of factors that may influence patients' desires and experiences in infertility care; culturally responsive providers should be wary of assuming that membership in any given cultural group is determinative of patients' preferences for care.

The impact of racism and bias can be experienced in areas as seemingly disparate as the interaction between two people and the air quality in the neighborhoods in which they each reside. Interventions to improve outcomes in fertility care for culturally diverse populations must therefore exist across multiple domains to target different aspects of inequity. Infertility care providers should be aware of the ways in which individual, systemic, and structural interventions can work in concert to mitigate these inequities and improve the experiences and treatment outcomes of minoritized patients in reproductive healthcare.

References

1. Bansal K. Timing, techniques, and troubleshooting in intrauterine insemination. Practical guide in infertility. 2018:p. 283.
2. Supramaniam PR, Mittal M. Assisted reproductive technology: where did the journey begin, and where are we today–a 40-year history. WJ Gynecol Women's Health. 2018;1(4).: WJGWH. MS. ID.;519.
3. Affairs (ASPA) AS for P. Fact sheet: in vitro fertilization (IVF) use across the United States. www.hhs.gov. 2024. https://www.hhs.gov/about/news/2024/03/13/fact-sheet-in-vitro-fertilization-ivf-use-across-united-states.html#:~:text=In%202021%2C%2086%2C146%20infants%20born,children%20at%20a%20later%20time.
4. Doulgeraki T, Iliodromiti S. Reproductive outcomes in women and men conceived by assisted reproductive technologies. BMJ Med. 2023;2(1):e000547. https://doi.org/10.1136/bmjmed-2023-000547. PMID: 37051027; PMCID: PMC10083816
5. Dongarwar D, Mercado-Evans V, Adu-Gyamfi S, Laracuente ML, Salihu HM. Racial/ethnic disparities in infertility treatment utilization in the US, 2011–2019. Syst Biol Reprod Med. 2022;68(3):180–9.
6. Almquist RG, Barrera CM, Fried R, Boulet SL, Kawwass JF, Hipp HS. Impact of access to care and race/ethnicity on IVF care discontinuation. Reprod Biomed Online. 2022;44(6):1159–68.
7. Seifer DB, Sharara FI, Jain T. The disparities in ART (DART) hypothesis of racial and ethnic disparities in access and outcomes of IVF treatment in the USA. Reprod Sci. 2022;29(7):2084–8.
8. Jain T. Racial disparities and in vitro fertilization (IVF) treatment outcomes: time to close the gap. Reprod Biol Endocrinol. 2020;18:112.
9. Kirubarajan A, Patel P, Leung S, Park B, Sierra S. Cultural competence in fertility care for lesbian, gay, bisexual, transgender, and queer people: a systematic review of patient and provider perspectives. Fertil Steril. 2021;115(5):1294–301.
10. Barnes L, Fledderjohann J. Reproductive justice for the invisible infertile: a critical examination of reproductive surveillance and stratification. Sociol Compass. 2020;14(2):e12745.
11. Merkison JM, Chada AR, Marsidi AM, Spencer JB. Racial and ethnic disparities in assisted reproductive technology: a systematic review. Fertil Steril. 2023;119(3):341–7.
12. Weiss MS, Marsh EE. Navigating unequal paths: racial disparities in the infertility journey. Obstet Gynecol. 2022:10–97.
13. Cebert-Gaitors M, Abdelnalbi S, Mantell E, Woodward A, Gonzalez-Guarda R, Stevenson EL. Multidimensional barriers and facilitators to treatment seeking for infertility among women in the United States: a systematic review. F&S Rev. 2022;3(1):76–89.
14. Cebert-Gaitors M, Shannon-Baker PA, Silva SG, Hart RE, Jahandideh S, Gonzalez-Guarda R, Stevenson EL. Psychobiological, clinical, and sociocultural factors that influence black women seeking treatment for infertility: a mixed-methods study. F&S Rep. 2022;3(2):29–39.
15. Portugal A, Kosturakis AK, Onyewuenyi TL, Rivera-Cruz G, Jimenez PT. Breaking down barriers: advancing toward health equity in fertility care for black and hispanic patients. Obstet Gynecol Clin. 2023;50(4):735–46.
16. Hoffman JR, Delaney MA, Valdes CT, Herrera D, Washington SL, Aghajanova L, Smith JF, Herndon CN. Disparities in fertility knowledge among women from low and high resource

settings presenting for fertility care in two United States metropolitan centers. Fertil Res Pract. 2020;6:1–9.
17. Jackson-Bey T, Morris J, Jasper E, Edwards DR, Thornton K, Richard-Davis G, Plowden TC. Systematic review of racial and ethnic disparities in reproductive endocrinology and infertility: where do we stand today? F&S Rev. 2021;2(3):169–88.
18. Moreta LE, Simpson AE, Ghidei L, Wiltshire AM. Sperm donor availability and selection based on race and ethnicity. Fertil Steril. 2022;118(4):e383–4.
19. Hobbs CL, Gadson AK, Sadikman S, Tsai S, Enemuo F, Raker C, Eaton JL. An investigation of racial and ethnic disparities in donor sperm availability in the United States. Fertil Steril. 2024;122:474–81.
20. Roediger D. Historical foundations of race. National Museum of African American History and Culture. Smithsonian; 2019. https://nmaahc.si.edu/learn/talking-about-race/topics/historical-foundations-race.
21. Vartija D. Revisiting enlightenment racial classification: time and the question of human diversity. Intellect Hist Rev. 2021;31(4):603–25.
22. Hudson N. From "nation" to "race": the origin of racial classification in eighteenth-century thought. Eighteenth Century Stud. 1996;29(3):247–64.
23. Jablonski NG. Skin color and race. Am J Phys Anthropol. 2021;175(2):437–47.
24. Reece RL. Whitewashing slavery: legacy of slavery and white social outcomes. Soc Probl. 2020;67(2):304–23.
25. Pierre J. Slavery, anthropological knowledge, and the racialization of Africans. Curr Anthropol. 2020;61(S22):S220–31.
26. Trawalter S, Hoffman KM. Got pain? Racial bias in perceptions of pain. Soc Personal Psychol Compass. 2015;9(3):146–57.
27. Hoffman KM, Trawalter S, Axt JR, Oliver MN. Racial bias in pain assessment and treatment recommendations, and false beliefs about biological differences between blacks and whites. Proc Natl Acad Sci. 2016;113(16):4296–301.
28. Lee E. The Chinese exclusion example: race, immigration, and American gatekeeping, 1882-1924. J Am Ethn Hist. 2002;21(3):36–62.
29. Gardaphé F. We weren't always white: race and ethnicity in Italian American literature. Lit. 2002;13(3):185–99.
30. Spickard P, Beltrán F, Hooton L. Almost all aliens: immigration, race, and colonialism in American history and identity. Routledge; 2022.
31. Mountain JL, Risch N. Assessing genetic contributions to phenotypic differences among 'racial' and 'ethnic' groups. Nat Genet. 2004;36(Suppl 11):S48–53.
32. Telles E, Flores R. Not just color: whiteness, nation, and status in Latin America. Hisp Am Hist Rev. 2013;93(3):411–49.
33. Davenport L. The fluidity of racial classifications. Annu Rev Polit Sci. 2020;23:221–40.
34. Zhao X, Hong F, Yin J, Tang W, Zhang G, Liang X, Li J, Cui C, Li X, China Multi-Ethnic Cohort (CMEC) Collaborative Group. Cohort profile: the China multi-ethnic cohort (CMEC) study. Int J Epidemiol. 2021;50(3):721–l.
35. Sue S, Sue D, Sue DW, Who are the Asian Americans? Commentary on the Asian American psychology special issue. Am Psychol. 2021;76(4):689–92.
36. Martínez DE, Gonzalez KE. "Latino" or "Hispanic"? The sociodemographic correlates of pan-ethnic label preferences among US Latinos/Hispanics. Sociol Perspect. 2021;64(3):365–86.
37. Thomson AM, McHugh TA, Oron AP, Teply C, Lonberg N, Tella VV, Wilner LB, Fuller K, Hagins H, Aboagye RG, Aboye MB. Global, regional, and national prevalence and mortality burden of sickle cell disease, 2000–2021: a systematic analysis from the global burden of disease study 2021. Lancet Haematol. 2023;10(8):e585–99.
38. Guo J, Garratt A, Hill A. Worldwide rates of diagnosis and effective treatment for cystic fibrosis. J Cyst Fibros. 2022;21(3):456–62.
39. Manica A, Prugnolle F, Balloux F. Geography is a better determinant of human genetic differentiation than ethnicity. Hum Genet. 2005;118:366–71.

40. Ortega VE, Meyers DA. Pharmacogenetics: implications of race and ethnicity on defining genetic profiles for personalized medicine. J Allergy Clin Immunol. 2014;133(1):16–26.
41. Flanagin A, Frey T, Christiansen SL, AMA Manual of Style Committee. Updated guidance on the reporting of race and ethnicity in medical and science journals. JAMA. 2021;326(7):621–7.
42. Guiso L, Sapienza P, Zingales L. Does culture affect economic outcomes? J Econ Perspect. 2006;20(2):23–48.
43. Cooper JE. The politics of (Jewish) revelation. Jew Q Rev. 2014;104(4):613–22.
44. Braun KL, Nichols R. Death and dying in four Asian American cultures: a descriptive study. Death Stud. 1997;21(4):327.
45. Chin JH. Malaysian Chinese funeral rituals: a study of special rituals for unnatural death 2023 (Doctoral dissertation).
46. Leigh IW, Andrews JF, Harris RL, Ávila TG. Deaf culture: exploring deaf communities in the United States. Plural Publishing; 2020.
47. Chapman M. Representation and resistance: a qualitative study of narratives of deaf cultural identity. Cult Psychol. 2021;27(3):374–91.
48. Abreu RL, Gonzalez KA, Arora S, Sostre JP, Lockett GM, Mosley DV. "Coming together after tragedy reaffirms the strong sense of community and pride we have:" LGBTQ people find strength in community and cultural values during the COVID-19 pandemic. Psychol Sex Orientat Gend Divers. 2023;10(1):140.
49. Hailey J, Burton W, Arscott J. We are family: chosen and created families as a protective factor against racialized trauma and anti-LGBTQ oppression among African American sexual and gender minority youth. J GLBT Fam Stud. 2020;16(2):176–91.
50. Allen KR, Lavender-Stott ES. The families of LGBTQ older adults: theoretical approaches to creative family connections in the context of marginalization, social-historical change, and resilience. J Fam Theory Rev. 2020;12(2):200–19.
51. Stubbe DE. Practicing cultural competence and cultural humility in the care of diverse patients. Focus. 2020;18(1):49–51.
52. Crenshaw KW. Mapping the margins: intersectionality, identity politics, and violence against women of color. In: The public nature of private violence. Routledge; 2013. p. 93–118.
53. Cho S, Crenshaw KW, McCall L. Toward a field of intersectionality studies: theory, applications, and praxis. Signs J Women Cult Soc. 2013;38(4):785–810.
54. Crenshaw K. 'Difference' through intersectionality 1. In: Dalit feminist theory. India: Routledge; 2019. p. 139–49.
55. Sue DW, Calle CZ, Mendez N, Alsaidi S, Glaeser E. Microintervention strategies: what you can do to disarm and dismantle individual and systemic racism and bias. John Wiley & Sons; 2020.
56. Banaji MR, Fiske ST, Massey DS. Systemic racism: individuals and interactions, institutions and society. Cogn Res. 2021;6(1):82.
57. Chung N. All you can ever know: a memoir of adoption. Pushkin Press; 2020.
58. James D. An initial framework for the study of internalized racism and health: internalized racism as a racism-induced identity threat response. Soc Personal Psychol Compass. 2022;16(11):e12712.
59. Roberson K, Pieterse AL. Internalized racism and self-esteem: do depressive symptoms matter? Cult Divers Ethn Minor Psychol. 2021;27(3):531.
60. James D. Health and health-related correlates of internalized racism among racial/ethnic minorities: a review of the literature. J Racial Ethn Health Disparities. 2020;7(4):785–806.
61. Gale MM, Pieterse AL, Lee DL, Huynh K, Powell S, Kirkinis K. A meta-analysis of the relationship between internalized racial oppression and health-related outcomes. Couns Psychol. 2020;48(4):498–525.
62. Elias A, Paradies Y. The costs of institutional racism and its ethical implications for healthcare. J Bioeth Inq. 2021;18(1):45–58.
63. Horner-Johnson W, Klein KA, Campbell J, Guise JM. Experiences of women with disabilities in accessing and receiving contraceptive care. J Obstet Gynecol Neonatal Nurs. 2021;50(6):732–41.

64. Bailey ZD, Feldman JM, Bassett MT. How structural racism works—racist policies as a root cause of US racial health inequities. N Engl J Med. 2021;384(8):768–73.
65. Adkins-Jackson PB, Chantarat T, Bailey ZD, Ponce NA. Measuring structural racism: a guide for epidemiologists and other health researchers. Am J Epidemiol. 2022;191(4):539–47.
66. American Medical Association. What is structural racism? American Medical Association; 2021. https://www.ama-assn.org/delivering-care/health-equity/what-structural-racism
67. Jilani MH, Javed Z, Yahya T, Valero-Elizondo J, Khan SU, Kash B, Blankstein R, Virani SS, Blaha MJ, Dubey P, Hyder AA. Social determinants of health and cardiovascular disease: current state and future directions towards healthcare equity. Curr Atheroscler Rep. 2021;23:1–1.
68. Majoka MA, Schimming C. Effect of social determinants of health on cognition and risk of Alzheimer disease and related dementias. Clin Ther. 2021;43(6):922–9.
69. Sullivan K, Thakur N. Structural and social determinants of health in asthma in developed economies: a scoping review of literature published between 2014 and 2019. Curr Allergy Asthma Rep. 2020;20:1–2.
70. Shim RS, Compton MT. The social determinants of mental health: psychiatrists' roles in addressing discrimination and food insecurity. Focus. 2020;18(1):25–30.
71. Office of Disease Prevention and Health Promotion. Social Determinants of Health—Healthy People 2030 | health.gov [Internet]. health.gov. 2023. https://health.gov/healthypeople/priority-areas/social-determinants-health.
72. Benda NC, Veinot TC, Sieck CJ, Ancker JS. Broadband internet access is a social determinant of health!. Am J Public Health 2020;110(8):1123–1125.
73. Sieck CJ, Rastetter M, McAlearney AS. Could telehealth improve equity during the COVID-19 pandemic? J Am Board Fam Med. 2021;34(Supplement):S225–8.
74. Linde S, Walker RJ, Campbell JA, Egede LE. Historic residential redlining and present-day social determinants of health, home evictions, and food insecurity within US neighborhoods. J Gen Intern Med. 2023;38(15):3321–8.
75. Bullock HE, Toolis EE, Sencion B, Cadenas MT. The high price of economic marginalization: low-income Latinas' experiences with mainstream banking and alternative financial services. Peace Confl J Peace Psychol. 2020;26(2):136.
76. Jbaily A, Zhou X, Liu J, Lee TH, Kamareddine L, Verguet S, Dominici F. Air pollution exposure disparities across US population and income groups. Nature. 2022;601(7892):228–33.
77. Kumar N, Singh AK. Impact of environmental factors on human semen quality and male fertility: a narrative review. Environ Sci Eur. 2022;34:1–3.
78. Katon JG, Plowden TC, Marsh EE. Racial disparities in uterine fibroids and endometriosis: a systematic review and application of social, structural, and political context. Fertil Steril. 2023;119(3):355–63.
79. Dykstra C, Laily A, Marsh EE, Kasting ML, DeMaria AL. "I think people should be more aware:" uterine fibroid experiences among women living in Indiana, USA. Patient Educ Couns. 2023;107:107584.
80. Don EE, Mijatovic V, Huirne JA. Infertility in patients with uterine fibroids: a debate about the hypothetical mechanisms. Hum Reprod. 2023;38(11):2045–54.
81. Namkung EH, Valentine A, Warner L, Mitra M. Contraceptive use at first sexual intercourse among adolescent and young adult women with disabilities: the role of formal sex education. Contraception. 2021;103(3):178–84.
82. Chen WA, Wu CL, Ho HY, Chang F, Yang JH, Kung FT, Chen MJ, Chen MJ. Social determinants of health that impact the time to diagnosis and treatment of infertility in Taiwan. J Formos Med Assoc. 2024.
83. Metzl JM, Hansen H. Structural competency: theorizing a new medical engagement with stigma and inequality. Soc Sci Med. 2014;103:126–33.
84. Hansen H, Metzl JM. New medicine for the US health care system: training physicians for structural interventions. Acad Med. 2017;92(3):279–81.

85. Lazzari E, Baffour B, Chambers GM. Residential proximity to a fertility clinic is independently associated with likelihood of women having ART and IUI treatment. Hum Reprod. 2022;37(11):2662–71.
86. Berga SL. Social determinants of infertility: beyond the obvious. Fertil Steril. 2016;105(6):1459–60.
87. Bagade T, Mersha AG, Majeed T. The social determinants of mental health disorders among women with infertility: a systematic review. BMC Womens Health. 2023;23(1):668.
88. Melino K. Structural competency in health care. Nurs Clin. 2022;57(3):433–41.

Chapter 2
Culturally Responsive Care in the Assisted Reproductive Community

Loree A. Johnson

Culturally responsive practices must be integrated into the core framework of healthcare for diverse populations. Individuals from diverse cultural backgrounds seeking reproductive healthcare often encounter substantial challenges, as patients' needs reveal disparities in access to and use of reproductive medical and mental health services and patient outcomes [1–5]. These disparities underscore inequities linked to cultural identity markers within the healthcare system. Addressing these intentionally or unintententionally racist and discriminatory systems requires a profound commitment to cultural responsiveness to ensure care is tailored to the cultural factors influencing patients' needs and experiences.

Cultural responsiveness involves individuals and organizations responding respectfully and effectively to people from diverse cultures, regardless of language, socioeconomic status, race, ethnic background, disabilities, religion, sexual identity/orientation, and other identity markers [6]. Therefore, it signifies an acknowledgment, affirmation, and valuing of the patient's worth. In addition, culturally responsive practices, essential alongside evidence-based treatments, play a crucial role in facilitating effective communication and understanding within the medical and mental health communities [7], which is the cornerstone of patient care. Rather than requiring the patient to adapt their needs, communication styles, and expressions of identity to conform to the demands of the healthcare setting, culturally responsive care places the onus on the healthcare provider to demonstrate an understanding of cultural variations, identify potential biases, and bridge differences rooted in cultural contexts distinct from their own [8–12].

Integrating culturally responsive practices positively impacts treatment outcomes, as established in clinical research [13–15] and serves as an agent of change in improving equity in the system. In this chapter, I explore the basic principles of

L. A. Johnson (✉)
Independent Practice, Hermosa Beach, CA, USA
e-mail: drloree@drloreejohnson.com

D. A. Kaplan (ed.), *Cultural Responsiveness in Assisted Reproductive Technology*, https://doi.org/10.1007/978-3-031-76204-8_2

cultural responsiveness and how to apply them to the assisted reproductive community. I accomplish this by examining the definition of cultural responsiveness and elucidating the progression toward increased cultural responsiveness by exploring the interrelated concepts of cultural awareness, competency, and humility in clinical practice. Additionally, in this chapter, I address the challenges associated with adopting a culturally responsive approach and present practical strategies and interventions to stimulate reflection and action at both individual and systemic levels within reproductive healthcare communities.

What Is Culture?

Delving into the fundamental definition of culture and its varied contextual interpretations is essential to enhance and clarify the concept of cultural responsiveness. Culture defies a singular definition and encompasses dynamic elements beyond traditional classifications. It is defined in various ways depending on the context, including the ideologies, practices, and rituals associated with the groups to which a person belongs [16]. While culture is often mistakenly limited to categories such as race, nationality, country of origin, religion, or gender, it extends far beyond these conventional identifiers to broader contextual factors such as politics and socioeconomic status. In the realm of reproductive health, culture operates as a silent but influential factor, guiding how stakeholders interpret and articulate their experiences of infertility and its treatment and influencing how providers influence the diagnostic frameworks and standards of care in the treatment of reproductive concerns.

Culture represents an intricate interweaving of the identifiers that directly or indirectly influence access to care. Social norms and cultural foundations influence an individual's experiences and determine how they perceive and are perceived by the world. Throughout history and within our social and political culture, differences in identity and the associated struggles for recognition and influence have been defining elements in creating a disproportionate stratification of privilege and power that belies the principle that all are created and treated equally. Cultivating culturally responsive care requires honoring the complexity of these identities to maintain integrity in work that is unavoidably embedded within an interconnected web of privilege and marginalization [17].

Despite the acknowledgment of diversity as a national value, the quest for common ground, mutual respect, and equity has posed significant challenges for nearly every racial, ethnic, religious, gender, sexual orientation, and disability group integrated into the fabric of this country. Generational experiences, shaped by society's exposure to colonialism, imperialism, racism, homophobia, ableism, religious discrimination, and patriarchy, confer power and privilege on dominant groups while marginalizing others. For example, some individuals might not recognize that being White, cisgender, heterosexual, middle-class, or Christian can bestow specific privileges or experiences, potentially to the detriment of others. Meanwhile, others may not view themselves as privileged because of their social or economic status but still reap the advantage of holding membership in a dominant group, even if often hidden or unrecognized.

The tension is particularly evident when those in the majority group or holding privilege become the group against which marginalized groups are measured. The current research in the assisted reproductive community illustrates this as the vast majority of researchers and research subjects are White, heterosexual individuals or couples. When disparities are identified and measured, researchers present findings in ways where the marginalized are measured according to the dominant group.

Culture can serve as the framework through which individuals derive meaning from information, comprehend their health status, interpret diagnoses, explore available treatment options, and understand their treatment [6]. Providers must contextualize their patients within a multilevel, multidimensional cultural framework that incorporates diverse communities' geographic, historical, social, and political realities. This framework not only shapes how individuals perceive the world and attribute meaning to their daily lives but also informs how patients engage with and are treated by the healthcare system.

Cultural Disparities

The cultural impact on the assisted reproductive health community is notably reflected in disparities related to access to care, the provision of care across diverse identities, and how those disparities are presented. Racial and ethnic disparities present in various ways.

Black patients are more likely to experience delays in accessing treatment in comparison to their White counterparts [18, 19] or experience worse outcomes after engaging in treatment. Black, Asian, and Latine women undergoing fertility treatment may experience reduced pregnancy and live birth rates compared to White women [20, 21]. Moreover, Native American women undergoing fertility treatment exhibit lower pregnancy rates compared to White women [22], and Black and Latine women using egg donors encounter lower pregnancy and live birth rates [23].

These challenges are heightened by economic disparities, where individuals facing financial disadvantages may encounter obstacles in accessing treatment due to increased costs [24–27]. Providers hold significant power and influence in the doctor–patient relationship regardless of their cultural identifiers. However, these relational gaps may be compounded in intercultural doctor–patient interaction due to the inherent cultural hierarchy embedded in this dynamic. In a study of infertility patients, Black women conveyed that physicians often lack an understanding of their cultural background when seeking treatment [28], a finding with implications for provider–patient communication. Negris et al.'s [29] research echoes this sentiment, revealing that when patients feel understood by providers, they are more likely to engage in meaningful conversations during visits. Feeling understood fosters the comfort needed to pose significant questions and receive the specialist referrals necessary for comprehensive fertility education. In this study, those who perceived their fertility physician as not understanding their cultural background were over 2.5 times more likely to believe inaccuracies about the connection between their infertility and stress compared to those who perceived their fertility physician as understanding their culture [29].

The disparities in access to care for patients of color, combined with discrepancies in the quality of care, contribute to inferior outcomes. The complex issues influencing healthcare delivery to vulnerable populations emphasize the need to develop or enhance a culturally responsive approach.

Why Is Cultural Responsiveness Important?

Cultural responsiveness is important because every medical encounter, therapeutic session, or counseling interaction is inherently cultural [30], involving two individuals with unique cultural backgrounds and experiences. This assertion acknowledges that culture is a dynamic and multifaceted aspect of identity, encompassing beliefs, values, and experiences that influence how people perceive themselves, others, and the world. While the patient and the provider may share cultural similarities, a power asymmetry often infuses the patient–provider relationship. Managing the power differential in the doctor–patient relationship is crucial, as it influences how both patients and providers experience their interactions, especially when their cultural contexts intersect. While shared cultural backgrounds can facilitate communication and strengthen rapport, they do not erase the fundamental hierarchical nature of the provider–patient relationship.

Cultural responsiveness is crucial from a patient's standpoint because healthcare providers must recognize that individuals from marginalized groups often face discrimination based on their cultural identity. This underscores the significance of engaging with patients in ways that actively counteract the perpetuation of marginalization, particularly within medical environments. Providers must also acknowledge the mechanisms through which marginalization operates within social hierarchies. These dynamics establish dominant groups or categories against which others are compared, highlighting the importance of addressing power differentials and promoting equity in healthcare interactions.

From the provider's perspective, cultural responsiveness is vital because it calls into awareness how their own insights and experiences impact their perception of the patient. It goes beyond being an add-on to medical or mental health interventions; rather, it acknowledges that culture, embedded within hierarchical systems that favor certain groups and disadvantage others, greatly influences the clinical concerns expressed by clients and their health outcomes. Additionally, cultural responsiveness underscores the significance of how the provider's experiences shape their understanding of the patient's presentation.

Starting the Process of Self-Examination

Culturally responsive care calls for the provider to wrestle with locating themselves within a society that confers privilege to some while intentionally or unintentionally marginalizing others. As providers consider the power differentials embedded in a cultural framework, initiating self-examination and cultivating awareness begins with evaluating personal cultural identity, including values, beliefs, and life experiences. Through this process, providers can be both challenged and empowered to address prevalent myths that impede the development of the provider–patient relationship. These include:

- The misconception that culture pertains exclusively to individuals of color.
- The idea that culture is pertinent in healthcare only when specific groups are involved.
- The belief that the provider's cultural identity and background are not essential aspects of the provider–patient relationship.
- The belief that culture and cultural distinctions do not hold significance without explicit indications from the client.
- The belief that patients will initiate discussions about cultural issues and highlight the cultural factors that are salient aspects of their experience.
- Overestimating patients' comfort with and willingness to broach cultural topics.
- The notion that discussing culture within the medical or mental health community is inherently "political."
- The belief that providers can effectively join and work only with patients from their own cultural background or from a background with which they have specialized expertise [10].

Dispelling these myths and weaving together the interconnected strands of cultural identity encourages an elevation and integration of social consciousness. Reassessing and integrating a social justice lens into clinical practices is seen as an opportunity rather than a mere obligation, encouraging the delivery of culturally responsive care. While this approach may seem unconventional and divergent from the traditionally neutral stance in clinical training, it can serve as a pivotal component of cultural responsiveness when starting to identify bias.

Implicit Bias

Implicit bias within the assisted reproductive community must be addressed in the context of healthcare disparities, as these biases can contribute to differential diagnoses and treatments, ultimately impacting patient outcomes in significant ways. Acknowledging implicit bias is a key factor in developing culturally sensitive practices, particularly as healthcare providers address misconceptions about cultural influence and location from both the provider and patient perspectives. Numerous studies [31–33] highlight unconscious attitudes that impact provider perceptions and, consequently, the delivery of care.

Bias is an unconscious process where involuntary attitudes or stereotypes influence individuals' understanding, actions, and decisions without conscious awareness [34]. This differs from explicit bias, where individuals are aware of their biases and may openly express them, showing a dislike for members of marginalized groups based on race, ethnicity, gender, or economic status. Implicit biases can develop over time and may not align with an individual's stated beliefs. Social pressures often make it challenging to identify or address implicit bias, as most people do not see themselves as prejudiced and recognize that harboring bias can be problematic. Because individuals absorb repeated messages, attitudes, and stereotypes from their environment, no one is immune to biases [31]. This phenomenon could explain the defensive reaction that can arise when confronted with potential biases.

Historically, medical education has perpetuated stereotypes about Black patients and reproductive health. In the early twentieth century, the identification and diagnostic characterization of endometriosis, a gynecological condition, were significantly shaped by the prevailing biases of that era related to sex, class, race, and cultural politics. Initial theories about the cause of endometriosis proposed that it resulted from contraceptive use and delayed childbearing [35, 36]. As a result, it was often perceived as a condition primarily affecting middle-class White women, a widespread belief propagated in various medical texts and popular culture that led to misdiagnosis or delays in diagnosis among Black women [37, 38]. Consequently, clinicians were less inclined to include endometriosis in their list of potential diagnoses for Black women presenting with pelvic pain and other symptoms indicative of the condition.

Research shows that racial biases among non-Black healthcare providers, especially in pain perception, are associated with biased pain treatment for Black patients, leading to potential misdiagnosis, diagnostic delays, or adverse reproductive outcomes [39–41]. Biased beliefs about Black patients' pain perception can lead to dismissive attitudes during clinical assessments [40, 41]. Unfortunately, the persistent myth that Black individuals experience less pain has historical origins in obstetrics, tracing back to the nineteenth century when enslaved Black women were subjected to gynecological surgical procedures without anesthesia. The conception of these women's pain as unimportant or nonexistent was rooted in a system based on dehumanizing the enslaved, which in turn justified their mistreatment. Further justification was found in the pseudoscience of the time, which falsely claimed that Africans and Black people did not experience pain in the same way as White people. These spurious findings, enshrined in medical history, led to the perpetuation of biases in medical education, research, and clinical care that extend to the assisted reproductive community.

Developing a Culturally Responsive Lens

Unlearning biases is achievable through intentional self-exploration [34]. By acknowledging and actively addressing implicit bias, the assisted reproductive community can make significant strides toward delivering equitable care that meets the diverse needs of all individuals. Developing a culturally responsive lens is an ongoing journey that requires a commitment to understanding the complexity of culture within the provider–patient relationship and addressing biases that could impact care. It involves meaningfully recognizing and addressing disparities within the assisted reproductive community rather than just acknowledging their existence. Developing a culturally responsive lens involves a deep personal transformation characterized by rigorous and intentional work, including self-exploration and self-reflection [10, 34]. This process informs cultural humility and enhances the ability to manage microaggressions effectively. By actively addressing implicit bias, the reproductive health community can progress toward providing truly equitable care centered around the diverse needs of all individuals.

Self-Exploration

Self-exploration entails curiosity in understanding our own cultural location and lifelong experiences that have shaped our cultural perspectives, attitudes, actions, and behaviors. Self-exploration is a lifelong process; however, formal exercises in self-exploration can be introduced during or after medical or graduate training [42].

Researchers suggest various avenues for self-exploration, such as the "iceberg" method, which posits that much of an individual's culture lies beneath the surface [43]. Therefore, recognition that what is visible may not fully represent the individual is crucial. This method suggests the existence of a hidden culture or cultural unconscious influenced by worldview, perception, and behavior. Unspoken rules, including norms regulating relationships, identity, boundaries, and emotional space, contribute to this hidden culture.

The questions in Example 1, adapted from Hardy [10] can assist in the self-exploration process. Additionally, a sample response is included to offer insight into how a reproductive healthcare professional might respond.

Example 1

How does your lived experience as a provider, both personal and professional, inform your work with others cross-culturally?

I grew up as a Black woman in an all-White suburban neighborhood in the heart of the Confederacy, where very few people looked like me. My education and lived experience were shaped by White Southern culture, and I rarely saw myself represented in the media or in my educational environment, which often minimized the experiences of my culture. During my clinical training, I gained an understanding of social justice and the power of my social location. However, I quickly realized that the theories and clinical applications I was taught were primarily conceptualized with White individuals in mind rather than people of color or those with marginalized identities. As a Southern Black woman, my lived experience of being othered has equipped me to work cross-culturally. However, I've also recognized that I am still susceptible to internalized systemic messages, which can make me blind to the marginalization of other groups and lead me to view their struggles as separate from my own. I am hyperaware and sensitive to feeling "othered," using it to stay curious and connect with those who may identify differently from me, while also being mindful of the tensions that can arise between marginalized groups, often pitting us against each other within the system.

What could potentially be an asset, and what would be harmful in these cross-cultural interactions?

I consider my willingness to learn about other cultures an asset—knowing what it feels like to feel different or othered, I can use that as a way to build rapport, validate and be curious about others who identify differently than me. I think there can also be a tendency to over-identify with culturally marginalized patients because of my sensitivity due to lived experience. This may cause me to miss cues from others and patients about their own lived experiences.

What cross-cultural experiences have you had as someone from a dominant or nondominant group?

My experiences, like my identity, are complex and intersectional. Visibly, I have always navigated the world as a member of nondominant groups, particularly in my identity as a Black woman. I constantly encounter racial nuances in cross-cultural relationships, facing overt discrimination and microaggressions, such as misdiagnosis by the medical community I am part of or having my experiences minimized through a racial lens. However, I also recognize that I hold certain privileges as a cisgender, heterosexual, middle-class woman.

How do you grapple with the ways in which the tension between your privilege and marginalization shows up?

Managing the tension is a constant struggle, but being aware of it feels like the most authentic place to start. I am aware that I have access to financial, social, and familial resources, AND I am tasked with advocating for myself and making sure I am seen.

Can you make a deliberate effort to empathize with members of marginalized groups by putting yourself in the other group's shoes? How does your clinical perspective shift? Or not?

For me, empathy is cultivated through exposure and understanding, and one of the most effective ways I gain insight into what I don't know is by immersing myself in it. While I've learned a great deal about relating to the dominant racial group in my community, I've made a deliberate effort to spend time with other groups I wasn't as familiar with. This approach has shaped my clinical perspective, reminding me to stay open to the learning process. I'm mindful not to treat any group as a monolith, as this can happen unintentionally. I also recognize the importance of seeking out and consulting with individuals from different groups as part of a proactive approach to my learning, which helps me explore and address any triggers that may arise.

Self-exploration involves examining our individual responses within and/or as a part of the dominant culture, fostering a deeper understanding through thoughtful introspection. Acknowledging resistance is part of countertransference and honoring what arises. Resistance [30] presents an opportunity to confront fears, explore feelings as a cultural being, and gain new insights into how these feelings and beliefs have shaped one's approach to care. For some healthcare providers, this may involve examining the experiences that lead them to engage in heteronormative or cisnormative practices, such as not honoring a nongestational partner in the room or making assumptions about participants' comfort with medical technologies based on their gender presentations [44, 45]. For others, it could mean making active efforts to use gender neutral language and preferred pronouns and avoid heteronormative assumptions. Recognizing resistance involves noticing intense feelings or challenging thoughts related to one's experience with a client or their identity. This recognition is the first step in embracing what emerges during the self-exploration journey.

Self-Reflection

Self-reflection marks the final step in the transformative process. Scholars argue that self-reflection serves as the cornerstone of action [10, 46–48]. Managing resistance during the self-reflection stage involves expanding our contextual understanding through awareness of the potential ways in which we as providers have engaged in or perpetuated blind spots involving patient care. Training in healthcare has evolved from a neutral stance or color-blind approach, as the exhortation to treat everyone "equally" has in fact led to inequitable practices in the delivery of healthcare. Self-reflection in reproductive care may, for example, involve asking yourself: What comes up for me when I think about working with queer/Black/poor/disabled individuals or couples? How can I use this internal experience to shape how I want to work? How can I ensure that my practice aligns with my values and reflects not just who I *want* to serve but who I think I *am* serving as well? Critical reflection on sociopolitical inequities affecting patients can significantly enhance awareness of these issues [49].

As noted by Decety [50], reflection enables healthcare providers to sustain openness and empathy toward understanding how sociopolitical structures influence their worldviews and intersecting identities. Heightened awareness and empathy, fostered by reflection, are vital in discerning whether a practice or provider reinforces or dismantles oppressive structures that contribute to disparities within the reproductive health field.

Cultural Humility

Self-exploration and reflection constitute an internal process through which healthcare providers understand themselves as cultural beings, learn to avoid stereotyping, manage power imbalances, and embody an understanding of cultural differences. In tandem with increased self-understanding, cultural humility plays a distinct role in guiding patient–provider interactions. Increased cultural humility allows us to shift from a performative action of displaying cultural awareness to embodying a sense of awareness [12]. It is described as a lifelong process involving three key elements: (a) the ongoing quest to comprehend oneself as a cultural being with intersecting identities; (b) a commitment to understanding individuals from their profound cultural perspective, avoiding stereotypical or generalized views; and (c) the active management of power imbalances within relationships with those who are culturally different, with a focus on cultivating mutually respectful connections [49, 51]. This continuous learning process acknowledges the limitations and barriers to intercultural understanding and emphasizes the distinction between an intellectual understanding of cultural differences and the embodiment of that understanding. Cultural humility extends beyond an individual's awareness of their assumptions, values, and biases; it involves scrutinizing their background and social context to understand how they embody their experiences in their interactions with others [52].

Client perception of providers' cultural humility has been associated with positive therapeutic alliance, therapy adherence, and treatment effectiveness [53], as well as favorable treatment outcomes [54–56]. It has also been associated with higher psychotherapist ratings [57], lower microaggression frequency and impact [58], lower color-blind racial attitudes [59], and an increase in clients' willingness to disclose religious beliefs [60]. These findings can be generalized to the relationships in medical settings, echoing Negris' et al.'s research [29].

Levi [61] proposes that cultural humility encourages individuals to identify and acknowledge biases, necessitating a deeper level of recognition. It goes beyond mere acknowledgment or sensitivity to differences, requiring individuals to take responsibility for their interactions with others. Cultural humility is instrumental in redressing power imbalances in clinical relationships and larger systems. When providers approach their interactions with patients by acknowledging assumptions and prejudices, they are more likely to maintain respect for clients, thereby correcting power imbalances. This humility cultivates patients' sense of trust in therapeutic relationships [53]. Patients who feel seen and respected are likelier to trust their providers and remain engaged in medical care.

Microaggressions

Even when an individual remains mindful of the complex experience of interactions through a cultural lens, microaggressions still occur and, when not tended to, can create a rupture in the relationship. Research on microaggressions is somewhat limited, but they are broadly defined as subtle communications reflecting insensitivity, disrespect, or insults based on cultural identity or background [62]. Microaggressions encompass everyday slights, put-downs, invalidations, and insults directed at culturally devalued group members. It is important to note that these actions are often perpetrated by well-intentioned individuals who may be unaware that their behaviors are biased and harmful. The cumulative impact of a lifetime of microaggressions can significantly harm victims' physical and psychological well-being [63–65], highlighting the importance of addressing them within the context of the provider–patient relationship.

Patients who have encountered discrimination based on race, ethnicity, sexual orientation, or gender identity reported avoiding seeking healthcare [64, 65]. Cruz et al. [66] observed that patients can discern when their healthcare providers hold negative stereotypes about their cultural backgrounds. A provider's attempt to either overly identify culturally or downplay concerns through a cultural lens, along with avoiding diversity discussions during medical encounters, triggers a heightened awareness for the patient of cultural dynamics in patient-provider interactions. This awareness is likely influenced by experiences with racism or discrimination as an ongoing stressor extending beyond isolated incidents, as discrimination is deeply rooted in society's collective unconscious and perpetuated through systemic and institutional practices. Consequently, providers who deny cultural differences or avoid discussions about individual distinctions may unintentionally support the oppressive ideology that fuels microaggressions, further marginalizing cultural groups with whom they wish to connect.

Within this context, effectively handling microaggressions demands that the provider adopt a culturally humble stance, acknowledging and addressing cultural factors within the provider–patient relationship to foster a deeper understanding of the patient [67]. Hook et al. [53] suggested that a patient's perception of a provider's cultural humility plays a mediating role in the relationship between encountered microaggressions and medical outcomes, reinforcing the importance of employing a culturally responsive approach.

Broaching Cultural Issues

Engaging in self-examination to acknowledge implicit bias and managing microaggressions are integral steps in developing a culturally responsive lens. Furthermore, addressing cultural factors and differences within the provider–patient relationship is crucial for enhancing connection and communication in healthcare interactions.

Researchers have highlighted the importance of adopting a client-centered approach that recognizes and addresses cultural differences and actively engages in discussions about them [67–69]. Healthcare providers can improve their approach by not only acknowledging cultural differences but also by actively ensuring that they understand the patient's perspective. This can be achieved by asking reflective questions, such as, "How does it feel to sit with someone who identifies differently culturally?" Additionally, providers should recognize that no amount of training can fully encompass lived experiences, so they should remain open to feedback if they make mistakes. Directly asking patients if there is anything they want the provider to know or if there are aspects of their experience that are often misunderstood can further demonstrate a commitment to validating the patient's perspective. Regular check-ins can also help assess how well the provider is attuned to the patient's needs and experiences.

Broaching cultural issues can occur in both covert and overt ways. Covert methods include being mindful of how one's office environment and paperwork reflect the provider's values. For example, providers should consider whether their staff reflects the diversity of the population they serve and whether their paperwork is inclusive. Overt methods involve directly acknowledging the differences that exist within the provider–patient relationship, which can give patients permission to discuss relevant topics. Recognizing that the provider–patient relationship is central to care is crucial in this context.

This proactive approach is vital for enhancing the provider–patient relationship and improving patient outcomes, especially within the assisted reproductive health community where marginalized communities may not feel adequately represented. Drinane et al. [70] demonstrated a link between avoiding cultural discussions and poorer treatment outcomes, while Singh et al. [71] advocated for providers to take the lead in facilitating conversations about culturally specific values, attitudes, beliefs, and experiences. This active involvement promotes cultural responsiveness and understanding within healthcare settings.

Holding Space for Hard Conversations

Addressing cultural factors in medical and therapeutic settings can be challenging, especially when providers adopt the "color-blind" approach often taught in clinical training programs. This approach, while aiming for neutrality, often lacks guidance on navigating cross-cultural relationships effectively. Failing to acknowledge differences or avoiding them under the guise of not seeing patients as "different" can lead to mistrust within the provider–patient relationship, impacting communication, information exchange, assessment, referral, treatment, and overall care delivery [29, 69].

Providers can deepen their self-examination process by identifying their approach to engaging in challenging conversations, particularly regarding cultural topics. Days-Vine [8, 68] outlined five styles for initiating discussions on such topics: avoidance, isolating, continuing/incongruent, integrated congruence, and infusing. These approaches help providers assess their comfort levels in embracing these conversations, recognizing that their approach may vary along a continuum. This continuum ranges from avoidance of cultural discussions to a style that integrates or infuses skills and comfort with cultural issues into the clinical conversation.

Avoidance Style: Providers employing an avoidance strategy tend to sidestep discussions on culture, focusing more on the presenting issues. Many members of groups considered the majority evade confronting ethnocentrism and acknowledging discrimination. They tend to shy away from discussing these issues due to feelings of guilt about the historical mistreatment of oppressed groups, fear of being accused of mistreating others, and apprehension about being labeled as prejudiced. Consequently, discomfort arises when issues of such as race emerge, leading to a tendency to back away, become defensive, assert innocence, express sympathy, or adopt a color-blind stance. "Rejecting and avoiding cultural topics" becomes a stance that allows the provider to maintain a self-image as a good, moral, decent human being who sees themselves as innocent of cultural bias or discrimination [30]. When working with patients from historically disenfranchised or marginalized groups, this approach may inadvertently hinder exploring crucial cultural aspects relevant to the client's concerns.

For example, a Latine patient in fertility counseling who discloses a history of feeling dismissed by medical providers might feel dismissed once again if their mental health provider offers an alternate explanation for a doctor's medical decision. The failure to validate this experience minimizes the patient's reports of how their racial identity has impacted their medical care and decreases the likelihood that the patient will feel free to disclose other painful experiences.

Isolating Style: Providers sometimes acknowledge a patient's comment about a cultural issue but redirect or minimize the discussion without delving deeper through a cultural lens. A provider may validate a patient's experience of being dismissed but may not explore the meaning of that dismissal for the client. This can result in the cultural context being isolated or downplayed, narrowing the clinical focus and signaling that this discussion is a box to check rather than a relevant aspect of the client's experience to be understood.

Continuing Incongruent Style: Providers using a continuing incongruent style may mechanically broach cultural topics, expressing discomfort and struggling with verbiage. A provider who treats LGBTQ and nonbinary patients may struggle using gender neutral language or pronouns that reflect the patient's identity. This mechanical approach may create a sense of unease, potentially affecting the therapeutic relationship and hindering authentic engagement on cultural issues.

Integrated Congruent Style: Providers employing an integrated and congruent strategy demonstrate ease in discussing cultural topics. The broaching is seamless, reflecting genuine comfort in addressing these issues. Providers may acknowledge the challenges patients face due to their identity. For Black patients, a physician may encourage bringing a family member or friend to appointments, understanding that they may have experienced doctors not listening to them in the past. This approach fosters a positive therapeutic environment, allowing for open and honest discussions about cultural markers.

Infusing Style: Providers seamlessly integrate discussions on cultural topics into medical and therapeutic interventions. The ease of discussing these issues translates into interventions that reflect the provider's knowledge and comfort with these discussions. This style promotes open dialogue and collaboration and ensures that interventions are informed by the provider's understanding of the client's cultural context. For example, a provider who has explored a patient's religious beliefs with regards to donor conception would reference this conversation as they explore additional treatment options should the patient not be able to conceive with their own gametes.

Each approach reflects varying levels of comfort along a developmental continuum, where healthcare providers assess their comfort level in addressing cultural issues within a clinical context. Like cultural humility and the evolution of a culturally responsive lens, the development of the provider's comfort with engaging patients in challenging conversations may be an on-going process.

Factors Affecting Broaching

Provider and patient factors significantly influence the process of broaching cultural topics. From the provider's perspective, beliefs about the importance or relevance of broaching, individual beliefs regarding the significance of discussing cultural topics, and past experiences with similar conversations all play a crucial role in shaping the provider's approach to broaching. The provider's comfort level, willingness to broach such topics, self-efficacy, and degrees of multicultural awareness and competency also contribute to their ability to initiate these discussions [8]. For instance, some providers may feel more at ease discussing issues related to race rather than gender. Others may be more proficient in addressing matters related to religion as opposed to sexual identity.

The patient's view of the provider's responsiveness to cultural issues plays a pivotal role in the provider's success in initiating discussions [53, 72]. This perception is shaped by the patient's cultural understanding, awareness, feeling of safety within the patient–provider relationship, and willingness to delve into and address cultural aspects of their experience. These factors collectively influence the patient's receptiveness to conversations about cultural topics.

The process of broaching sensitive topics involves a dynamic interaction between the perspectives of the healthcare provider and the patient. This interaction encompasses beliefs, experiences, comfort levels, skills, multicultural awareness, and comfort with specific topics. The success of broaching conversations depends on how these factors align and influence the communication between the provider and the patient.

Conclusion

A culturally responsive approach in the assisted reproductive community prioritizes the patient's cultural context and lived experience. It involves recognizing and considering the impact of both the patient's and the provider's cultural backgrounds on the patient–provider relationship, as well as on the assessment, diagnosis, and treatment of reproductive conditions. This approach ensures that treatment methods and care provision respect and align with patients' cultural identities. Cultural responsiveness also entails acknowledging the inherent power dynamics within the clinical relationship. Persistent inequities emphasize the need to identify cultural nuances, understand the repercussions of neglecting these discussions, recognize the provider's role in facilitating culturally sensitive conversations, and remain mindful of the complex dynamics of power, privilege, and oppression within the patient–provider relationship.

References

1. Armstrong A, Plowden TC. Ethnicity and assisted reproductive technologies. Clin Pract (Lond). 2012;9(6):651.
2. Bell AV. Beyond (financial) accessibility: Inequities within the medicalisation of infertility. Sociol Hum Illn. 2010;32(4):631–46.
3. Dieke AC, Zhang Y, Kissin DM, Barfield WD, Boulet SL. Disparities in assisted reproductive technology utilization by race and ethnicity, United States, 2014: a commentary. J Women's Health. 2017;26(6):605–8.
4. Inhorn MC, Fakih MH. Arab Americans, African Americans, and infertility: Barriers to reproduction and medical care. Fertil Steril. 2006;85(4):844–52.
5. Mikhael S, Gaidis A, Gavrilova-Jordan L. Regional disparities in access to assisted reproductive technology: assessment of patient satisfaction when employing modern technology to close the gap. J Assist Reprod Genet. 2021;38(4):889–94.
6. Nielsen-Bohlman LT. Institute of Medicine. Health literacy: a prescription to end confusion. Washington, DC: National Academies Press; 2004.
7. Cabassa LJ, Baumann AA. A two-way street: bridging implementation science and cultural adaptations of mental health treatments. Implement Sci. 2013;8:1–4.
8. Day-Vines NL, Holcomb-McCoy C. Broaching the subjects of race, ethnicity, and culture as a tool for addressing diversity in counselor education classes. Teaching in counselor education: Engaging students in learning. 2013: pp. 151–166.
9. Day-Vines NL, Cluxton-Keller F, Agorsor C, Gubara S. Strategies for broaching the subjects of race, ethnicity, and culture. J Couns Dev. 2021;99(3):348–57.
10. Hardy KV. Racial trauma: clinical strategies and techniques for healing invisible wounds. WW Norton & Company; 2023.
11. Hays PA. Addressing cultural complexities in practice: a framework for clinicians and counselors. American Psychological Association; 2001.
12. Holyoak D, Johnson W, Garcia M, Johnson DJ. I see you: addressing diversity in clinical practice through therapist's way-of-being. Contemp Fam Ther. 2020;42:131–9.
13. López CM, Shealy KM, Rheingold AA. Empirically supported trauma treatment for an adult Latino man diagnosed with PTSD: overcoming barriers to engagement. Clin Case Stud. 2014;13(5):436–52.
14. McCarthy-Keith DM, Schisterman EF, Robinson RD, O'Leary K, Lucidi RS, Armstrong AY. Will decreasing assisted reproduction technology costs improve utilization and outcomes among minority women? Fertil Steril. 2010;94(7):2587–9.
15. Handtke O, Schilgen B, Mösko M. Culturally competent healthcare–A scoping review of strategies implemented in healthcare organizations and a model of culturally competent healthcare provision. PLoS One. 2019;14(7):e0219971.
16. Harper FD, McFadden J. Culture and counseling: new approaches. Pearson; 2003.
17. Watts-Jones TD. Location of self: opening the door to dialogue on intersectionality in the therapy process. Fam Process. 2010;49(3):405–20.

18. Gadson AK, Sauerbrun-Cutler MT, Eaton JL. Racial disparities in fertility care: a narrative review of challenges in the utilization of fertility preservation and ART in minority populations. J Clin Med. 2024;13(4):1060.
19. Jackson-Bey T, Morris J, Jasper E, Edwards DR, Thornton K, Richard-Davis G, Plowden TC. Systematic review of racial and ethnic disparities in reproductive endocrinology and infertility: where do we stand today? F&S Rev. 2021;2(3):169–88.
20. Humphries LA, Chang O, Humm K, Sakkas D, Hacker MR. Influence of race and ethnicity on in vitro fertilization outcomes: systematic review. Am J Obstet Gynecol. 2016;214(2):212–e1.
21. McQueen DB, Schufreider A, Lee SM, Feinberg EC, Uhler ML. Racial disparities in in vitro fertilization outcomes. Fertil Steril. 2015;104(2):398–402.e1.
22. Craig LB, Weedin EA, Walker WD, Janitz AE, Hansen KR, Peck JD. Racial and ethnic differences in pregnancy rates following intrauterine insemination with a focus on American Indians. J Racial Ethn Health Disparities. 2018;5:1077–83.
23. Zhou L, Wang L, Geng Q, Zhang H, Xu S, Diao L, Zeng Y, Mo M, Li L. Endometriosis is associated with a lowered cumulative live birth rate: a retrospective matched cohort study including 3071 in vitro fertilization cycles. J Reprod Immunol. 2022;151:103631.
24. Adashi EY, Dean LA. Access to and use of infertility services in the United States: framing the challenges. Fertil Steril. 2016;105(5):1113–8.
25. Bedrick BS, Anderson K, Broughton DE, Hamilton B, Jungheim ES. Factors associated with early in vitro fertilization treatment discontinuation. Fertil Steril. 2019;112(1):105–11.
26. Bitler M, Schmidt L. Health disparities and infertility: impacts of state-level insurance mandates. Fertil Steril. 2006;85(4):858–65.
27. Feinberg EC, Larsen FW, Wah RM, Alvero RJ, Armstrong AY. Economics may not explain Hispanic underutilization of assisted reproductive technology services. Fertil Steril. 2007;88(5):1439–41.
28. Galic I, Negris O, Warren C, Brown D, Bozen A, Jain T. Disparities in access to fertility care: who's in and who's out. F&S Rep. 2021;2(1):109–17.
29. Negris O, Lawson A, Brown D, Warren C, Galic I, Bozen A, Swanson A, Jain T. Emotional stress and reproduction: what do fertility patients believe? J Assist Reprod Genet. 2021;38(4):877–87.
30. Sue DW, Sue D, Neville HA, Smith L. Counseling the culturally diverse: theory and practice. John Wiley & Sons; 2022.
31. Amodio DM. The neuroscience of prejudice and stereotyping. Nat Rev Neurosci. 2014;15(10):670–82.
32. Banaji MR, Greenwald AG. Blindspot: hidden biases of good people. Bantam; 2016.
33. FitzGerald C, Hurst S. Implicit bias in healthcare professionals: a systematic review. BMC Med Ethics. 2017;18:1–8.
34. Jones-Smith E. Culturally responsive strengths-based therapy: the journey. In: Jones-Smith E, editor. Culturally diverse counseling: theory and practice. Sage Publications, Inc.; 2019.
35. Brzezinski A, Koren Z, Kedar S. Contribution to the problem of the etiology of endometriosis. Isr Med J. 1962;21:111–7.
36. Bougie O, Healey J, Singh SS. Behind the times: revisiting endometriosis and race. Am J Obstet Gynecol. 2019;221(1):35–e1.
37. Novak E, Jones G, Novak E. Endometriosis. In: Novak E, editor. Textbook of gynecology. 6th ed; 1961. p. 247–50.
38. Kistner R. Endometriosis. In: Kistner R, editor. Gynecology: principles and practice. 2nd ed. Mosby; 1971. p. 432–56.
39. Gillette-Pierce KT, Richards-McDonald L, Arscott J, Josiah N, Duroseau B, Jacques K, Wilson PR, Baptiste D. Factors influencing intrapartum health outcomes among Black birthing persons: a discursive paper. J Adv Nurs. 2023;79(5):1735–44.
40. Hoffman KM, Trawalter S, Axt JR, Oliver MN. Racial bias in pain assessment and treatment recommendations, and false beliefs about biological differences between blacks and whites. Proc Natl Acad Sci. 2016;113(16):4296–301.

41. Saluja B, Bryant Z. How implicit bias contributes to racial disparities in maternal morbidity and mortality in the United States. J Women's Health. 2021;30(2):270–3.
42. Comas-Díaz L. Multicultural care: a clinician's guide to cultural competence. American Psychological Association; 2012.
43. Weaver GR. Understanding and coping with cross-cultural adjustment stress,[w:] Cross—cultural orientation: new conceptualizations and applications, red. Lanham: RM Paige; 1986.
44. Kirubarajan A, Patel P, Leung S, Prethipan T, Sierra S. Barriers to fertility care for racial/ethnic minority groups: a qualitative systematic review. F&S Rev. 2021;2(2):150–9.
45. Craven C. Reproductive losses: challenges to LGBTQ family-making. Routledge; 2019.
46. Bolgatz J. Talking race in the classroom. Teachers College Press; 2005.
47. Ford KA. Shifting White ideological scripts: the educational benefits of inter-and intraracial curricular dialogues on the experiences of white college students. J Divers High Educ. 2012;5(3):138.
48. Freire P. Pedagogy of the oppressed. In: Toward a sociology of education. Routledge; 2020. p. 374–86.
49. Gallardo ME, editor. Developing cultural humility: Embracing race, privilege and power. Sage Publications; 2013.
50. Decety J. Empathy in medicine: what it is, and how much we really need it. Am J Med. 2020;133(5):561–6.
51. Mosher DK, Hook JN, Captari LE, Davis DE, DeBlaere C, Owen J. Cultural humility: a therapeutic framework for engaging diverse clients. Pract Innov. 2017;2(4):221.
52. Yeager KA, Bauer-Wu S. Cultural humility: essential foundation for clinical researchers. Appl Nurs Res. 2013;26(4):251–6.
53. Hook JN, Davis DE, Owen J, Worthington EL Jr, Utsey SO. Cultural humility: measuring openness to culturally diverse clients. J Couns Psychol. 2013;60(3):353.
54. Kivlighan DM III, Adams MC, Drinane JM, Tao KW, Owen J. Construction and validation of the multicultural orientation inventory—group version. J Couns Psychol. 2019;66(1):45.
55. Owen J, Jordan TA, Turner D, Davis DE, Hook JN, Leach MM. Therapists' multicultural orientation: client perceptions of cultural humility, spiritual/religious commitment, and therapy outcomes. J Psychol Theol. 2014;42(1):91–8.
56. Owen J, Tao KW, Drinane JM, Hook J, Davis DE, Kune NF. Client perceptions of therapists' multicultural orientation: cultural (missed) opportunities and cultural humility. Prof Psychol Res Pract. 2016;47(1):30.
57. DeBlaere C, Shodiya-Zeumalt S, Hinger C, Cobourne L, Davis DE, Zelaya DG, Chadwick CN, Zeligman M, Hook JN, Owen J. Cultural humility with religious and spiritually diverse women of color clients: a psychometric analysis. J Psychol Theol. 2019;47(2):87–99.
58. Hook JN, Farrell JE, Davis DE, DeBlaere C, Van Tongeren DR, Utsey SO. Cultural humility and racial microaggressions in counseling. J Couns Psychol. 2016;63(3):269.
59. Stewart SH. Psychotherapy task-based assessment of therapists' multicultural orientation: a measurement development study (Doctoral dissertation, University of Denver).
60. Judd K. Doctrinal dialogues: factors influencing client willingness to discuss religious beliefs. Men Health Reli Cult. 2019;22(7):711–23.
61. Levi A. The ethics of nursing student international clinical experiences. J Obstet Gynecol Neonatal Nurs. 2009;38(1):94–9.
62. Pierce CM, Carew JV, Pierce-Gonzalez D, Wills D. An experiment in racism: TV commercials. Educ Urban Soc. 1977;10(1):61–87.
63. Turner J, Higgins R, Childs E. Microaggression and implicit bias. Am Surg. 2021;87(11):1727–31.
64. Casey LS, Reisner SL, Findling MG, Blendon RJ, Benson JM, Sayde JM, Miller C. Discrimination in the United States: experiences of lesbian, gay, bisexual, transgender, and queer Americans. Health Serv Res. 2019;54:1454–66.
65. Slaughter-Acey JC, Sneed D, Parker L, Keith VM, Lee NL, Misra DP. Skin tone matters: racial microaggressions and delayed prenatal care. Am J Prev Med. 2019;57(3):321–9.

66. Cruz D, Rodriguez Y, Mastropaolo C. Perceived microaggressions in health care: a measurement study. PLoS One. 2019;14(2):e0211620.
67. Comas-Díaz L, Jacobsen FM. Ethnocultural transference and countertransference in the therapeutic dyad. Am J Orthopsychiatry. 1991;61(3):392–402.
68. Day-Vines NL, Cluxton-Keller F, Agorsor C, Gubara S, Otabil NA. The multidimensional model of broaching behavior. J Couns Dev. 2020;98(1):107–18.
69. Grocher K, Gerrits T. A racially and culturally sensitive approach to fertility counseling. Fertility counseling: clinical guide. 2022: p. 183.
70. Drinane JM, Owen J, Tao KW. Cultural concealment and therapy outcomes. J Couns Psychol. 2018;65(2):239.
71. Singh AA, Nassar SC, Arredondo P, Toporek R. The past guides the future: implementing the multicultural and social justice counseling competencies. J Couns Dev. 2020;98(3):238–52.
72. Chang DF, Berk A. Making cross-racial therapy work: a phenomenological study of clients' experiences of cross-racial therapy. J Couns Psychol. 2009;56(4):521.

Chapter 3
Implicit Bias in Healthcare Professionals Beyond Implicit Association Tests: A Neuroscientific Understanding

Jacquelyn Doran Cunningham

The landmark release of *Unequal Treatment* by the Institute of Medicine in 2003 provided the first and the most comprehensive account of racial and ethnic inequities in healthcare in the United States [1]. Findings introduced healthcare providers, policymakers, and the public to the potential role of medical professionals' implicit bias in contributing to medical disparities, bringing widespread attention to the idea that healthcare professionals could make decisions that affect quality of care based on unconscious stereotypes. Unlike explicit biases that individuals can easily articulate, implicit biases have been described as unconsciously held stereotypes that are sometimes antithetical to an individual's beliefs and produce unintentional discriminatory behavior [2, 3].

For example, high levels of implicit racial bias in physicians are related to increased physician control of discussions, less patient-focused dialogue during a consultation, and shorter visits with Black compared to White patients [4, 5]. Patients who perceive bias are more likely to express reduced levels of trust, confidence, and satisfaction in their medical care and simultaneously less likely to adhere to medical advice and/or more likely to delay seeking treatment [4, 6, 7]. Moreover, Black, Hispanic, Asian American patients, and nonnative English speakers who perceive bias within the patient–provider relationship are more likely than White patients to believe they would receive better treatment if they were of a different race [7].

Awareness of implicit bias arose from a growing body of research beginning with Greenwald and Banaji's [8] introduction of the term "implicit social cognition" to describe the automatic, unconscious effects of previous encounters on social cognitive constructs such as attitudes and stereotypes (for a review of implicit social cognition, (see [9]). In 1998, Greenwald and colleagues introduced the Implicit

J. Doran Cunningham (✉)
Westfield Mental Health Specialists, Westfield, NJ, USA
e-mail: jdcphd@westfieldmentalhealth.com

D. A. Kaplan (ed.), *Cultural Responsiveness in Assisted Reproductive Technology*, https://doi.org/10.1007/978-3-031-76204-8_3

Association Test (IAT) (see Box 3.1: Implicit Association Tests) as a method to gauge "implicit attitudes by measuring their underlying automatic evaluation" ([10], p. 1464). The initial IAT assessed implicit bias about racially stereotyped attitudes; since then, IATs have been adapted for use in a multitude of social categories (e.g., gender, suicidality, and political affiliation) and various settings. By 2021, over 3000 peer-reviewed research articles had used IATs [11].

Box 3.1: Implicit Association Tests (IATs)

The most widely used assessment of implicit bias, the Implicit Association Test (IAT) was developed by Greenwald and colleagues in 1998. In contrast to norm-referenced tests with standardized content, IATs use a psychological assessment method with a standardized procedure for administration and scoring. For example, a race-based IAT may require participants to sort Black and White faces and evaluative words (e.g., *adore*, *cherish*, *dirty*, and *selfish*) into categories that corresponded with societal stereotypes (e.g., White/good, Black/bad) and counter to societal stereotypes (e.g., White/bad, Black/good). Scores are summarized in one metric that reflect reaction time to associate categories with traits.

Over the years, there has been considerable debate about the psychometric properties of IATs, including an issue of *Perspectives on Psychological Science* devoted to discussing the validity of IATs ([12–15]; also see [16]). Although a complete analysis of the debate is beyond the scope of this chapter, given the extensive use of IATs in research and bias reduction efforts for more than 20 years, it is critical to examine some of the questions raised about what IATs measure and the statistical evidence for those conclusions.

Construct Validity

The primary concern raised about IATs involve whether they actually measure what they purport to measure, which is the automatic, unconscious associations between specific concepts such as social groups or identities and emotional judgements (e.g., good or bad; [10]). Some researchers question whether they truly assess implicit attitudes or simply reflect unrelated associative processes. For example, Schimmack [12] found no validity evidence for the stereotype IAT and self-esteem IAT as measures of implicit constructs distinct from explicit measures of those constructs. Additionally, researchers question the degree to which IATs are a measure of automatic judgment that assesses implicit attitudes and the degree to which results are influenced by conscious, controlled processing [14, 17].

Finally, Schimmack [12] notes that Greenwald and colleagues have adjusted their original description of IATs being able to tap into unconscious aspects of mental processes not assessed by self-report [18] to measures of associative strength ([19]; also see [11, 20]). Overall, ambiguity about construct validity has the potential to complicate the interpretation of IATs for researchers and practitioners, who may draw conclusions about the meaning of IAT scores when there is no statistical evidence for those interpretations.

Predictive Validity

Three meta-analyses examined the predictive validity of the IAT with respect to implicit stereotypes and intergroup discrimination [21–23]. Collectively, these studies showed only modest validity correlations of the stereotype IAT's ability to predict intergroup discrimination, which likely reflects the influence of other factors contributing to discriminatory judgments and behaviors [24]. For example, when individuals attribute behaviors of a stigmatized group to external factors such as discrimination or economic disparity, negative stereotype IAT scores may reflect empathy [25]. Influences such as these impact the construct validity of IATs and the meaningfulness of an IAT score.

Although Greenwald et al.'s [26] statistical evidence showing that smaller effect sizes than those established in the three metanalyses "were large enough to explain discriminatory impacts that are societally significant either because they can affect many people simultaneously or because they can repeatedly affect single persons" (p. 553), the meaningfulness of the stereotype IAT's prediction of discriminatory impact becomes ambiguous if the overall construct validity (i.e., the construct the test measures and the psychometric properties that support the accuracy of that measurement) of the IAT is low.

Indeed, the stereotype IAT was used in the majority of studies included in various systematic reviews of implicit bias in healthcare providers over the past decade [27–31]. It has also been used in bias-reduction efforts for individuals and groups with the goal of altering biased behaviors and improving outcomes for racial groups. For example, medical education and training programs have used the stereotype IAT both as an exercise to increase awareness of implicit bias among healthcare professionals and as an efficacy measure of interventions with the goal of reducing implicit bias [32].

Despite the popularity of IATs in academia and the media (e.g., [33, 34]), IATs remain a controversial tool for both assessment and intervention due to concerns about their construct validity and overall psychometric properties. Many researchers assert that IATs have utility despite these problems. This chapter challenges that view by discussing how, in addition to psychometric concerns, the stereotype IAT measures only one aspect of bias that does not account for neuroscientific advances in how intergroup biases are formed, enacted, and reinforced, which complicates its overall clinical utility. As an alternative, this chapter proposes that bias mitigation efforts in healthcare should focus on patient—provider communication and patient—provider interactions guided by the neuroscientific understanding of intergroup biases. Further, by integrating a critical analysis of the stereotype IAT with social neuroscience, this chapter provides a comprehensive and contextual account of bias that reinforces the necessity for overall structural changes in the healthcare system.

Systemic Biases in Healthcare

Viewed systemically, individual biases interact with broader social, cultural, and economic institutions, such as the healthcare system, that have their own discriminatory practices and intergroup biases that exacerbate inequities [35, 36]. Health inequities are systematic differences that result in certain groups attaining less than optimal health outcomes [37, 38]. These differences in health outcomes, often referred to as health disparities, largely stem from inequities resulting from the societal structures that allocate resources and opportunities disproportionately (e.g., housing, education, employment [37, 39]).

In one such model of health disparities, Vela et al. [40] discuss the reciprocal interactions of racial implicit bias in healthcare providers with structural determinants of bias. According to the model, implicit biases of healthcare providers are activated and reinforced by structural factors such as lack of diversity in the workforce and exposure to biased curricula and training in medical education and practice settings. For example, race-based clinical guidelines may link specific races or ethnicities with certain diseases, essentially pathologizing race by implying that inherent racial characteristics result in a disposition for high-risk diseases rather than explaining the interplay of race and structural health disparities[1] [41]. Other factors in the model include time constraints during the medical professional's workday and cognitive overload when making medical decisions.

Vela et al.'s [40] model posits that these types of structural factors collectively and differentially impact the quality of healthcare providers' communication with marginalized patients in ways that often (unintentionally) reflect this structural bias. Patient perception of provider bias results in distrust of the healthcare system, poor adherence to treatment recommendations, and reinforcement of both the provider's biases and the cycle of disparities through poor patient outcomes. Noting challenges associated with individual and often short-term interventions in reducing implicit bias, Vela et al. [40] concluded that "interruption of this cycle is possible only through an overall shift toward favorable structural influences on implicit bias" (p. 495). To understand why altering bias at the structural level is so critical to enacting enduring change throughout healthcare systems, it is important to understand how implicit bias functions at individual and group levels and the mediators of bias that are most amenable to change.

---

[1] For example, statistics that refer to the higher rates of hypertension among Black men may fail to consider the impact of economic and geographic factors that influence the availability of healthy dietary choices for those living in poorer communities. Both dietary factors and hypertension have also been linked to the development of uterine fibroids, suggesting that their increased prevalence in Black women is at least in part a downstream effect of structural inequities.

Social Neuroscience

In the early 2000s, along with the introduction of IATs to assess implicit social cognition, an interdisciplinary field termed social neuroscience [42] emerged. This field used neuroimaging technology to investigate how neurobiological structures shape and are shaped by social behavior, and how an individual's neurobiology influences and is influenced by relationships and larger social systems [43]. A sub-speciality developed within social neuroscience dedicated to examining the neural correlates of implicit attitudes, prejudice, and intergroup differences in how people perceive and respond to their own group (ingroup) versus an external group (out-group) based on classifications such as race and gender, among other categories (e.g., [44–46]).

Although recent research examining bias in healthcare has broadened to include biases such as weight, age, and disability status, much of the earlier bias research focused on gender and racial biases [31]. This chapter discusses the most commonly available data with respect to White–Black racial bias, with the understanding that other experiences of bias may be different, and multiple biases may be (and often are) experienced simultaneously throughout the healthcare sector by patients who hold more than one marginalized identity.

Semantic Memory

Both implicit social cognition and social neuroscience have their roots in information-processing models of cognitive psychology that rely on semantic memory. For over 40 years, social psychologists have posited that biased judgments and stereotypes utilize a dual-processing approach to social cognition [47]. According to dual-processing models, information can be processed as automatic (rapid, intuitive, associative, and requiring little conscious effort) or controlled (deliberate, reflective, analytical, and goal directed) [48].

Semantic memory consists of concepts, facts, and general knowledge about the world, including accumulated societal knowledge and beliefs about various social groups [49]. Functional magnetic resonance imaging (fMRI) evidence points to the anterior temporal lobe as a global neural hub for semantic knowledge that supports social cognition through retrieval of conceptual social information [50]. Within associative network theory, unrelated concepts have little to no association in semantic memory, while highly related concepts are strongly linked in an interconnected network [51]. Activation of one concept automatically triggers the activation of related concepts through a process called spreading activation [51]. Consequently, stereotyping can result from attempts to utilize cognitive resources efficiently by applying broad, generalized traits encoded in semantic memory to various social categories while minimizing specific individual attributes [52].

In her seminal research, Devine [53] investigated how automatic and controlled processes function with respect to prejudice and stereotype activation. For her first study, White participants completed a self-report measure of prejudice and listed characteristic descriptors with which Black individuals are frequently stereotyped. Individuals with both high and low levels of prejudice possessed stereotype knowledge, which she attributed to the pervasiveness of stereotypes in everyday culture. Her second study used stereotype priming (i.e., briefly flashing stereotyped words interspersed with letters on a screen as either 80% or 20% of the content) before participants evaluated a vignette of a person of unspecified race and behavioral intentions. Regardless of prejudice status, ratings of behavioral hostility were higher in the 80%, compared to the 20%, stereotype priming condition, indicating that stereotype activation can influence judgment even in individuals who self-report low levels of prejudice. A third study asked participants to anonymously list their perceptions of Black people. Individuals with high levels of prejudice provided more negative descriptions, while individuals with low levels of prejudice listed more positive traits. Thus, despite both high and low prejudice individuals possessing stereotype knowledge, those identifying as non-prejudiced could inhibit prejudicial responses when given the opportunity for reflection during list making. Although motivation for providing non-prejudicial responses was not assessed in this study, these participants may have held egalitarian beliefs and/or did not want to appear prejudiced to others.

Hinton [54] discussed how stereotypical associations are acquired through frequent encounters in everyday social interactions and accessed by a "predictive brain." Because the predictive brain sets expectations based on probabilities from past experience, the automaticity of stereotype generation presents challenges to making non-stereotypical judgments or evaluations even for those with egalitarian goals. Hinton [54] further asserted "that the predictive brain operates on the state of the world *as it is experienced* and not on the state of the world *as we believe it should be*" (p. 6). The term implicit bias, as understood within the cognitive bias framework, implies an individual flaw and is inconsistent with the universality of societal stereotypes. Instead, Hinton [54] argues for use of the term "implicit stereotype," to reflect a wider cultural issue instead of a personal cognitive shortcoming. Although stereotype knowledge is stored in an individual's semantic memory, Hinton's perspective situates stereotypes as a societal problem that reflects the necessity for structural changes to address the ramifications of deeply entrenched stereotypes.

Indeed, computational modeling and behavioral studies suggest that statistically regular co-occurrences of language and visual information strongly influence semantic development [55]. This can be seen with neural patterns found on the stereotype IAT. For stereotype congruent (e.g., White/good, Black/bad) and stereotype incongruent (e.g., White/bad, Black/good) blocks of the IAT, there is a great deal of overlap in neural activation for both semantic representation and automatic processing [56, 57]. However, distinct neural patterns emerge for each IAT condition. Stereotype congruent associations on the IAT activated several brain regions that have been implicated in processing simple associations between related concepts [56–58], whereas counter-stereotypic associations activated brain regions often implicated in situations that require conscious effort and control [56, 58]. Moreover, compared to the more efficient neural processing and activation patterns within the stereotype congruent condition, Forbes et al. [56] proposed that the less efficient neural processing of the counter-stereotypic condition may reflect weaker associations learned from less statistically frequent encounters with societal counter-stereotypes.

Memory Systems Model of Intergroup Bias

In addition to semantic memory, the memory systems model of intergroup bias ([59]; also see [35, 47, 60, 61, 62]) incorporates the interactions of multiple memory systems for social information learned through affective and instrumental learning. Considering these neurocognitive influences enhances understanding of how biases are differentially formed, enacted, reinforced, and altered over time.

Pavlovian Aversive Conditioning

During Pavlovian aversive conditioning, a neutral stimulus evokes a reflexive, involuntary fear response when consistently paired with a negative stimulus. A form of prejudice resulting in amygdala activation and behaviors such as freezing, vigilance, and avoidance in intergroup interactions was initially proposed to result from this type of aversive conditioning [35, 46, 59–61]. In their seminal study, Cunningham et al. [63] used fMRI to examine the neural systems activated by White participants when they were shown Black and White faces very briefly (30 ms). Participants demonstrated increased amygdala activation in response to Black compared to White faces, suggesting a heightened emotional response. After a longer exposure (525 ms), the amygdala response significantly diminished and was accompanied by activation of the control, regulation, and inhibition regions of the prefrontal cortex and anterior cingulate, regions of the brain associated with emotion regulation, cognitive control, and decision making. Based on this pattern, Cunningham et al. [63] concluded that individuals can override their initial, automatic biased responses to Black faces.

However, although early fMRI studies indicated an amygdala response to racial outgroups and suggested potential avenues for intervention (e.g., [64, 65]), later work found mixed support for a racially based threat-related response in the amygdala [66]. Rather than a purely aversively conditioned fear response, Chekroud et al. [66] proposed that the amygdala may be responding to culturally learned associations to threat. Another possibility may involve a Pavlovian-to-Instrumental transfer, whereby a learned association between racial outgroup members and social threats (Pavlovian conditioning) affects later decisions and behaviors towards those groups [35, 67, 68].

Instrumental Learning

Instrumental learning occurs when voluntary behaviors are strengthened (through reinforcement) or weakened (through punishment or a lack of response from the environment) because of their consequences. Based on repeated positive or negative behavioral feedback, individuals learn and internalize associations between actions and their value, actively making choices about the conditions under which those actions are worth repeating in the future [69, 70]. Within this framework, prejudiced attitudes and willingness to enact prejudiced behaviors can be reinforced by positive outcomes (e.g., social approval and personal gain) or discouraged by negative outcomes (e.g., social disapproval and personal loss) [59, 70].

Behavioral studies support an instrumental learning model of social interaction. Hackel et al. [71] found that in an experiment in which participants were given the opportunity to change partners over repeated interactions, individuals adapted their choice of partner based on the amount and proportion of money each partner shared during an interaction. Participants ultimately selected partners who gave larger rewards and showed higher levels of generosity. Hackel et al. [70] expanded this work, finding that differing levels of rewarding interactions with one individual generalized to perceptions of reward value for other members of the same social group. Although participants interacted with only one group member, the transfer of reward value to nonparticipating group members generalized to overall attitudes toward the group, perceptions of group generosity, and decisions to interact with or avoid new members of the same group. Similarly, Lindstrom et al. [72] found that previously formed associations of racial bias affected the rate at which individuals learned to avoid threatening outgroup faces, with those higher in racial bias forming avoidance behaviors toward threatening out-group members more rapidly than toward in-group members or less threatening faces.

Prior associations to race can influence interaction preference even when the interactional reward value is equal. Using a money sharing game, Traast et al. [73] found that White participants developed a stronger behavioral preference for interacting with White compared to Black players, despite both groups sharing an equal amount of reward and despite participants perceiving the shared reward value as equivalent between groups. This race effect was stronger for individuals with high levels of explicit prejudice and low internal motivation for providing non-prejudiced responses. Computation modeling results showed that race not only predisposed White participants to hold different initial expectations for player behavior but also differentially impacted learning rate patterns which adjusted reward expectations for players from each group (i.e., participants updated their expectations for receiving a reward after a positive interaction more quickly with White players compared to Black players who provided an equal reward). Thus, prior associations to race can preemptively shape associations developed through direct social interactions with individual members of a group.

Brain imaging studies show that the neural mechanisms for race-based evaluations differ from those for stereotypes stored in semantic memory. Gilbert et al. [74]

compared neural representations of implicit evaluations of others (as assessed by questions such as "Who would you befriend?") and stereotype traits ("Who is more likely to enjoy athletic activities?") when White participants viewed pairs of Black and White faces. The researchers then mapped these fMRI images onto participants' responses to an IAT for evaluative words and an IAT for stereotyped words. Stereotype traits for Black, but not White, individuals activated the anterior temporal lobe and medial prefrontal cortex, suggesting simple semantic processing between related concepts [58]. Social friendship evaluation of Black, but not White, individuals activated the anterior temporal lobe and orbitofrontal cortex, suggesting that individuals may have been assessing the reward value of befriending an outgroup member [75, 76].

In addition to social outcomes, the emotions individuals experience during social interactions may serve as a reward or punishment that influences the estimated reward value of future interactions. Proposing a multiprocess theory of motivational and emotional states, Rolls [76] described motivational states as performing goal-directed actions to seek rewards or avoid punishments and affective states as emotions resulting from whether a reward or punishment was given or denied. The affective responses learned from the associations between actions and emotions (e.g., I feel happy, I feel afraid) are themselves interpreted as a reward or punishment that shape future actions.

Affective responses are directly linked to the evaluation of social situations because they enable real-time emotional assessment and help individuals adapt their behavior to achieve social goals such as gaining acceptance or avoiding conflict. For example, Amodio and Hamilton [77] examined whether anxiety about an impending interracial interaction (assessed via a state affect checklist) influenced performance on assessments of implicit racial evaluation and stereotyping. After viewing a Black or White male face with a neutral expression, participants completed two IATs adapted from Amodio and Devine [78] where they classified words as pleasant or unpleasant in an evaluative condition and mental or physical in a stereotype condition. Results indicated that higher levels of anticipatory anxiety about the interracial interaction increased negative racial evaluations but not stereotyping. Thus, heightened anxiety may have amplified negative evaluations of outgroup members, potentially to mentally prepare for or avoid anticipated negative outcomes in the interaction.

Community Level Bias

Given that social neuroscience investigates the interaction between an individual's neurobiology and their relationships with larger social systems, it is critical to examine bias within a social context. Although research regarding the interaction of individual bias with communities is notably limited, one study by Hatzenbuehler et al. [79] adopted a social neuroscience approach to investigate whether levels of community-reported bias corresponded with neural responses to racial outgroup members. Results indicated that residing in areas with greater, compared to reduced, levels of explicit racial prejudice correlated with the intensity of Whites' neural responses to Black, but not White, faces. Contrary to their hypothesis, this neural pattern was not associated with community-level implicit bias.

Applying a neuroscientific model of learning and memory systems [47, 59] alongside a critical analysis of the IAT provides a dynamic account of the neurobehavioral and environmental mechanisms that potentially explain these findings. The next section offers an in-depth review of the study within these frameworks, as this conceptualization has implications for understanding the interaction between individual biases in healthcare providers and the overall healthcare system.

Description of the Study

Hatzenbuehler et al. [79] employed spatial meta-analysis to analyze the neural activations of participants in 22 fMRI studies as well as aggregated data of explicit and implicit bias for the communities in which the fMRI studies were conducted. Implicit and explicit data were obtained from Project Implicit, which has state- and county-linked datasets freely available in the public domain. Explicit racial attitude data consisted of aggregated self-report responses to 20 items (e.g., "It would not bother me if my new roommate was Black"). Implicit racial attitude data consisted of county-level, aggregated scores from a stereotype IAT that required participants to sort Black and White faces and evaluative words into stereotype congruent and stereotype incongruent categories.

Differentiating Constructs in Bias Measurement

The assessment of attitudes and stereotypes warrants further exploration, as it is possible Hatzenbuehler et al.'s [79] aggregated explicit bias variable reflects evaluative attitudes. Specifically, their classification of the item "It would not bother me if my new roommate was Black" as an explicit measure of bias aligns with Gilbert et al.'s [74] evaluative use of "Who would you befriend?" in response to Black and White faces. Further, Amodio and Devine [78] identified stereotyping and evaluation as distinct constructs by demonstrating the independence of two adaptations of the IAT: a stereotyped IAT (based in a semantic memory system) and a racial evaluation IAT (based in an emotional/instrumental memory system). Moreover, using an adaptation of these measures, Amodio and Hamilton [77] found that anxiety about an interracial interaction (which they posited to be associated with the amygdala) correlated with high levels of implicit negative racial evaluations but not stereotyping. Consequently, Hatzenbuehler et al. [79] may not find an association between amygdala activation and the stereotype IAT if the stereotype IAT is an assessment of semantic knowledge. What was originally intended to be a measure of participants' own *unacknowledged attitudes and beliefs* about stereotyped groups may in fact more accurately reflect an *easily accessible body of knowledge* about stereotypes commonly applied to members of these groups (see Box 3.2: Caution Against Conflating the IAT with Implicit Bias).

Memory Systems Approach to Understanding Community Racial Bias

A neuroscientific model of learning and memory systems [47, 59] might further elucidate the findings from Hatzenbuehler et al. [79]. Individuals in the study may have had varying levels of cultural stereotype knowledge in their semantic memory. However, neural activation in response to interracial encounters may have only occurred when they resided in areas where they were exposed to high levels of negative racial evaluations. This may be attributed to the interactive processing of emotional salience and evaluative biases within an instrumental memory system, which may include the amygdala responding to an emotional association with race. Thus, experiencing environments with high levels of racial evaluation may trigger these neural pathways based on learned evaluative racial biases that are unrelated to stereotype knowledge.

Other explanations for these results are possible, including those delineated by Hatzenbuehler et al. [79]. Nonetheless, adopting a memory systems model of intergroup bias that differentiates and accounts for the interaction between semantic, affective, and instrumental memory systems could provide insights into Hatzenbuehler et al.'s [79] community-based findings. This approach not only aids in interpreting the results but also has implications for improving the utility of IATs, informing instrumental and reward-based bias reduction strategies, and addressing overall systemic biases.

Box 3.2: Caution Against Conflating the IAT with Implicit Bias

Despite the efforts of Greenwald and colleagues to clarify what IATs measure and how well they measure it (e.g., [9, 11, 20, 24]), at times researchers and practitioners conflate the IAT with the construct of implicit bias (i.e., viewing the IAT method as equivalent to the concept of implicit bias rather than as one method for measuring implicit bias). Conflation of the construct of implicit bias with the IAT is problematic for several reasons. First, all tests contain measurement error and are not a "pure" representation of even the most clearly defined construct. Thus, interpretation of IAT scores should occur while understanding the limits of the method, particularly given concerns raised about the overall psychometric properties of IATs.

Second, the stereotype IAT is intended to assess one aspect of implicit bias: associative knowledge [20]. Conflating the IAT with implicit bias is problematic because neurocognitive models suggest multiple pathways for biased learning and behavioral responding. Amodio and Cikara [60] state "that a prejudiced response may occur for multiple reasons, each associated with a different underlying process [46]. For example, a person may fail to detect the conflict between their biased response tendency and either their egalitarian goals or normative antiprejudice social cues.... Alternatively, they may have trouble inhibiting a biased response, despite having detected it.... Or they may have trouble identifying and implementing a desired egalitarian response." (p. 459–460).

Finally, conflating the stereotype IAT with implicit bias may obscure research findings and undermine intervention efforts to address bias and prejudice. For example, Forscher et al. [80] evaluated the effectiveness of various procedures to change implicit bias through a network metanalysis of 494 studies that examined implicit bias (predominantly assessed by the stereotype IAT), explicit bias, and behavior ratings. Interventions resulted in only modest changes in implicit bias. Moreover, changes in implicit bias did not produce changes in explicit bias or behavior. Challenging a core premise in implicit bias research, the researchers concluded that automatically retrieved associations may not cause behavior but instead reflect exposure to social and environmental interactions. Consequently, the researchers cautioned that intervention efforts focusing on altering automatically retrieved biased associations in order to reduce behaviors would be misdirected and ineffective in a structurally biased environment with ongoing stereotype exposure.

Indeed, Greenwald et al.'s [20] review of bias reduction interventions found minimal efficacy for both individual treatment (e.g., exposure to counter stereotypical exemplars and intergroup contact) and group-administered training methods such as raising awareness about the existence and pervasiveness of implicit bias and offering strategies to mitigate its impact. As Greenwald and Lai [9] stated, "there is no reason to expect that diversity trainers can reduce implicit biases when researchers cannot reliably produce such effects empirically" (p. 435). Instead, Greenwald et al. [20] advocate for a public health approach to addressing discriminatory bias, including the use of preventative measures that disrupt the connection between implicit bias and biased outcomes, and disparity-finding methods that detect and correct inequities in systems and practices that differentially affect various groups.

Implications for Healthcare Interventions and Future Directions

Much of this chapter has been dedicated to discussing the limitations of the IAT, largely because it forms the foundation for the majority of research and many interventions directed at addressing implicit bias in healthcare. The following section will use a social neuroscientific framework to provide insight about findings from multiple systematic reviews of studies of implicit racial bias in medical providers while considering these limitations.

Levels of Implicit Bias in Healthcare Providers

Somewhat shockingly at the time of publication, most studies showed that healthcare professionals exhibited levels of implicit bias comparable to the general population [27–31]. Considering the IAT as a measure of semantic knowledge of societal stereotypes in one's environment, however, can explain this finding. Medical professionals are not immune to the influence of societal prejudices even with their bioethical training. Therefore, interventions that address healthcare professionals' individual levels of semantic stereotype knowledge will be ineffective if they are continuously exposed to structural biases within the medical system. Interventions that reduce structural bias are imperative for breaking this cycle (see Chaps. 1 and 18; also see [40]).

Communication and Quality Interventions

Across reviews, a negative association emerged between implicit bias as assessed by the stereotype IAT and the quality of patient–provider interactions [28, 30], suggesting that implicit semantic stereotypes may mediate medical professionals' communication with patients. This finding is important because interventions improving communication quality could address a key component of healthcare delivery that affects patient satisfaction, trust, and adherence to medical advice to address disparities [40, 81, 82]. Moreover, widespread use of artificial intelligence for diagnosis and treatment recommendations (e.g., [83]) may amplify the importance of healthcare providers' ability to communicate test results and treatment recommendations empathically as an essential skill of relationship-centered care.

One avenue for intervention involves nonverbal communication. Lloyd and Hugenberg [84] proposed that a sensitivity deficit in accurately perceiving nonverbal expressions of emotional states across race may contribute to racial disparities. For example, they noted that while doctors' biased perceptions of Black patients having increased pain tolerance in general may result in undertreatment of pain, a sensitivity deficit of doctors' ability to accurately perceive the pain levels of individual Black patients may explain both over- and under-treatment of medical concerns.

Indeed, Fini et al. [85] found that greater implicit bias as assessed by the IAT was associated with a decreased ability to remap observations of an outgroup member's body onto the participant's own body. In contrast, a participant's ability to mentalize and integrate an outgroup member's facial features with their own facial features increased after viewing an outgroup member's face being touched while simultaneously experiencing the touch on their own face. This effect, which was more pronounced for individuals with higher levels of implicit bias, may be explained in part through a reduction of perceived visual differences in outgroup members [85] and neural synchronization.

According to Prochazkova and Kret [86], perceptual input from an individual's facial expressions, gestures, and physiological responses activates corresponding mirror neuron and emotional systems in the perceiver. Specifically, mimicry and "brain-to-brain coupling" between two individuals synchronizes the mirror neuron system (areas implicated in mimicking others' actions and understanding their intentions) with the limbic system (associated with emotions) and the hypothalamic-pituitary-axis (involved in the stress response). Emotional contagion through sensorimotor perception and neural synchronization may allow individuals to understand and share the feelings of others as a foundational component of empathy. For example, Goldstein et al. [87] investigated how movement synchronization and artificially imposed group membership affected pain perception and patient trust in the clinician during simulated pain-inducing medical procedures. Higher movement synchronization predicted higher levels of trust and lower levels of pain. Further, movement synchrony, which was higher in the ingroup versus outgroup pairs, fully mediated the relationship between group membership and pain and trust.

Similarly, Hamel et al. [88] found that levels of nonverbal synchrony between oncologists and their patients were associated with the communication quality indicators of informativeness, supportiveness, and partnership building. Interestingly, however, racially discordant (White-Black) physician—patient dyads demonstrated greater nonverbal synchrony than racially concordant (White-White) dyads. Although not assessed, the researchers hypothesized that internal motivation for bias control may have played a role in physician nonverbal communication and synchronization. Indeed, empathy toward outgroup members elicits activation of motor activity and executive functions in the prefrontal cortex, suggesting that communication of empathy toward outgroup members may involve an interaction between effortful control and sensorimotor activity [89]. Based on these findings, healthcare professionals should receive training in nonverbal communication techniques, such as maintaining appropriate eye contact, a similar tone and rhythm of speech to those used by their patients, and mirroring body language (e.g., leaning forward or using hand gestures in a similar rhythm as their patients).

Finally, another avenue for intervention involves direct observation and feedback on verbal communication skills during the clinical encounter. Gonzalez et al. [90] developed a realistic simulation of a clinical encounter that included cognitive stressors such as interruptions and time constraints. Findings indicated that physician stereotype IAT scores corresponded with (simulated) patient ratings of physician communication by race, such that physicians with greater implicit bias were rated higher by White patients and lower by Black patients. The researchers proposed using this type of simulation for intervention and efficacy research to improve communication. Further, interventions might focus on the use of affiliative language and building emotional connections to improve verbal communication. In a review of the literature, Forsey and colleagues [91] highlighted strategies such as healthcare providers using "we" instead of "I" (e.g., "We're going to run some blood tests today"), asking hearer-oriented questions ("You're not experiencing any pain right now, are you?"), and engaging in casual conversation as ways to enhance feelings of interpersonal connection through relationship-centered care.

These and other explicit communication interventions present opportunities to combat implicit bias within the healthcare encounter; in contrast, the stereotype IAT poses psychometric concerns and presenting healthcare providers with their IAT results has demonstrated minimal efficacy in decreasing bias-driven behavior. Nonetheless, investigation of the impact of how medical professionals' semantic knowledge of societal stereotypes may mediate verbal and nonverbal communication warrants further consideration (see Box 3.3: Future Directions for the IAT). A less explored avenue for intervention could examine the neural correlates of nonverbal communication, including the use of nonverbal synchronization, to improve qualities such as trust and empathy in racially discordant dyads and overall care.

Box 3.3: Future Directions for the IAT

Controversy remains regarding the construct validity of the IAT and whether it measures semantic, associative knowledge of societal stereotypes. Critics contend that either its psychometric properties render the IAT an invalid tool or direct ratings might provide a better assessment of the construct it assesses [12]. Two possible factors may be contributing to measurement error and systematic method variance on the IAT.

First, stereotype congruent (e.g., White/good and Black/bad) and stereotype incongruent (e.g., White/bad, Black/good) blocks of the IAT are summarized in the same metric. Neural activation patterns and computational modeling suggest that examining these scores separately may provide useful information about the cognitive processes used to complete each block of the IAT (e.g., spreading activation of simple associations, weaker associations learned from less statistically frequent encounters with societal counter stereotypes; [55, 56, 58]). Future research could determine whether assessing cognitive processes separately reduces measurement error and systematic method variance to strengthen the overall construct validity of the stereotype IAT as a measure of sematic associative knowledge about racial groups.

Second, scores on the stereotype version of the IAT may summarize both evaluative and conceptual aspects of racial implicit bias in one metric, although theoretical and measurement findings support semantic stereotyping and racial evaluation as independent constructs [77, 78]. Indeed, Greenwald et al. [11] caution against confounding stereotypes and emotional valence, noting that development of a stereotype IAT should ensure that the traits being compared are neutral so that the test accurately measures the stereotype itself without the results being skewed by the participants' feelings about the traits.

Nonetheless, avoiding the confounding of stereotype traits with emotional valence can be challenging because language often carries inherent biases, cultural contexts of traits may vary, and participants may have their own preconceptions and emotional responses to traits. Future research could further delineate best practices for assessing semantic stereotyping and racial evaluation as independent constructs on a stereotype IAT, perhaps within a neurocognitive framework.

As it stands, researchers and practitioners are urged to consider the additive value of utilizing the IAT for research and intervention efforts. Research findings from the stereotype IAT may not capture important aspects of implicit racial bias within a clearly defined construct. Further, continued use of the stereotype IAT in its current form could sow distrust of implicit racial bias interventions by skeptics and divert the commitment of those eager for change into ineffective solutions. This commitment to change may be better served by public health [20] and neurobehavioral approaches to ameliorating discriminatory bias.

Clinical Decision Making and Treatment Outcomes

Systematic healthcare reviews found that implicit bias, as assessed by the stereotype IAT, did not conclusively impact clinical decision-making and treatment recommendations [27, 30]. Rather than evidence of bias not impacting these areas, the inconclusive findings may reflect a differentiated role for neurocognitive types of bias that impact clinical decision-making and treatment recommendations within the healthcare system. This can be illustrated by applying the research reviewed in this chapter to Vela et al.'s [40] model of bias in healthcare.

Within Vela et al.'s [40] model, medical professionals may be primed by the ubiquity of societal stereotypes [53, 54] and structural factors within healthcare systems such as provider time constraints during the workday, cognitive overload when making medical decisions, and lack of workforce diversity. Even for medical professionals with egalitarian goals, the automaticity of stereotype generation presents challenges to making nonstereotypical judgments or evaluations [53, 54] due to the statistically regular co-occurrences of stereotyped language and visual information [55] encountered within medical education and practice.

Because different types of semantic information activate different neural systems (e.g., processing simple associations between related concepts, activating conscious effort and control to navigate complex environmental demands; [58]), semantic stereotype knowledge differentially contributes to patient interactions and medical decision-making. Working memory overload may increase medical professionals' use of computationally efficient learning, such as associative semantic stereotypes [52]. Consequently, the communication quality of medical professionals, who also may have a sensitivity deficit in accurately perceiving nonverbal expressions of emotional states across race [84], can (unintentionally) reflect bias in verbal [28–30], and nonverbal [87, 88] medical interactions.

Moreover, healthcare professionals who reside or work in areas with greater, compared to reduced, degrees of community-level explicit racial prejudice may be primed by neural activation of the amygdala during clinical encounters with out-group members [79]. A Pavlovian-to-Instrumental transfer of learned social threats might influence these healthcare professionals' behavior during clinical interactions with racial outgroup members [35, 67, 68].

Further, patient perception of bias may result in distrust of the healthcare system and poor adherence to treatment recommendations. Applying Traast et al.'s [73] instrumental learning findings to the clinical setting, patient race may predispose White medical professionals to differ in their initial expectations for White and Black patient adherence to treatment recommendations. Medical professionals, especially those with high levels of explicit prejudice and low internal motivation for providing non-prejudiced responses, may be slower to update their perceptions of Black, compared to White, patients even with similar rates of treatment adherence.[2] Consequently, poor patient adherence to treatment recommendations and *perceptions* of poor adherence to treatment recommendations could result in reinforcement of the provider's biases through poor patient outcomes.

Finally, physician feelings of reward and treatment-related satisfaction may play a role in successful medical encounters [92]. Indeed, patient ratings of positive interactions with physicians during medical examinations were correlated with physician self-report of empathic concern and reward- and compassion-related activation of specific brain regions [93]. Thus, the deleterious effects of the cycle of disparities might also influence both healthcare provider and patient experiences of reward and treatment-related satisfaction and lead to negative outcomes that further perpetuate the cycle.

Given the neurocognitive complexity of the multiple pathways for biased learning and behavioral responding [46, 60], interventions that rely on semantic stereotype knowledge to interrupt the cycle of health disparities are ineffective [20, 80]. Therefore, in addition to the recommendations mentioned above, future research and bias reduction efforts should also consider the influence of emotional and instrumental learning of bias on patient—provider interactions, such as healthcare professionals' expectations for treatment outcomes, internal motivation for providing non-prejudiced responses, and feelings of reward and treatment-related satisfaction, in addition to the interactive effects of hospital and community level variables (e.g., medical education curricula and guidelines, high levels of explicit racial prejudice in the community).

[2] Because this type of bias is associated with instrumental learning rather than semantic knowledge, it would not be expected to correlate with the stereotype IAT. Indeed, Traast et al. [79] found no association between the race effects of instrumental leaning and IAT scores.

Conclusion

This chapter proposed how bias might be learned, encoded, and enacted from the perspective of the healthcare provider. It also will be important to understand these issues from the perspective of the patient, including patients' neural patterns associated with perceived bias, the impact of these neural responses on patient stress levels and health outcomes, and patient formation of expectations for future medical encounters. Overall, adopting a multifaceted framework that integrates social neuroscience advances the understanding of implicit bias in healthcare systems, responding to the call of *Unequal Treatment* to "explore how social cognitive processes may operate to influence patients' and providers' conscious and unconscious perceptions of each other and affect the structure, processes, and outcomes of care" ([1], p. 236–237). Moreover, it encourages new methods for bias reduction at the individual, group, and systemic levels with the ultimate goal of ameliorating disparities and providing equitable healthcare for all groups.

References

1. Smedley BD, Stith AY, Nelson AR. Unequal treatment: confronting racial and ethnic disparities in health care. Washington, DC: National Academies Press; 2003.
2. Fiske ST. Stereotyping, prejudice, and discrimination. In: Gilbert DT, Fiske ST, Lindzey G, editors. The handbook of social psychology. McGraw-Hill; 1998. p. 357–411.
3. Greenwald AG, Krieger LH. Implicit bias: scientific foundations. Calif Law Rev. 2006;94(4):945. https://doi.org/10.2307/20439056.
4. Cooper LA, Roter DL, Carson KA, Beach MC, Sabin JA, Greenwald AG, et al. The associations of clinicians' implicit attitudes about race with medical visit communication and patient ratings of interpersonal care. Am J Public Health. 2012;102(5):979–87. https://doi.org/10.2105/ajph.2011.300558.
5. Hagiwara N, Penner LA, Gonzalez R, Eggly S, Dovidio JF, Gaertner SL, et al. Racial attitudes, physician–patient talk time ratio, and adherence in racially discordant medical interactions. Soc Sci Med. 2013;87:123–31. https://doi.org/10.1016/j.socscimed.2013.03.016.
6. Blair IV, Steiner JF, Fairclough DL, Hanratty R, Price DW, Hirsh HK, et al. Clinicians' implicit ethnic/racial bias and perceptions of care among black and Latino patients. Ann Fam Med. 2013;11(1):43–52. https://doi.org/10.1370/afm.1442.
7. Blanchard J, Lurie N. R-E-S-P-E-C-T: patient reports of disrespect in the health care setting and its impact on care. J Fam Pract. 2004;53(9):721–30.
8. Greenwald AG, Banaji MR. Implicit social cognition: attitudes, self-esteem, and stereotypes. Psychol Rev. 1995;102(1):4–27. https://doi.org/10.1037/0033-295x.102.1.4.
9. Greenwald AG, Lai CK. Implicit social cognition. Annu Rev Psychol. 2020;71(1):419–45. https://doi.org/10.1146/annurev-psych-010419-050837.
10. Greenwald AG, McGhee DE, Schwartz JLK. Measuring individual differences in implicit cognition: the implicit association test. J Pers Soc Psychol. 1998;74(6):1464–80. https://doi.org/10.1037/0022-3514.74.6.1464.
11. Greenwald AG, Brendl M, Cai H, Cvencek D, Dovidio JF, Friese M, et al. Best research practices for using the implicit association test. Behav Res Methods. 2022;54(3):1161–80. https://doi.org/10.3758/s13428-021-01624-3.

12. Schimmack U. The implicit association test: a method in search of a construct. Perspect Psychol Sci. 2021;16(2):396–414. https://doi.org/10.1177/1745691619863798.
13. Kurdi B, Ratliff KA, Cunningham WA. Can the implicit association test serve as a valid measure of automatic cognition? A response to Schimmack (2021). Perspect Psychol Sci. 2021;16(2):422–34. https://doi.org/10.1177/1745691620904080.
14. Vianello M, Bar-Anan Y. Can the Implicit Association Test measure automatic judgment? The validation continues. Perspect Psychol Sci. 2021;16(2):415–21. https://doi.org/10.1177/1745691619897960.
15. Schimmack U. Invalid claims about the validity of Implicit Association Tests by prisoners of the implicit social-cognition paradigm. Perspect Psychol Sci. 2021;16(2):435–42. https://doi.org/10.1177/1745691621991860.
16. Röhner J, Iliescu D. On the death of implicit association tests (IATs). Eur. J Psychol Assess. 2023;39(5):317–22. https://doi.org/10.1027/1015-5759/a000778.
17. Pennington CR, Ploszajski M, Mistry P, NgOmbe N, Back C, Parsons S, et al. Relationships between the race implicit association test and other measures of implicit and explicit social cognition. Front Psychol. 2023;14:1197298. https://doi.org/10.3389/fpsyg.2023.1197298.
18. Banaji MR, Greenwald AG. Blindspot: Hidden biases of good people. New York, NY: Random House; 2013.
19. Cvencek D, Meltzoff AN, Maddox CD, Nosek BA, Rudman LA, Devos T, et al. Meta-analytic use of balanced identity theory to validate the implicit association test. Pers Soc Psychol Bull. 2021;47(2):185–200. https://doi.org/10.1177/0146167220916631.
20. Greenwald AG, Dasgupta N, Dovidio JF, Kang J, Moss-Racusin CA, Teachman BA. Implicit-bias remedies: Treating discriminatory bias as a public-health problem. Psychol Sci Public Interest. 2022;23(1):7–40. https://doi.org/10.1177/15291006211070781.
21. Greenwald AG, Poehlman TA, Uhlmann EL, Banaji MR. Understanding and using the implicit association test: III. Meta-analysis of predictive validity. J Pers Soc Psychol. 2009;97(1):17–41. https://doi.org/10.1037/a0015575.
22. Kurdi B, Seitchik AE, Axt JR, Carroll TJ, Karapetyan A, Kaushik N, et al. Relationship between the implicit association test and intergroup behavior: a meta-analysis. Am Psychol. 2019;74(5):569–86. https://doi.org/10.1037/amp0000364.
23. Oswald FL, Mitchell G, Blanton H, Jaccard J, Tetlock PE. Predicting ethnic and racial discrimination: a meta-analysis of IAT criterion studies. J Pers Soc Psychol. 2013;105(2):171–92. https://doi.org/10.1037/a0032734.
24. Greenwald AG, Brendl M, Cai H, Cvencek D, Dovidio J, Friese M, et al. The implicit association test at age 20: what is known and what is not known about implicit bias. PsyArXiv. 2020; https://doi.org/10.31234/osf.io/bf97c.
25. Andreychik MR, Gill MJ. Do negative implicit associations indicate negative attitudes? Social explanations moderate whether ostensible "negative" associations are prejudice-based or empathy-based. J Exp Soc Psychol. 2012;48(5):1082–93. https://doi.org/10.1016/j.jesp.2012.05.006.
26. Greenwald AG, Banaji MR, Nosek BA. Statistically small effects of the implicit association test can have societally large effects. J Pers Soc Psychol. 2015;108(4):553–61. https://doi.org/10.1037/pspa0000016.
27. Dehon E, Weiss N, Jones J, Faulconer W, Hinton E, Sterling S. A systematic review of the impact of physician implicit racial bias on clinical decision making. Acad Emerg Med. 2017;24(8):895–904. https://doi.org/10.1111/acem.13214.
28. FitzGerald C, Hurst S. Implicit bias in healthcare professionals: a systematic review. BMC Med Ethics. 2017;18(1):1–8. https://doi.org/10.1186/s12910-017-0179-8.
29. Hall WJ, Chapman MV, Lee KM, Merino YM, Thomas TW, Payne BK, et al. Implicit racial/ethnic bias among health care professionals and its influence on health care outcomes: a systematic review. Am J Public Health. 2015;105(12):e60–76. https://doi.org/10.2105/ajph.2015.302903.

30. Maina IW, Belton TD, Ginzberg S, Singh A, Johnson TJ. A decade of studying implicit racial/ethnic bias in healthcare providers using the implicit association test. Soc Sci Med. 2018;199:219–29. https://doi.org/10.1016/j.socscimed.2017.05.009.
31. Meidert U, Dönnges G, Bucher T, Wieber F, Gerber-Grote A. Unconscious bias among health professionals: a scoping review. Int J Environ Res Public Health. 2023;20(16):6569. https://doi.org/10.3390/ijerph20166569.
32. Sukhera J, Watling CJ, Gonzalez CM. Implicit bias in health professions: from recognition to transformation. Acad Med. 2020;95(5):717–23. https://doi.org/10.1097/acm.0000000000003173.
33. Mason B, Knowable Magazine. Making people aware of their implicit biases doesn't usually change minds. But here's what does work. PBS NewsHour. 2020 [cited 2024 May 11]. https://www.pbs.org/newshour/nation/making-people-aware-of-their-implicit-biases-doesnt-usually-change-minds-but-heres-what-does-work
34. Vedantam S. The mind of the village: understanding our implicit biases. NPR. 2020 Jun 20 [cited 2024 May 11]; https://www.npr.org/2020/06/20/880379282/the-mind-of-the-village-understanding-our-implicit-biases
35. Amodio DM, Berg JJ. The neural underpinnings of intergroup bias. In: Molenberghs P, editor. The neuroscience of intergroup relations. New York, NY: Routledge; 2022.
36. Sabin JA. Tackling implicit bias in health care. N Engl J Med. 2022;387(2):105–7. https://doi.org/10.1056/nejmp2201180.
37. Braveman P. Health disparities and health equity: concepts and measurement. Annu Rev Public Health. 2006;27(1):167–94. https://doi.org/10.1146/annurev.publhealth.27.021405.102103.
38. Braveman P. What are health disparities and health equity? We need to be clear. Public Health Rep. 2014;129(1_suppl2):5–8. https://doi.org/10.1177/00333549141291S203.
39. Bailey ZD, Krieger N, Agénor M, Graves J, Linos N, Bassett MT. Structural racism and health inequities in the USA: evidence and interventions. Lancet. 2017;389(10077):1453–63. https://doi.org/10.1016/s0140-6736(17)30569-x.
40. Vela MB, Erondu AI, Smith NA, Peek ME, Woodruff JN, Chin MH. Eliminating explicit and implicit biases in health care: evidence and research needs. Annu Rev Public Health. 2022;43(1):477–501. https://doi.org/10.1146/annurev-publhealth-052620-103528.
41. Amutah C, Greenidge K, Mante A, Munyikwa M, Surya SL, Higginbotham E, et al. Misrepresenting race—the role of medical schools in propagating physician bias. N Engl J Med. 2021;384(9):872–8. https://doi.org/10.1056/NEJMms2025768.
42. Cacioppo JT, Berntson GG, Sheridan JF, McClintock MK. Multilevel integrative analyses of human behavior: social neuroscience and the complementing nature of social and biological approaches. Psychol Bull. 2000;126(6):829–43. https://doi.org/10.1037/0033-2909.126.6.829.
43. Cacioppo JT, Berntson GG, Decety J. Social neuroscience and its relationship to social psychology. Soc Cogn. 2010;28(6):675–85. https://doi.org/10.1521/soco.2010.28.6.675.
44. Molenberghs P. The neuroscience of in-group bias. Neurosci Biobehav Rev. 2013;37(8):1530–6. https://doi.org/10.1016/j.neubiorev.2013.06.002.
45. Cikara M, Van Bavel JJ. The neuroscience of intergroup relations: an integrative review: an integrative review. Perspect Psychol Sci. 2014;9(3):245–74. https://doi.org/10.1177/1745691614527464.
46. Amodio DM. The neuroscience of prejudice and stereotyping. Nat Rev Neurosci. 2014;15(10):670–82. https://doi.org/10.1038/nrn3800.
47. Amodio DM. Social cognition 2.0: an interactive memory systems account. Trends Cogn Sci. 2019;23(1):21–33. https://doi.org/10.1016/j.tics.2018.10.002.
48. Stanovich KE, West RF, Toplak MJ, Sherman B, Gawronski Y. Rationality, intelligence, and the defining features of Type 1 and Type 2 processing. In: Dual-process theories of the social mind. New York, NY: Guilford Press; 2014. p. 80–91.
49. Yee E, Jones MN, McRae K. Semantic memory. In: Stevens' handbook of experimental psychology and cognitive neuroscience. Wiley; 2018. p. 1–38. https://doi.org/10.1002/9781119170174.epcn309.

50. Balgova E, Diveica V, Walbrin J, Binney RJ. The role of the ventrolateral anterior temporal lobes in social cognition. Hum Brain Mapp. 2022;43(15):4589–608. https://doi.org/10.1002/hbm.25976.
51. Bodenhausen GV, Macrae CN, Hugenberg K. Social cognition. Handbook of psychology. Wiley; 2003. p. 255–82. https://doi.org/10.1002/0471264385.wei0511.
52. Contreras JM, Banaji MR, Mitchell JP. Dissociable neural correlates of stereotypes and other forms of semantic knowledge. Soc Cogn Affect Neurosci. 2012;7(7):764–70. https://doi.org/10.1093/scan/nsr053.
53. Devine PG. Stereotypes and prejudice: their automatic and controlled components. J Pers Soc Psychol. 1989;56(1):5–18. https://doi.org/10.1037/0022-3514.56.1.5.
54. Hinton P. Implicit stereotypes and the predictive brain: cognition and culture in "biased" person perception. Palgrave Commun. 2017;3(1):1–9. https://doi.org/10.1057/palcomms.2017.86.
55. Unger L, Fisher AV. The emergence of richly organized semantic knowledge from simple statistics: a synthetic review. Dev Rev. 2021;60(100949):100949. https://doi.org/10.1016/j.dr.2021.100949.
56. Forbes CE, Cameron KA, Grafman J, Barbey A, Solomon J, Ritter W, et al. Identifying temporal and causal contributions of neural processes underlying the implicit association test (IAT). Front Hum Neurosci. 2012;6:320. https://doi.org/10.3389/fnhum.2012.00320.
57. Healy GF, Boran L, Smeaton AF. Neural patterns of the implicit association test. Front Hum Neurosci. 2015;9:605. https://doi.org/10.3389/fnhum.2015.00605.
58. Davey J, Thompson HE, Hallam G, Karapanagiotidis T, Murphy C, De Caso I, et al. Exploring the role of the posterior middle temporal gyrus in semantic cognition: integration of anterior temporal lobe with executive processes. Neuroimage. 2016;137:165–77. https://doi.org/10.1016/j.neuroimage.2016.05.051.
59. Amodio DM, Ratner KG. A memory systems model of implicit social cognition. Curr Dir Psychol Sci. 2011;20(3):143–8. https://doi.org/10.1177/0963721411408562.
60. Amodio DM, Cikara M. The social neuroscience of prejudice. Annu Rev Psychol. 2021;72(1):439–69. https://doi.org/10.1146/annurev-psych-010419-050928.
61. Rösler IK, Amodio DM. Neural basis of prejudice and prejudice reduction. Biol Psychiatry Cogn Neurosci Neuroimaging. 2022;7(12):1200–8. https://doi.org/10.1016/j.bpsc.2022.10.008.
62. Amodio DM, Berg JJ. Toward a multiple memory systems model of attitudes and social cognition. Psychol Inq. 2018;29(1):14–9. https://doi.org/10.1080/1047840x.2018.1435620.
63. Cunningham WA, Johnson MK, Raye CL, Gatenby JC, Gore JC, Banaji MR. Separable neural components in the processing of Black and White faces. Psychol Sci. 2004;15(12):806–13. https://doi.org/10.1111/j.0956-7976.2004.00760.x.
64. Lieberman MD, Hariri A, Jarcho JM, Eisenberger NI, Bookheimer SY. An fMRI investigation of race-related amygdala activity in African-American and Caucasian-American individuals. Nat Neurosci. 2005;8(6):720–2. https://doi.org/10.1038/nn1465.
65. Phelps EA, O'Connor KJ, Cunningham WA, Funayama ES, Gatenby JC, Gore JC, et al. Performance on indirect measures of race evaluation predicts amygdala activation. J Cogn Neurosci. 2000;12(5):729–38. https://doi.org/10.1162/089892900562552.
66. Chekroud AM, Everett JAC, Bridge H, Hewstone M. A review of neuroimaging studies of race-related prejudice: does amygdala response reflect threat? Front Hum Neurosci. 2014;8:179. https://doi.org/10.3389/fnhum.2014.00179.
67. Selbing I, Sandberg D, Olsson A, Lindström B, Golkar A. The transfer of social threat learning to decision making is robust to extinction. Emotion. 2024;24(7):1689–96. https://doi.org/10.1037/emo0001392.
68. da Costa RQM, Furukawa E, Hoefle S, Moll J, Tripp G, Mattos P. An adaptation of Pavlovian-to-instrumental transfer (PIT) methodology to examine the energizing effects of reward-predicting cues on behavior in young adults. Front Psychol. 2020:11, 195. https://doi.org/10.3389/fpsyg.2020.00195.
69. Schmid PC, Hackel LM, Amodio DM. Power effects on instrumental learning: evidence from the brain and behavior. Motiv Sci. 2018;4(3):206–26. https://doi.org/10.1037/mot0000088.

70. Hackel LM, Mende-Siedlecki P, Loken S, Amodio DM. Context-dependent learning in social interaction: trait impressions support flexible social choices. J Pers Soc Psychol. 2022;123(4):655–75. https://doi.org/10.1037/pspa0000296.
71. Hackel LM, Doll BB, Amodio DM. Instrumental learning of traits versus rewards: dissociable neural correlates and effects on choice. Nat Neurosci. 2015;18(9):1233–5. https://doi.org/10.1038/nn.4080.
72. Lindström B, Selbing I, Molapour T, Olsson A. Racial bias shapes social reinforcement learning. Psychol Sci. 2014;25(3):711–9. https://doi.org/10.1177/0956797613514093.
73. Traast IJ, Schultner DT, Doosje B, Amodio DM. Race effects on impression formation in social interaction: an instrumental learning account. J Exp Psychol Gen. 2024; https://doi.org/10.1037/xge0001523.
74. Gilbert SJ, Swencionis JK, Amodio DM. Evaluative vs. trait representation in intergroup social judgments: distinct roles of anterior temporal lobe and prefrontal cortex. Neuropsychologia. 2012;50(14):3600–11. https://doi.org/10.1016/j.neuropsychologia.2012.09.002.
75. Petersen KJ, Donahue MJ, Claassen DO. Mapping the orbitofrontal cortex using temporal fluctuations in cerebral blood flow. Brain Behav. 2021;11(3):e02034. https://doi.org/10.1002/brb3.2034.
76. Rolls ET. Emotion, motivation, decision-making, the orbitofrontal cortex, anterior cingulate cortex, and the amygdala. Brain Struct Funct. 2023;228(5):1201–57. https://doi.org/10.1007/s00429-023-02644-9.
77. Amodio DM, Hamilton HK. Intergroup anxiety effects on implicit racial evaluation and stereotyping. Emotion. 2012;12(6):1273–80. https://doi.org/10.1037/a0029016.
78. Amodio DM, Devine PG. Stereotyping and evaluation in implicit race bias: evidence for independent constructs and unique effects on behavior. J Pers Soc Psychol. 2006;91(4):652–61. https://doi.org/10.1037/0022-3514.91.4.652.
79. Hatzenbuehler ML, Mclaughlin KA, Weissman DG, Cikara M. Community-level explicit racial prejudice potentiates whites' neural responses to black faces: a spatial meta-analysis. Soc Neurosci. 2022;17(6):508–19. https://doi.org/10.1080/17470919.2022.2153915.
80. Forscher PS, Lai CK, Axt JR, Ebersole CR, Herman M, Devine PG, et al. A meta-analysis of procedures to change implicit measures. J Pers Soc Psychol. 2019;117(3):522–59. https://doi.org/10.1037/pspa0000160.
81. Hagiwara N, Elston Lafata J, Mezuk B, Vrana SR, Fetters MD. Detecting implicit racial bias in provider communication behaviors to reduce disparities in healthcare: challenges, solutions, and future directions for provider communication training. Patient Educ Couns. 2019;102(9):1738–43. https://doi.org/10.1016/j.pec.2019.04.023.
82. Hagiwara N, Dovidio JF, Stone J, Penner LA. Applied racial/ethnic healthcare disparities research using implicit measures. Soc Cogn. 2020;38(Supplement):s68–97. https://doi.org/10.1521/soco.2020.38.supp.s68.
83. Alowais SA, Alghamdi SS, Alsuhebany N, Alqahtani T, Alshaya AI, Almohareb SN, et al. Revolutionizing healthcare: the role of artificial intelligence in clinical practice. BMC Med Educ. 2023;23(1):689. https://doi.org/10.1186/s12909-023-04698-z.
84. Lloyd EP, Hugenberg K. Beyond bias: response bias and interpersonal (in)sensitivity as a contributors to race disparities. Eur Rev Soc Psychol. 2021;32(2):201–34. https://doi.org/10.1080/10463283.2020.1820699.
85. Fini C, Cardini F, Tajadura-Jiménez A, Serino A, Tsakiris M. Embodying an outgroup: the role of racial bias and the effect of multisensory processing in somatosensory remapping. Front Behav Neurosci. 2013;7:165. https://doi.org/10.3389/fnbeh.2013.00165.
86. Prochazkova E, Kret ME. Connecting minds and sharing emotions through mimicry: a neurocognitive model of emotional contagion. Neurosci Biobehav Rev. 2017;80:99–114. https://doi.org/10.1016/j.neubiorev.2017.05.013.
87. Goldstein P, Losin EAR, Anderson SR, Schelkun VR, Wager TD. Clinician-patient movement synchrony mediates social group effects on interpersonal trust and perceived pain. J Pain. 2020;21(11–12):1160–74. https://doi.org/10.1016/j.jpain.2020.03.001.

88. Hamel LM, Moulder R, Ramseyer FT, Penner LA, Albrecht TL, Boker S, et al. Nonverbal synchrony: an indicator of clinical communication quality in racially-concordant and racially-discordant oncology interactions. Cancer Control. 2022;29:107327482211139. https://doi.org/10.1177/10732748221113905.
89. Merritt CC, MacCormack JK, Stein AG, Lindquist KA, Muscatell KA. The neural underpinnings of intergroup social cognition: an fMRI meta-analysis. Soc Cogn Affect Neurosci. 2021;16(9):903–14. https://doi.org/10.1093/scan/nsab034.
90. Gonzalez CM, Ark TK, Fisher MR, Marantz PR, Burgess DJ, Milan F, et al. Racial implicit bias and communication among physicians in a simulated environment. JAMA Netw Open. 2024;7(3):e242181. https://doi.org/10.1001/jamanetworkopen.2024.2181.
91. Forsey J, Ng S, Rowland P, Freeman R, Li C, Woods NN. The basic science of patient–physician communication: a critical scoping review: a critical scoping review. Acad Med. 2021;96(11S):S109–18. https://doi.org/10.1097/acm.0000000000004323.
92. Jensen KB, Petrovic P, Kerr CE, Kirsch I, Raicek J, Cheetham A, et al. Sharing pain and relief: neural correlates of physicians during treatment of patients. Mol Psychiatry. 2014;19(3):392–8. https://doi.org/10.1038/mp.2012.195.
93. Jensen K, Gollub RL, Kong J, Lamm C, Kaptchuk TJ, Petrovic P. Reward and empathy in the treating clinician: the neural correlates of successful doctor–patient interactions. Transl Psychiatry. 2020;10(1):17. https://doi.org/10.1038/s41398-020-0712-2.

Chapter 4
Bias in Reproductive Medicine

Danielle A. Kaplan, R. Raoul Meyer, and Torie C. Plowden

Introduction

Health disparities and inequities in healthcare exist widely across all fields of medicine [1]. There are many factors that influence this phenomenon, including implicit bias in clinicians. Indeed, there is evidence that biases about patients' race or ethnicity as well as other identity-based characteristics can impact healthcare providers' diagnostic and treatment decisions [1]. Clinician implicit bias is not limited to racial or ethnic minority patients; members of gender and sexual minority groups and people with disabilities (PWDs) are equally subjected to its impact. Bias at the level of the individual clinician can interact with and magnify systemic and structural factors that disadvantage minoritized patients across categories. The result is a reproductive healthcare system in which patients who are not White, heterosexual, cisgender, and neurotypical or able-bodied are often deprived of timely and accessible reproductive care to the detriment of their physical health and reproductive potential. In this chapter, we provide a broad overview of the impact of individual, legal, and systemic bias on the reproductive care of marginalized populations. Our focus is on patients from Black, Latinx, and LGBTQ+ communities and those with disabilities, as the reproductive health of members of these groups has been significantly impacted by providers' perceptions of their sexuality and the desirability of their reproduction.

D. A. Kaplan (✉)
Department of Psychiatry, NYU Langone Medical Center, New York, NY, USA

R. R. Meyer
Independent Practice, New York, NY, USA

T. C. Plowden
Walter Reed National Military Medical Center, Bethesda, MD, USA

D. A. Kaplan (ed.), *Cultural Responsiveness in Assisted Reproductive Technology*, https://doi.org/10.1007/978-3-031-76204-8_4

Intersectionality refers to the concept that people who belong to multiple minoritized groups have a unique set of experiences that collude to increase the likelihood of oppression and inequitable treatment [2, 3]. For example, the experiences of individuals who identify as Black sexual minority women have overlapping identities that may compound their experience of discrimination and be different than those of people occupying only one of these identities [4–6]. People holding intersectional marginalized identities must overcome racism, sexism, ableism, and homophobia to access reproductive health care and their unique reproductive issues have not been centered in policy development or research initiatives [7].

Black Women and Bias in Reproductive Medicine

The experiences of Black patients across the continuum of medical care are discussed at length throughout this volume (see especially Chaps. 6, 9, and 13), and therefore the current chapter provides only an episodic discussion of these experiences. Both historically and currently, Black women have been subject to inequitable treatment in medical care that leads to worse outcomes in their general health and their experiences of infertility and pregnancy care. Racism and bias, both implicit and explicit, significantly and negatively impact the outcomes Black women face in reproductive healthcare [8–10]. Many principles and advances seen in modern-day obstetrics and gynecology were predicated on experimental surgeries of Black enslaved women. These advances have come at the cost of perpetuating myths about Black women's pain tolerance and reproductive anatomy and of decreasing the trust of Black patients in the medical system [9, 11, 12].

Reproductive Autonomy and Slavery

Historically, systems of racial oppression have hindered Black women's reproductive autonomy. As early as 1662, the legal doctrine of *partus sequitur ventrem* (literally, "offspring follows womb") dictated that any child born of an enslaved mother would themselves automatically inherit the legal status of an enslaved person regardless of the legal status of their fathers. This doctrine both promoted the creation of a permanent enslaved class in the colonies and created a system in which Black women's essential value was tied to their reproductive capacity [13]. During his term as President of the United States, Thomas Jefferson (himself the father of several enslaved children) was reputed to have said, "I consider a slave woman who can give birth to a child every 2 years as more profitable than the best man on the farm" ([11], p. 106). The valuing of enslaved Black women for their ability to have children also gave rise to the myth that Black women were hypersexual and that (particularly White) men were vulnerable to being coerced into sexual relationships with them—a damaging stereotype that would soon have implications for the State's interest in their reproduction.

State-Sponsored Sterilization

As legalized slavery was ended, Black women's reproductive capacity went from being viewed as essential to the creation of a permanent involuntary labor force to being seen by many in power as a threat to the racial and moral purity and economic stability of the nation. The growth of the eugenics movement in nineteenth- and early twentieth-century America promoted the belief that reproductive capacity should be tied to intellectual and moral fitness to parent—qualities that Black women were widely believed to lack. Eugenicist policies in America have historically targeted women of color and those with mental illness [14–16]; the impact of eugenics on the reproductive potential of minoritized patients is a recurring theme in American history and therefore of this chapter.

State-sponsored sterilization programs, reflecting the biases of policy makers and medical professionals, have disproportionately targeted Black women for permanent contraception (see Box 4.1). Agents of both the state and the medical establishment feared that the supposed hyperfertility and low socioeconomic status of Black women would contribute to their having too many children, thus creating a drain on the resources of the state. Proponents of curtailing the reproductive potential of Black women sought to bolster their position by calling the inherent parental competency of these women into question, raising the specter of creating an "embryonic criminal class" if Black mothers were allowed to parent unchecked ([17], p. 57).

It is important to note that some of these issues are not relegated to a remote past. Black women continue to be counseled toward permanent sterilization at higher rates than White women [18]. Ironically, among women *desiring* permanent sterilization after childbirth, both White women with private insurance and those on Medicaid are more likely to have their request honored than are Black women, speaking yet again to the overall lack of reproductive autonomy afforded to Black women regardless of their fertility desires [19].

Box 4.1: The Relf Sisters

The most egregious examples of bias affecting women's reproductive choices occur when states enact policies that enforce sterilization. These policies disproportionately have ensnared Black women and other people of color, as well as people with intellectual and physical disabilities. The Relf sisters are a particularly tragic example of how bias and policies interact to destroy marginalized women's reproductive rights. In 1972, the Relf family—Lonnie, Minnie and their six children—were living in a cardboard shack in a field in Montgomery, Alabama. A social worker, Jessie Bly, worked hard to find the Relfs a place in public housing, secure clothes for the family, and get the children into school. She made sure that Mary Alice, who had been born without one of her hands, was tested for eligibility for special education services, at which point it was determined that she was developmentally disabled and recommended for the McInnis School for Retarded Children. The family also received food stamps, welfare, and disability payments for Lonnie, who was unable to work because of an earlier accident. The Relf family was deeply enmeshed in state and federal social safety net programs, which is likely what brought them to the attention of the Family Planning Clinic of the Montgomery Community Action Committee [20].

At the Family Planning clinic, the Relfs' oldest daughter Katie was the first member of the family to be given injections of the Depo-Provera contraceptive, which at the time was not FDA approved for use in adults or teenagers. Neither Katie nor her mother gave the staff permission to administer the contraceptive. In March 1973, 17-year-old Katie was brought to the clinic to have an IUD inserted, again without her permission, after the FDA determined that Depo-Provera was too dangerous. In June, employees of the clinic picked up Mary Alice and Minnie Lee, the two youngest Relf daughters, and brought them in for what their mother believed would be more shots. Mrs. Relf was given a consent form to sign, but it was clear that she didn't understand that she was giving permission for her daughters to be surgically sterilized. Mrs. Relf, unable to sign her full name, marked the piece of paper with an "X." Clinic employees returned to the Relf home for Katie, but the older girl, knowing that something untoward was happening to her little sisters, refused to go. After speaking with Katie, Jessie Bly went to the clinic where she found the two younger girls huddled in pain [20]. At the time they were sterilized, Minnie Lee Relf was 14 years old. Mary Alice was twelve.

With Bly's help, the Relf family secured the services of the newly-founded Southern Poverty Law Center and filed a lawsuit in federal district court. The case, *Relf v. Weinberger*, claimed that the Departments of Health Education and Welfare (HEW) and Health and Human Services (HHS) had knowingly funded experimental drugs and sterilization procedures for poor, Black women who received government benefits. The case received national attention, even inspiring Senator Ted Kennedy to hold Congressional hearings at which Minne and Lonnie Relf testified that they were unaware that their daughters were undergoing procedures that would make it impossible for them ever to have children. The couple testified that, had they known, they would never have allowed it [21].

The *Relf v. Weinberger* case and accompanying publicity brought to light the fact that between 100,000 and 150,000 mostly poor, Black women had been sterilized each year pursuant to federal programs. The case did result in the federal government changing its policies, with HEW withdrawing its regulation that authorized funding for forced sterilization and creating new procedures for obtaining informed consent. This provided little comfort to the Relf family, however, and they brought a civil damages suit against the government claiming five million dollars in damages. The case was dismissed on a technicality in 1977. Mary Alice and Minnie Lee Relf continued to live in public housing, often yearning for the babies that they would never be able to have [22].

Infertility Care

Black women face pervasive stereotypes regarding their fertility. The pernicious myth that Black women are hyperfertile began during slavery in the United States. This long-held belief persists into the present day [23, 24], despite existing evidence that Black women experience infertility at higher rates than their White counterparts [25]. Some people in Black communities believe this stereotype is true, and have reported feelings of shame, guilt and isolation when faced with infertility [23]. More significantly, the long-standing misbelief that Black women do not suffer fertility issues impacts the way they are treated by medical professionals.

The experiences of Black women denote a lack of empathetic encounters with physicians and other health care providers, particularly in reproductive health settings [26]. Black women suffering from infertility have encountered health care providers who assume they can't afford treatment, are unmarried or are sexually promiscuous [23]. In one study, a high proportion of high-income, educated Black women patients still reported having a lack of support at infertility clinics [27]. Perhaps reflecting the hyperfertility myth, Black women are less likely to be referred for infertility treatment by their physicians and more likely to self-refer for care or present for infertility treatment at the urging of a friend or relative [27]. Taken together, these studies indicate that bias may be at play in the decreased rate of referral for Black patients and the use of less effective forms of ART treatment for those who are referred [28]. The negative consequences of physician bias include both physical and emotional harm. In a review of qualitative research, women from underserved communities experienced psychological distress when experiencing bias from healthcare providers, ultimately leading them to feel judged rather than heard and have an overall lack of trust toward the physician [29].

Individual and structural suggestions for ameliorating the impact of bias on the reproductive lives of Black women are discussed at length throughout this volume. It is important to note, however, that the inequities in reproductive care for Black women are inextricably tied to the United States' unique history of slavery and anti-Black racism. To remedy these inequities, then, requires us to reckon with systems that were built on the idea of Black bodies as qualitatively different from and less worthy than White bodies, and the downstream effects of those systems on Black patients' reproductive health.

LGBTQ+ Patients in Reproductive Medicine

Individual and systemic biases result in many sub-optimal healthcare outcomes for members of the LGBTQ+ community. Disparities in reproductive healthcare and health literacy for LGBTQ+ individuals begin long before considerations of parenthood. Most school-based sexual education curricula are heteronormative; although 70% of adolescents report receiving some form of sex education at school, only eleven states require a curriculum that comprises an inclusive discussion of sexual orientation and gender identity. Almost as many require the opposite; as of 2024, six states mandated that school curricula comprise only negative information about homosexuality and gender diversity [30]. When issues of sexual orientation are raised in the curriculum, it is often exclusively in the context of HIV prevention.

A lack of inclusive sex education puts LGBTQ+ adolescents and young adults at risk. Education that focuses exclusively on penile-vaginal intercourse is insufficient to provide gay, lesbian, and transgender students with accurate relevant information about safe sex practices [31]. The absence of accurate information about their sexuality increases these adolescents' risk of STDs and intimate partner violence [32], both of which have implications for their reproductive futures and their physical and emotional well-being.

When seeking medical care, LGBTQ+ patients may again find themselves working with providers who provide limited information. Both sexual minority women and transmasculine men are less likely to be provided with adequate contraception than are heterosexual and cisgender women. As both of these populations are able to and often do become pregnant, rates of unintended pregnancy among both teens and adults are higher for these groups than they are for their heterosexual and cisgender peers [33, 34].

Among adults, sexual orientation and gender identity alone are not determinative of the desire for parenthood. Internationally, many LGBTQ+ individuals report the desire to parent either alone or with a partner [35, 36]. Studies that do document lower levels of desire for parenthood among LGBTQ+ individuals often tie this finding to fears about social stigma and lower rates of expectation that they will achieve their desired life outcomes across all domains, including education, employment, and housing [37, 38].

If they desire a biologically related child, LGBTQ+ individuals often need medical assistance to create their families. Many lesbian couples are choosing to pursue assisted reproductive technology (ART) treatments in which one or both partners participate in conceiving or carrying a child or children [39]. Gay men who desire parenthood often require the collaboration of both an egg donor and a gestational carrier. In fact, in recent years, there has been a substantial increase in the use of

ART among members of the LGBTQ+ community [40]. Simultaneously, there has been a recognition by the ART community that, contrary to stereotypical perception, sexual orientation and gender identity are not determinative of patients' desire for parenthood or the well-being of their children; the most recent ASRM Ethics Committee Opinion exhorts programs to "treat all requests for assisted reproduction equally, without regard to marital status, sexual orientation, or gender identity" [41, 42].

Yet patients in the LGBTQ+ community report not feeling well supported by their healthcare team. One systematic review examined studies that commented on either the patients' or the providers' perspective of cultural competence in reproductive healthcare [43]. Patients reported not feeling welcomed, noting that standardized forms were heteronormative and excluded LGBTQ+ individuals. They also experienced a lack of information specifically geared toward same-sex couples, leaving them unsure of what their treatment options were [43]. Some patients reported experiencing frank discrimination and having negative interactions with fertility clinics [43]. A qualitative study conducted in Canada sought to better understand the lived experience of lesbian patients attempting to build their families. Those interviewed in this study expressed a desire for additional support navigating access to treatment as well as the actual process of undergoing treatment [44].

The LGBTQ+ community may have different concerns when building their families than heterosexual couples [44]. Members of this community express that many physicians and other healthcare providers lack a fundamental understanding of their community's reproductive health priorities [45]. Healthcare providers have also recognized that LGBTQ+ fertility patients face barriers including a lack of tailored information [43]. In a small survey of 169 currently practicing board-certified obstetricians/gynecologists, less than half reported training in caring for lesbian, gay, bisexual, transgender and gender- nonconforming individuals [46].

In the past, the assumption was that most transgender people did not want to have children [47], but studies indicate that a large portion of transgender individuals are open to parenthood [48], and many transgender individuals are already parents [47]. In recent years, more transgender patients are undergoing referral to a reproductive endocrinologist to discuss fertility preservation options [49]. However, transgender individuals may face more barriers to fertility care than other in the LGBTQ+ community. In a survey of over 1600 transgender, nonbinary and gender expansive people, 70% reported at least one negative interaction with a healthcare provider in the past year [50]. Further, as recently as 2021, a review of records suggested that between 45 and 77% of patients received no counseling about fertility preservation prior to initiating gender-affirming medical treatment [51]. Another study that focused on the perspective of the provider noted that providers were fearful of using incorrect pronouns or otherwise offending their transgender patients [52]. In that qualitative study, providers recognized the need to "unlearn cisnormativity" to improve their ability to care for transgender patients [52].

It should also be noted that the traditional diagnosis of infertility, which forms the basis for insurance coverage for infertility care, presumes that couples have attempted to conceive through penile-vaginal intercourse. By definition, this diagnosis excludes same-sex couples and some couples in which one partner is transgender, making them ineligible for insurance-subsidized care [53]. For many LGBTQ+ patients, then, lack of provider cultural competence is secondary to a lack of access to fertility care based solely on the prohibitively high costs of unsubsidized treatment.

The treatment of sexual and gender minority patients across the continuum of reproductive healthcare and education is at odds with the aspirational principle of providing equitable services to all patients. Improved patient and provider education and changes in clinic forms and policies are needed to ensure that medical advances in fertility care for LGBTQ+ patients are accompanied by similar advances in these patients' experience of care.

Latinx Patients in Reproductive Medicine

As is true for many racialized and minoritized groups, the reproductive potential of Latinx men and women has often been viewed as a problem to be curtailed rather than a possibility to be facilitated. Throughout the history of reproductive medicine, the conflation of Latinx identity with poverty, criminality, foreignness, and incompetence has served as justification for reproductive treatment of Latinx men and women that emphasizes contraception and sterilization over fertility preservation and infertility care.

Contraception Policy

In the 1950s, Katherine McCormick, one of the early financial backers of the oral contraceptive Enovid, lamented the difficulties of finding a "cage of ovulating females" on which to conduct large-scale studies of the efficacy and side effects of the drug ([54], p. 208). The belief in the need to control birth rates and decrease poverty in Puerto Rico led researchers to conclude that the island was an ideal location in which to find this cage. Small-scale oral contraceptive field trials began in 1953 with female nurses and psychiatric inpatients in Worcester, Massachusetts, and medical students in Puerto Rico. However, one of the first large-scale trials was conducted in Rio Piedras, a public housing project that was home to many women who had recently been relocated from a shanty town on the island [55].

Enrollment in the field trials was voluntary; however, echoing the intersection of poverty and race that was present in the Relf case (see Box 4.1), the women of Rio Piedras were considered uniquely unlikely to leave because of their desire to remain in safe and affordable housing. Nevertheless, many of the women in Rio Piedras ultimately discontinued participation in the trials, in large part because of the severity of nausea, vomiting, dizziness, and blood clots caused by the medication, which contained over 100 times the concentration of estrogen and progesterone that constitutes acceptable dosing by today's standards [56]. Informed consent protocols have changed significantly since the initiation of the Enovid trials in 1955. Nevertheless, the question remains of whether the women in Rio Piedras were given sufficient information to be considered truly voluntary participants in the study and whether their continued participation constituted ethical research practice given the pervasiveness and severity of the side effects they experienced.

Interest in limiting the reproductive potential of Latina women was not limited to contraceptive drug trials (see Box 4.2). Around the time that the Enovid trials were being conceived, concerns about overpopulation on the island led to the rampant adoption of permanent contraception in Puerto Rico. Sterilization of reproductive-aged women, colloquially known in Puerto Rico as "*la operación,*" was viewed by public health officials and healthcare providers alike as a sensible means of population control among people who were thought to be unfit to use contraception reliably. In the words of one doctor writing at the time, "A drastic measure by American standards, it is a godsend to a population not sufficiently educated and motivated to practice systematic birth control" ([57], p. 8). By 1952, 66% of practicing physicians in Puerto Rico endorsed sterilization for reasons of poverty. By 1954, approximately 16% of reproductive-aged women in Puerto Rico had been sterilized, effectively creating a population that was surgically rendered infertile at rates that mirror medical infertility in the general population [58].

Box 4.2: The Sterilization of Dolores Madrigal

In 1909, the state of California passed the third eugenic sterilization law in the United States. The law allowed for medical superintendents in state homes and hospitals to order the involuntary sterilization of patients whom they believed to be "feebleminded" or have medical or psychiatric conditions that were likely to be heritable by their descendants. From the law's inception through the mid-1950s, California was responsible for one-third of the nation's eugenic sterilizations [75]. During this period, Latinos in California, who were primarily Mexican American, were at a higher risk of compulsory sterilization than any other racial or ethnic group; Latino men were 23% more likely to be sterilized without their informed consent and Latina women were at 59% higher risk [76]. In language that disturbingly replicates the rationale for the involuntary sterilization of Carrie Buck and her mother (see Box 4.3), doctors who ordered the sterilization of Latina women during this period often justified this by noting in their charts the women's status as "sex delinquents" ([77], p. 6), conflating false beliefs about Latina promiscuity and hyperfertility with cognitive impairment.

Laws permitting sterilization without full consent persisted well into the latter half of the twentieth century. In 1978 a lawsuit, *Madrigal v Quilligan*, was filed by a group of ten Chicana women against the Los Angeles County/USC Medical Center and the head of its obstetrics department, Dr. Edward J. Quilligan [78]. All of the women had been admitted to USC Medical Center to give birth, and all of them were coerced into consenting to tubal ligation while they were in labor.

The lead plaintiff, Dolores Madrigal, was admitted to the Medical Center to give birth to her second child. She refused numerous attempts to obtain her consent to medical sterilization and only signed a consent form in English, which she could not read, after overhearing a nurse tell her husband that she would die if she were to have another child. Like other members of the Madrigal Ten, Dolores believed that having her "tubes tied" was an easily reversible procedure. As with the other women who filed the suit, Dolores Madrigal was pressured to sign a consent form that she did not understand while she was experiencing contractions. After finding out that she had been sterilized and that the procedure was irreversible, Madrigal experienced severe depression and PTSD symptoms [60].

Other women testified to having been sterilized without their consent, being given verbal or written information about sterilization only in English, or being given inaccurate information about the ease with which the procedure could be reversed [60]. Another of the plaintiffs, Estella Benavides, was also told that she would die if she were to become pregnant again, and later explained that she was "not thinking of anything since the doctors had told me that they were protecting me" ([78], p. 6). Multiple members of the group who gave birth via cesarean section were told, falsely, that California did not permit any woman to have more than three cesarean births. Almost all reported that pain medication was withheld in order to obtain their consent to sterilization, a common practice described by medical student Karen Benker, who witnessed it firsthand. Benker reported: "The doctor would hold a syringe in front of the mother who was in labor pain and ask her if she wanted a pain killer; while the woman was in the throes of a contraction the doctor would say, "Do you want the pain killer? Then sign the papers. Do you want the pain to stop? Do you want to have to go through this again? Sign the papers" ([78], p. 10).

Madrigal v. Quilligan was resolved in two phases, decided by two different judges because the first, Judge Elisha Avery Crary, died in the middle of the proceedings. Judge Crary ruled in favor of the Madrigal plaintiffs' motion for a preliminary injunction against California. He also signed off on a settlement agreement whereby California agreed to implement enhanced sterilization consent procedures based on new guidelines issued as a result of the *Relf v. Weinberger* decision (see Box 4.1). These included the use of consent forms in Spanish written at a sixth grade level, rather than the previous 12th grade level. The second phase of rulings on damages, made by Judge Jesse W. Curtis, did not go as well for the Madrigal Ten. Judge Curtis credited the physicians' belief that the plaintiffs had given their consent. In his ruling, the judge sided with the hospital, stating that the "atypical cultural traits" of the Chicana patients "created a linguistic barrier to communication that their providers could not be expected to overcome" ([79], p. 1). Additionally, the judge indicated that the plaintiffs' Mexican culture placed an unusually high value on their fertility that doctors could not easily grasp:

> The plaintiffs are Mexican Americans who have a culture somewhat foreign to ours which highly values the woman's ability to procreate and the size of the family is a matter of great concern; this is a cultural belief these people are entitled to enjoy. [However] there is a big segment of people in this country who believe that the prime causes of our social and economic problems are big families where the parents are not able to either socially or economically support them…so I do not think it is surprising that you might find a doctor who believes that people who have big families shouldn't and I cannot see anything wrong with the doctor having suggested or convinced the patient [of sterilization] ([80], p. 823).

The plaintiffs in *Madrigal v Quilligan* were ultimately not granted monetary relief by a court that overtly endorsed the prevailing stereotypes of the time. Given the severe psychological repercussions most of the Madrigal Ten experienced, it is unlikely that any damage award could have ever made them whole. Eventually, however, public outrage at the ruling became instrumental in actions by women's and Chicano rights groups that ultimately led to the reversal of California sterilization laws and the implementation of mandatory waiting periods and revised consents for sterilization [60]. Because of their efforts and those of their dedicated attorneys, the Madrigal Ten helped ensure that future generations of Latinas would not have their reproductive futures determined by a medicolegal system that questioned the legitimacy of their desires for parenthood.

Bias and Latinx Reproductive Care

The history of prioritizing the control of Latinx fertility over its promotion is inextricably tied to healthcare provider biases and attitudes toward Latinx patients. Latinx identity is often conflated with foreignness, with Latinx characters on television or in the movies often portrayed with heavy accents or speaking nonstandard English. Compared to non-Hispanic White characters, Latinx characters are also more likely to be depicted as unintelligent, criminals, or employed in low-status occupations [59].

Biased portrayals of Latinx people in the popular imagination are mimicked in the assumptions of the healthcare providers who treat them. Latinx patients are viewed by providers as more likely to be noncompliant with treatment recommendations and less likely to comprehend treatment instructions—a belief that places the onus on the patient to comprehend rather than on the provider to communicate information in an understandable way [60; see also Box 4.2]. Perhaps in consequence of these assumptions, healthcare providers have been shown to take up a greater amount of talk time when meeting with Latinx patients than with non-Hispanic White patients, to leave less room for patient questions and feedback, and to use more direct and simplified language [61].

Provider assumptions that Latina patients are noncompliant and unable to participate fully in their treatment often lead to disparities in Latinas' experience of reproductive healthcare. Although Latina women are more likely than non-Hispanic White women to experience vulvar pain, for example, their pain is routinely underdiagnosed and inadequately treated. This may be due in part to the vocabulary that they use to describe their pain—providers appear to have difficulty hearing beyond the descriptors they expect (for example, "burning" vs. "aching") and refrain from asking adequate follow-up questions that would enable them to arrive at accurate diagnoses [62]. Gynecological oncology diagnoses are on average made later in Latina patients than in non-Hispanic White patients, leading to worse treatment outcomes [63]. Latina patients are also offered minimally invasive gynecologic surgery at lower rates and therefore have longer recovery times and higher risk of complications [64]. They also report less structural and social support during post-surgical recovery, a factor that further complicates the healing process [65].

The impact of biases in reproductive care are even more likely to be in evidence among providers caring for lower-income Latinas, who are routinely stereotyped as uneducated, unmotivated, and incapable of future-oriented planning. In consequence, low-income Latina patients are often viewed as being unable to imagine a life trajectory beyond early and frequent childbearing [66]. As is the case for many minoritized groups, Latinx patients are routinely counseled towards permanent contraception at higher rates than White patients [18]. In a study of simulated patients, gynecologists recommended tubal ligation more frequently for Latina patients if they were portrayed as being of lower socioeconomic status [67]. Irrespective of their actual financial resources and insurance coverage, however, Latinx patients are often presumed to be unable to afford costly healthcare and may therefore be offered treatment based on their providers' assumptions about the kinds of care they can afford [68].

Disparities in the experience of care also exist among Latinx pregnant and birthing people. Latina women routinely report significantly higher rates of procedures during pregnancy, birth, and the postpartum period for which they did not provide full- or any-consent [69]. Although non-Hispanic White women are more likely to have their labor induced due to individual risk factors (for example, gestational diabetes), evidence suggests that the increase in labor induction rates among Latina women may be due not to actual individual risk factors, but to the biased assumption that Latinas' pregnancies are inherently high risk [70].

Unsurprisingly, the impact of bias-driven disparities persists among Latinas experiencing infertility. Although infertility occurs among Latinx patients at rates that are equal to or greater than those experienced by non-Hispanic white patients, Latinx patients have the lowest rate of uptake of infertility care [71]. This is partly a function of structural barriers; Latinx patients are less likely to have insurance that covers infertility diagnosis and treatment [71]. They also report greater structural barriers to accessing care, including a dearth of geographically accessible clinics and less support from employers and supervisors for attending appointments [72].

Provider biases also decrease the likelihood that Latina patients will be referred for infertility care. Latina women are significantly more likely to self-refer for an infertility workup than are non-Hispanic White women, whose referrals are more likely to be facilitated by a reproductive healthcare provider [72]. They also report greater difficulty obtaining an appointment for infertility care than do non-Hispanic

White women [73]. Among those who are able to obtain appointments, Latina patients are less likely to be offered genetic carrier screenings and access to the full complement of diagnostic procedures [74]. Ultimately, then, it is unsurprising that Latinx patients experiencing infertility are less likely to pursue infertility treatment even when a diagnosis and care plan are established [71].

People with Disabilities

People with disabilities (PWDs) are part of the largest minority in the United States. Most membership in a minoritized group is conferred at birth and, for those who maintain their natal sex, immutable. Disability status, however, is a group identity that can emerge at any point in a person's lifespan; anyone can become disabled at birth, in old age, or at any point in between [81]. At any given time, approximately 15% of the world's population lives with a condition that impairs their functioning and limits their access to full participation in daily activities [82]. Disabilities can take many forms and vary in their visibility and duration. Disability status comprises impairment in vision, hearing, cognition, mobility, self-care, or other factors impeding independent living. It should be noted that disability status is an interaction between a person's physical or cognitive characteristics and an environment that either facilitates or hampers their optimal functioning [82]; the degree to which a person is impaired by their physical or cognitive status depends in part on whether they live in a setting that recognizes the barriers to their full participation in activities of daily living and provides the necessary accommodations. As is evident from the history and current state of reproductive care, the attitudes and behaviors of healthcare providers can facilitate or impede the reproductive health of people with disabilities.

Like other minoritized groups, people with disabilities are impacted by stereotypes and implicit biases. Atypically, however, they exist at the intersection of competing and contradictory narratives. In a culture that valorizes struggle and overcoming difficulties, people with disabilities are often assumed to be brave, noble, and admirable [83]. In popular culture and media representations, characters with disabilities often serve as metaphors for personal growth or overcoming obstacles [84]. However, this characterization coexists with stereotypes and biases about people with disabilities that promote dislike and marginalization. Nursing and occupational therapy students given the Disability Implicit Associations Test have been shown to demonstrate a preference for ablebodiedness [85, 86], and a meta-analysis of healthcare providers' attitudes toward patients with disabilities showed evidence for providers' perception of patients with disabilities as cold, childlike, and incompetent [81]. In contrast to racist or prejudicial attitudes about other minoritized groups, which may be based on overt dislike of the minoritized person, belief that they are responsible for their own misfortune, or principled objection to equitable practices, attitudes toward people with disabilities are often a function of "aversive ableism"—the simultaneous belief that people with disabilities are deserving of assistance and a reluctance to engage in active efforts to provide it ([84], p. 109).

Reproductive Care and People with Disabilities

Competing narratives also exist when it comes to provider beliefs about the fertility of people with disabilities. On the one hand, PWDs are often assumed to be asexual and therefore unlikely to desire or have children [87]. A co-occurring narrative, however, casts people with disabilities as hypersexual and uniquely likely to become pregnant unintentionally.

Both among parents and caregivers, there may be more acceptance of sexuality in men with intellectual disabilities than in adult women, a finding that is perhaps related to the concern that women with intellectual disabilities are more likely to be victimized [88]. Expressed support for the sexuality of people with disabilities often ends when the possibility of parenthood is considered [89, 90]. Women with disabilities routinely report lack of caregiver and healthcare provider support for their desire to parent [91] and report being counseled toward abortion on the assumption that their pregnancies are unintended and undesired [92]. The belief that people with physical and especially intellectual disabilities are constitutionally unable to parent has a long history in the eugenics movement and has for long stretches in history been codified into United States law (see Box 4.3).

Box 4.3: Buck v. Bell

The American medical establishment has a long and troubled history of enacting a bias against people with disabilities in the arena of childbearing. From the late nineteenth century through the 1930s, American elites were enthralled by eugenics and terrified at the prospect that the American spirit was being diluted and diminished by an influx of inferior genetic material. The most well-known and far-reaching policies that were rooted in genetic ideas were the laws restricting immigration that Congress passed in 1921 and 1924. In addition to fear of predominantly Catholic and Jewish immigrants from southern and eastern Europe, the American government, along with medical experts and psychology professionals, was on guard against people with diseases or disabilities, including intellectual disabilities, which popular science posited were caused by heredity. These fears were reified and ratified by the United States Supreme Court in one of its most infamous cases, *Buck v. Bell*, decided in 1927 by an 8–1 majority [119].

Carrie Buck was 3 years old when the state of Virginia took her away from her mother, Emma, and placed her in foster care. She was seventeen when her foster family petitioned the state to have Carrie committed to the Colony for Epileptics and the Feeble-minded near Lynchburg. Despite Carrie's having completed sixth grade with good marks prior to her foster family taking her out of school so she could do more chores, the Charlottesville Commission of Feeblemindedness determined that Carrie was mentally defective and ordered her to the Colony. There, a Binet-Simon intelligence test would determine that

Carrie was a "middle grade moron," but she would be reunited with her birth mother, Emma, who had been committed to the Colony 4 years earlier in 1920. Carrie was not at all feebleminded; she was at the Colony because at 17 she had become pregnant, probably as the result of a sexual assault by one of her foster parents' relatives [120].

The *Buck v. Bell* lawsuit came about because Virginia wanted to test the constitutionality of its newly enacted law that allowed the state to sterilize individuals it determined to be "defective." A board of experts could determine that a patient was defective if they were "insane, idiotic, imbecile, feeble-minded, or epileptic, and by the laws of heredity is the probably potential parent of socially inadequate offspring likewise afflicted" [121]. Carrie Buck was the perfect test case. She and her mother had been judged feebleminded, and soon her daughter Vivian would also be determined to be defective despite achieving decent grades in school before her untimely death at age 8. Emma, Carrie and Vivian Buck were the "three generations of imbeciles" that Oliver Wendell Holmes Jr. decreed should be "enough," in the Buck v. Bell decision. After the ruling, the administrators at the Virginia colony sterilized Carrie Buck.

To be clear, neither Carrie nor Emma Buck had an intellectual disability. The state decided that they were defective because of their perceived lack of morals or control over their sexuality. Emma Buck had five children with three different men before she was committed, and Carrie was pregnant out of wedlock at 17. In the eyes of the male doctors and legislators of Virginia, their supposed promiscuity equated to feeblemindedness, and it needed to be curtailed in the most efficient way possible. Institutionalization was one answer, but sterilization was more permanent, less expensive, and the preferred choice of Virginia and thirty-one other states.

Biased assumptions about the sexuality and parenting fitness of people with disabilities have led to wide discrepancies in sexuality and fertility education, contraceptive counseling, and access to infertility care. It should also be noted that people with disabilities can exist at the intersection of more than one minoritized identity. People with disabilities who also belong to racial or sexual minority groups are at increased risk of marginalization and of receiving suboptimal reproductive healthcare [93, 94].

Experiences in Reproductive Healthcare

The majority of people with disabilities of reproductive age are both sexually active and fertile [95]. Women with disabilities desire children at the same rate as members of nondisabled populations [93, 96]. In contrast to nondisabled women, however, women with disabilities are less certain of their ultimate fertility intentions and anticipate a greater gap between the number of children they would ideally want and those they will actually have. Some of the factors that lead women with disabilities to anticipate a smaller than desired family size are medical; women may anticipate medical complications or having to stop taking a health-promoting medication during pregnancy. Others are economic; people with disabilities experience higher rates of unemployment than the general population and often have a lower standard of living [97, 98]. Additionally, however, women with disabilities frequently report feeling actively discouraged from having children by their healthcare providers and, as will be discussed below, have different experiences of gynecological care and preconception counseling than do their nondisabled counterparts [99].

All reproductive healthcare, including routine GYN exams, contraceptive counseling, and mammograms, requires patients to be able to access care. Across the range of reproductive healthcare, people with disabilities face a range of systemic and attitudinal biases that compromise their ability to access and act as full participants in their treatment. As Horner-Johnson suggests, the "process and infrastructure of …care [are] based on an able-bodied norm" ([100], p. 732). In a 2014 survey, up to 40% of gynecology practices were found to be physically inaccessible to women with disabilities [101]. The absence of wheelchair-accessible facilities, the height and positioning of exam tables and stirrups, the requirement to be examined while lying flat on a table, and the sensory and reading requirements for completing needed paperwork can all act as barriers for women with disabilities to compete their annual gynecological exam [102]. In one national survey, only 40–45% of women with disabilities over the age of 35 reported ever having had a mammogram due to the limited accessibility of rooms and equipment that could accommodate them [103]. Women with intellectual, rather than physical, disabilities are often offered HPV vaccines and cervical cancer screening at lower rates than their nondisabled counterparts of the same age [104]. Limited access to preventative care can lead to late or missed diagnoses that compromise patients' eventual physical or reproductive health.

Even among those patients who can physically access gynecologic care, people with disabilities routinely report barriers to contraceptive access and shared decision making [105]. Many women with disabilities report the perception that their providers are uncomfortable discussing issues of sexuality and contraceptive care with them, particularly if they are accompanied to appointments by caregivers who provide assistance for their physical, sensory, or comprehension needs [102, 105]. Women with disabilities also report less discussion of contraceptive side effects and perceive their providers as uncomfortable with or inadequately trained to have discussions about contraception and routine gynecological management.

Notably, the perceptions of women with disabilities are strikingly similar to those of the providers who care for them. In a survey of reproductive healthcare providers, almost 95% of those who provided contraceptive counseling reported initiating conversations about contraception more often with patients without disabilities. Further, although the majority of providers acknowledged that patients with disabilities required specific modifications to their gynecologic and contraceptive care, only 17% of providers surveyed reported having received any training or information about how to provide such care [106].

The combination of access to care difficulties, assumptions about the sexuality and parental competence of people with disabilities and limited provider training leads to wide discrepancies in the kinds of contraception that people with disabilities can access. Compared to women without disabilities, same-aged women with both physical and intellectual disabilities are almost 60% more likely to be sterilized [107–109]. In contrast, they are less likely to use oral contraception and more likely to report that they use no contraception at all [107]. This last finding may be due in part to the lack of contraceptive and sexuality education provided to young PWDs of reproductive age. Although half of all high school girls with disabilities are thought to be sexually active, adolescent girls with disabilities are less likely to receive any formal sexual health education and, concomitantly, are less likely to use contraception at the time of first intercourse [110, 111].

Issues in Infertility Care

The Ethics Committee of the American Society for Reproductive Medicine has repeatedly affirmed the right to the provision of accessible care for those who desire parenthood, including patients with medical complexities [112]. However, women with disabilities who are infertile may seek and receive care less frequently than infertile women without disabilities [95]. The reasons for the lower rates of uptake of infertility care mirror those that prevent women with disabilities from getting adequate reproductive healthcare in general.

Assumptions about the sexuality, parenting competence, and risks of pregnancy for people with disabilities may lead providers to assess for conditions that impair fertility and refer patients for evaluation and treatment at lower rates [91, 113]. Like providers of routine GYN care, providers of infertility treatment often have offices, equipment, and methods of information delivery that render their services functionally inaccessible to people with disabilities. The underemployment and lower socioeconomic status of people with disabilities also means that they are less likely to be able to access either out-of-pocket infertility healthcare or have insurance that covers infertility treatment.

Increasingly, people with disabilities are creating communities based on shared cultural identities and self-advocacy. The desire to preserve these identities may be at odds with prevailing practices in reproductive medicine, where the emphasis is on mitigating the risk of passing on disabilities or significant health concerns. For example, carrier screenings for genes likely to result in deafness may contrast with the desires of some members of the Deaf community to raise Deaf children who have full access to Deaf languages and culture [114, 115].

Even less is known about the experiences and desires of neurodivergent people in reproductive healthcare and infertility treatment. A literature search using the terms "IVF" and "ADHD" or "Autism" yields copious research on the rates of neurodivergence in children conceived via assisted reproductive technology [116–118]. Neurodivergent adults work, marry, and desire children, yet virtually nothing has been written about access to reproductive care for neurodivergent adults or ways to improve their experience of receiving care. With this awareness comes a growing need for research aimed at understanding their experiences of reproductive healthcare and best practices for accommodating their needs in treatment.

Summary and Conclusions

For many marginalized patients, the impact of clinician and systemic bias on their reproductive health is evident long before they contemplate family building. Members of racial, sexual, and gender minority groups are often faced with a lack of inclusive sexual health education, counseling that emphasizes contraception over procreation for some groups and misses the need for contraceptive care for others, and healthcare systems that fail to take their unique physical and socioemotional needs into account.

This chapter outlines the historical and current inequities in reproductive care for Black, Latinx, LGBTQIA+ patients, and patients with disabilities. It is important to note, however, that these are far from the only groups whose experience in reproductive care has been impacted by clinicians' assumptions—either explicitly stated or unexpressed—about who can, wants to, or deserves to parent. We invite you to look beyond the specific stories and statistics in this chapter to the broader questions they raise about whose sexuality, desire for parenthood, and needs in treatment are recognized by the medical system and whose are curtailed rather than fostered.

References

1. Smedley BD, Stith AY, Nelson AR. Racial and ethnic disparities in diagnosis and treatment: a review of the evidence and a consideration of causes. Unequal treatment: Confronting racial and ethnic disparities in health care. 2003.
2. Crenshaw KW. Mapping the margins: intersectionality, identity politics, and violence against women of color. The public nature of private violence 2013. Routledge. p. 93–118.
3. Bowleg L. The problem with the phrase women and minorities: intersectionality—an important theoretical framework for public health. Am J Public Health. 2012;102(7):1267–73.
4. Bowleg L. When black+ lesbian+ woman≠ black lesbian woman: the methodological challenges of qualitative and quantitative intersectionality research. Sex Roles. 2008;59:312–25.
5. Lett E, Dowshen NL, Baker KE. Intersectionality and health inequities for gender minority blacks in the US. Am J Prev Med. 2020;59(5):639–47.
6. Yette EM, Ahern J. Health-related quality of life among black sexual minority women. Am J Prev Med. 2018;55(3):281–9.
7. Tam MW. Queering reproductive access: reproductive justice in assisted reproductive technologies. Reprod Health. 2021;18(1):164.
8. Crear-Perry J, Correa-de-Araujo R, Lewis Johnson T, McLemore MR, Neilson E, Wallace M. Social and structural determsinants of health inequities in maternal health. J Women's Health. 2021;30(2):230–5.
9. Owens DC, Fett SM. Black maternal and infant health: historical legacies of slavery. Am J Public Health. 2019;109(10):1342–5.

10. Saluja B, Bryant Z. How implicit bias contributes to racial disparities in maternal morbidity and mortality in the United States. J Women's Health. 2021;30(2):270–3.
11. Brown HL, Small MJ, Clare CA, Hill WC. Black women health inequity: the origin of perinatal health disparity. J Natl Med Assoc. 2021;113(1):105–13.
12. Owens DC. Medical bondage: race, gender, and the origins of American gynecology. University of Georgia Press; 2017.
13. Morgan JL. Partus sequitur ventrem: law, race, and reproduction in colonial slavery. Small Axe. 2018;22(1):1–7.
14. Smaw ED. Uterus collectors: the case for reproductive justice for African American, native American, and Hispanic American female victims of eugenics programs in the United States. Bioethics. 2022;36(3):318–27.
15. Gonullu DC, Huang XM, Robinson LG, Walker CA, Ayoola-Adeola M, Jameson R, Yim D, Awonuga A. Tubal factor infertility and its impact on reproductive freedom of African American women. Am J Obstet Gynecol. 2022;226(3):379–83.
16. Harris LH, Wolfe T. Stratified reproduction, family planning care and the double edge of history. Curr Opin Obstet Gynecol. 2014;26(6):539–44.
17. Campbell C. Medical violence, obstetric racism, and the limits of informed consent for black women. J Race L. 2021;47
18. Kathawa CA, Arora KS. Implicit bias in counseling for permanent contraception: historical context and recommendations for counseling. Health Equity. 2020;4(1):326–9.
19. Amalraj J, Arora KS. Ethics of a mandatory waiting period for female sterilization. Hastings Cent Rep. 2022;52(4):17–25.
20. Villarosa L. Under the skin: the hidden toll of racism on American lives. Anchor; 2022.
21. Calibey KA. Nonconsensual sterilization of the mentally retarded—analysis of standards for judicial determinations. West New Engl Law Rev. 1981;3(4):689.
22. Webb S. The push for contraceptives on African American women and the effects it causes. 2020.
23. Ceballo R, Graham ET, Hart J. Silent and infertile: an intersectional analysis of the experiences of socioeconomically diverse African American women with infertility. Psychol Women Q. 2015;39(4):497–511.
24. Greil AL, McQuillan J, Shreffler KM, Johnson KM, Slauson-Blevins KS. Race-ethnicity and medical services for infertility: stratified reproduction in a population-based sample of US women. J Health Soc Behav. 2011;52(4):493–509.
25. Committee on Women in Psychology. Infertility and BIPOC (Black, Indigenous, and People of Color) Women. [Internet] American Psychological Association. Retrieved 4/16/24. https://www.apa.org/pi/women/committee/infertility-bipoc.
26. Logan RG, Daley EM, Vamos CA, Louis-Jacques A, Marhefka SL. "When is health care actually going to be care?" The lived experience of family planning care among young black women. Qual Health Res. 2021;31(6):1169–82.
27. Cebert-Gaitors M, Shannon-Baker PA, Silva SG, Hart RE, Jahandideh S, Gonzalez-Guarda R, Stevenson EL. Psychobiological, clinical, and sociocultural factors that influence black women seeking treatment for infertility: a mixed-methods study. F&S Rep. 2022;3(2):29–39.
28. Wiltshire A, Ghidei L, Dawkins J, Phillips K, Licciardi F, Keefe D. Primary ovarian insufficiency: a glimpse into the racial and socioeconomic disparities found within third-party reproduction. F&S Rep. 2022;3(2):62–5.
29. Lawson AK, Marsh EE. Hearing the silenced voices of underserved women: the role of qualitative research in gynecologic and reproductive care. Obstet Gynecol Clin. 2017;44(1):109–20.
30. Rabbitte M, Enriquez M. Factors that impact assigned female sexual minority individuals health care experiences: a qualitative descriptive study. Am J Sex Educ. 2024;19(1):97–120.
31. Hobaica S, Schofield K, Kwon P. "Here's your anatomy… good luck": transgender individuals in cisnormative sex education. Am J Sex Educ. 2019;14(3):358–87.
32. Bodnar K, Tornello SL. Does sex education help everyone? Sex education exposure and timing as predictors of sexual health among lesbian, bisexual, and heterosexual young women. J Educ Psychol Consult. 2019;29(1):8–26.

33. Hudson GM. Factors influencing contraception use in sexual minority women: a systematic literature review. 2021.
34. Charlton BM, Reynolds CA, Janiak E, DiVasta AD, Jones RK, Chavarro JE, Sarda V, Austin SB. Sexual orientation-related differences in contraceptive use: a brief report based on a cohort of adolescent and young women. Contraception. 2021;103(3):195–8.
35. Lasio D, Serri F, Ibba I, Manuel De Oliveira J. Hegemony and heteronormativity: homonormative discourses of LGBTQ activists about lesbian and gay parenting. J Homosex. 2019;66(8):1058–81.
36. Maříková H, Vohlídalová M. To be or not to be a parent? Parenting aspiration of men with non-normative sexual identities in Czechia. LGBTQ+ Family. 2022;18(2):101–18.
37. Lasio D, Lampis J, Spiga R, Serri F. Lesbian and gay individual parenting desires in heteronormative contexts. Eur J Psychol. 2020;16(2):210.
38. Yee S, Mamone AA, Fatima M, Sharon-Weiner M, Librach CL. Parenthood desire, perceived parenthood stigma, and barriers to achieving parenthood in childless sexual minority men. J Assist Reprod Genet. 2024;41:1739–53.
39. Carpinello OJ, Jacob MC, Nulsen J, Benadiva C. Utilization of fertility treatment and reproductive choices by lesbian couples. Fertil Steril. 2016;106(7):1709–13.
40. Aktoz F, Loreti S, Darici E, Leunens L, Tournaye H, De Munck N, Blockeel C, Roelens C, Mackens S. IVF with reception of oocytes from partner in lesbian couples: a systematic review and SWOT analysis. Reprod Biomed Online. 2023;48:103411.
41. Ethics Committee of the American Society for Reproductive Medicine. Access to fertility treatment irrespective of marital status, sexual orientation, or gender identity: an ethics committee opinion. Fertil Steril. 2021;116(2):326–30.
42. Ethics Committee of the American Society for Reproductive Medicine. Access to fertility services by transgender and nonbinary persons: an ethics committee opinion. Fertil Steril. 2021;115(4):874–8.
43. Kirubarajan A, Patel P, Leung S, Park B, Sierra S. Cultural competence in fertility care for lesbian, gay, bisexual, transgender, and queer people: a systematic review of patient and provider perspectives. Fertil Steril. 2021;115(5):1294–301.
44. Gregory KB, Mielke JG, Neiterman E. Building families through healthcare: experiences of lesbians using reproductive services. J Patient Exp. 2022;9:23743735221089459.
45. Wingo E, Ingraham N, Roberts SC. Reproductive health care priorities and barriers to effective care for LGBTQ people assigned female at birth: a qualitative study. Womens Health Issues. 2018;28(4):350–7.
46. Mehta PK, Easter SR, Potter J, Castleberry N, Schulkin J, Robinson JN. Lesbian, gay, bisexual, and transgender health: obstetrician–gynecologists' training, attitudes, knowledge, and practice. J Women's Health. 2018;27(12):1459–65.
47. Raja NS, Russell CB, Moravek MB. Assisted reproductive technology: considerations for the nonheterosexual population and single parents. Fertil Steril. 2022;118(1):47–53.
48. Morong JJ, Class QA, Zamah AM, Hinz E. Parenting intentions in transgender and gender-nonconforming adults. Int J Gynecol Obstet. 2022;159(2):557–62.
49. Cooper HC, Long J, Aye T. Fertility preservation in transgender and non-binary adolescents and young adults. PLoS One. 2022;17(3):e0265043.
50. Inman EM, Obedin-Maliver J, Ragosta S, Hastings J, Berry J, Lunn MR, Flentje A, Capriotti MR, Lubensky ME, Stoeffler A, Dastur Z. Reports of negative interactions with healthcare providers among transgender, nonbinary, and gender-expansive people assigned female at birth in the United States: results from an online, cross-sectional survey. Int J Environ Res Public Health. 2023;20(11):6007.
51. Choi JY, Kim TJ. Fertility preservation and reproductive potential in transgender and gender fluid population. Biomedicines. 2022;10(9):2279.
52. Erbenius T, Gunnarsson PJ. Unlearning cisnormativity in the clinic: enacting transgender reproductive rights in everyday patient encounters. J Int Women's Stud. 2018;20(1):27–39.

53. American Society for Reproductive Medicine. Definition of infertility: a committee opinion. asrm.org. https://www.asrm.org/practice-guidance/practice-committee-documents/denitions-of-infertility/. Accessed 29 Apr 2024.
54. Marks L. "A 'cage of ovulating females": the history of the early oral contraceptive pill clinical trials, 1950–1959. Molecularizing Biology and Medicine: New Practices and Alliances, 1920s to 1970s. 2003: p. 208.
55. Lankford KD. More than a way station: ground-level experiences in the field trials of oral contraceptives and IUDs in Puerto Rico, 1956–1966. Michigan State University; 2021.
56. Contraceptive trials in Puerto Rico, lo que debes saber. scientiaen.com. https://scientiaen.com/Contraceptive_trials_in_Puerto_Rico.
57. Stycos JM. Female Sterilization in Puerto Rico. Eugen Q. 1954;1(2):3–9.
58. Lazar A. La operación: coerced sterilization of Puerto Rican women in the 20th century. 2021.
59. Shafer J, Rivadeneyra R. The impact of televised stereotypes on the state self-esteem of Latino/a emerging adults: the moderating role of ethnic–racial identity. Emerg Adulthood. 2022;10(2):335–41.
60. Menchaca HJ. "Ya Acabó La Canción:" reproductive injustice and chicana testimonio as resistance in Madrigal V. *Quilligan*. Doctoral dissertation, San Diego State University. 2022.
61. Wolsiefer KJ, Mehl M, Moskowitz GB, Cagno CK, Zestcott CA, Tejeda-Padron A, Stone J. Investigating the relationship between resident physician implicit bias and language use during a clinical encounter with hispanic patients. Health Commun. 2023;38(1):124–32.
62. Labuski CM. A black and white issue? Learning to see the intersectional and racialized dimensions of gynecological pain. Soc Theory Health. 2017;15:160–81.
63. Torres TK, Chase DM, Salani R, Hamann HA, Stone J. Implicit biases in healthcare: implications and future directions for gynecologic oncology. Am J Obstet Gynecol. 2022;227(1):1–9.
64. Barnes WA, Carter-Brooks CM, Wu CZ, Acosta DA, Vargas MV. Racial and ethnic disparities in access to minimally invasive gynecologic surgery for benign pathology. Curr Opin Obstet Gynecol. 2021;33(4):279–87.
65. Philp L, Alimena S, Sullivan M, Del Carmen M, Bregar A, Eisenhauer E, Goodman A, Sisodia RC. Black and hispanic women have less support during cancer evaluation and treatment: results from a prospective patient reported outcomes program in gynecologic malignancy. Int J Gynecol Cancer. 2023;33(5):770–7.
66. Carvajal DN, Zambrana RE. Challenging stereotypes: a counter-narrative of the contraceptive experiences of low-income Latinas. Health Equity. 2020;4(1):10–6.
67. DiCenzo N, Brandi K, Getz K, Matthews G. Characteristics associated with physician bias in contraceptive recommendations. Womens Health Issues. 2024;34(1):51–8.
68. Kirubarajan A, Patel P, Leung S, Prethipan T, Sierra S. Barriers to fertility care for racial/ethnic minority groups: a qualitative systematic review. F&S Rev. 2021;2(2):150–9.
69. Logan RG, McLemore MR, Julian Z, Stoll K, Malhotra N, Vedam S, s. Coercion and non-consent during birth and newborn care in the United States. Birth. 2022;49(4):749–62.
70. Masters RK, Tilstra AM, Simon DH, Coleman-Minahan K. Differences in determinants: racialized obstetric care and increases in US state labor induction rates. J Health Soc Behav. 2023;64(2):174–91.
71. Komorowski AS, Jain T. A review of disparities in access to infertility care and treatment outcomes among Hispanic women. Reprod Biol Endocrinol. 2022;20(1):1.
72. Cebert-Gaitors M, Abdelnalbi S, Mantell E, Woodward A, Gonzalez-Guarda R, Stevenson EL. Multidimensional barriers and facilitators to treatment seeking for infertility among women in the United States: a systematic review. F&S Rev. 2022;3(1):76–89.
73. Merkison JM, Chada AR, Marsidi AM, Spencer JB. Racial and ethnic disparities in assisted reproductive technology: a systematic review. Fertil Steril. 2023;119(3):341–7.
74. McQueen DB, Warren CM, Xiao AH, Shulman LP, Jain T. Disparities among infertility patients regarding genetic carrier screening, sex selection, and gene editing. J Assist Reprod Genet. 2021;38(9):2319–25.

75. Lira N, Stern AM. Mexican Americans and eugenic sterilization: resisting reproductive injustice in California, 1920–1950. Aztlán. 2014;39(2):9–34.
76. Novak NL, Lira N, O'Connor KE, Harlow SD, Kardia SL, Stern AM. Disproportionate sterilization of Latinos under California's eugenic sterilization program, 1920–1945. Am J Public Health. 2018;108(5):611–3.
77. Alonso P. Autonomy revoked: the forced sterilization of women of color in 20th century America. J Agric Appl Econ. 2020:13.
78. Manian M. The story of Madrigal v. Quilligan: coerced sterilization of Mexican-American women. Quilligan: Coerced Sterilization of Mexican-American Women (March 1, 2018). Forthcoming in Melissa Murray, Kate Shaw, & Reva Siegel, eds., Reproductive Rights and Justice Stories (Foundation Press, 2019), Univ. of San Francisco Law Research Paper. 2018 (2018–04).
79. Hood CA. "A better life with fewer children": assimilation, eugenics, and sterilization abuse in 1970s Los Angeles. 2021.
80. Benker Testimony. Carlos Velez-Ibanez Sterilization Papers, UCLA Chicano Studies Research Center, University of California, Los Angeles, Box: Madrigal v Quilligan. 1978: pp. 823–825.
81. Antonopoulos CR, Sugden N, Saliba A. Implicit bias toward people with disability: a systematic review and meta-analysis. Rehabil Psychol. 2023;68(2):121.
82. World Health Organization. Global report on health equity for persons with disabilities. World Health Organization; 2022.
83. Cameron L, Knezevic I, Hanes R. Inspiring people or perpetuating stereotypes?: the complicated case of disability as inspiration. In Disability representation in film, TV, and print media. Routledge; 2021. p. 108–27.
84. Friedman C. Mapping ableism: a two-dimensional model of explicit and implicit disability attitudes. Can J Dis Stud. 2019;8(3):95–120.
85. Lum J, Morean W, Maccarrone A, Carpenter TP, Aaberg V, Bentley JA. Implicit associations related to physical disability among nursing students. Disabil Health J. 2021;14(4):101150.
86. Feldner HA, VanPuymbrouck L, Friedman C. Explicit and implicit disability attitudes of occupational and physical therapy assistants. Disabil Health J. 2022;15(1):101217.
87. Pebdani RN, Tashjian A. An analysis of the attitudes of the general public towards the sexuality of individuals with disabilities through a systematic literature review. Sex Disabil. 2022;40(1):21–55.
88. Correa AB, Castro Á, Barrada JR. Attitudes towards the sexuality of adults with intellectual disabilities: a systematic review. Sex Disabil. 2022;40(2):261–97.
89. Tamas D, Brkic Jovanovic N, Rajic M, Bugarski Ignjatovic V, Peric Prkosovacki B. Professionals, parents and the general public: attitudes towards the sexuality of persons with intellectual disability. Sex Disabil. 2019;37:245–58.
90. McConnell D, Aunos M, Pacheco L, Hahn L. Reconsidering sexuality, relationships, and parenthood for adults with intellectual disability. 2021.
91. Francis LP, Silvers A, Badesch B. Women with disabilities: ethics of access and accommodation for infertility care. Ethical issues in women's healthcare: practice and policy (2019). University of Utah College of Law Research Paper; 2019.
92. Wu JP, McKee MM, Mckee KS, Meade MA, Plegue M, Sen A. Female sterilization is more common among women with physical and/or sensory disabilities than women without disabilities in the United States. Disabil Health J. 2017;10(3):400–5.
93. Horner-Johnson W, Dissanayake M, Wu JP, Caughey AB, Darney BG. Pregnancy intendedness by maternal disability status and type in the United States. Perspect Sex Reprod Health. 2020;52(1):31–8.
94. Fuentes K, Hsu S, Patel S, Lindsay S. More than just double discrimination: a scoping review of the experiences and impact of ableism and racism in employment. Disabil Rehabil. 2024;46(4):650–71.
95. Ha S, Martinez V. Associations between disability and infertility among US reproductive-aged women. Int J Environ Res Public Health. 2021;18(6):3202.

96. Bloom TL, Mosher W, Alhusen J, Lantos H, Hughes RB. Fertility desires and intentions among US women by disability status: findings from the 2011–2013 National Survey of family growth. Matern Child Health J. 2017;21:1606–15.
97. Friedman C. The relationship between disability prejudice and disability employment rates. Work. 2020;65(3):591–8.
98. Houtenville A, Bach S, Paul S. Annual report on people with disabilities in America: 2023. Institute on Disability, University of New Hampshire; 2023.
99. Pebdani RN. Rehabilitation counselor knowledge, comfort, approach, and attitude toward sex and disability. Rehabil Res Policy Educ. 2013;27:27(1).
100. Horner-Johnson W, Klein KA, Campbell J, Guise JM. Experiences of women with disabilities in accessing and receiving contraceptive care. J Obstet Gynecol Neonatal Nurs. 2021;50(6):732–41.
101. Sonalkar S, Chavez V, McClusky J, Hunter TA, Mollen CJ. Gynecologic care for women with physical disabilities: a qualitative study of patients and providers. Womens Health Issues. 2020;30(2):136–41.
102. Alhusen JL, Bloom T, Laughon K, Behan L, Hughes RB. Perceptions of barriers to effective family planning services among women with disabilities. Disabil Health J. 2021;14(3):101055.
103. Schopp LH, Sanford TC, Hagglund KJ, Gay JW, Coatney MA. Removing service barriers for women with physical disabilities: promoting accessibility in the gynecologic care setting. J Midwifery Womens Health. 2002;47(2):74–9.
104. Carter A, Strnadová I, Watfern C, Pebdani R, Bateson D, Loblinzk J, Guy R, Newman C. The sexual and reproductive health and rights of young people with intellectual disability: a scoping review. Sexuality research and social. Policy. 2021;19:1–9.
105. Horner-Johnson W, Klein KA, Campbell J, Guise JM. "It would have been nice to have a choice": barriers to contraceptive decision-making among women with disabilities. Womens Health Issues. 2022;32(3):261–7.
106. Taouk LH, Fialkow MF, Schulkin JA. Provision of reproductive healthcare to women with disabilities: a survey of obstetrician–gynecologists' training, practices, and perceived barriers. Health Equity. 2018;2(1):207–15.
107. Mosher W, Hughes RB, Bloom T, Horton L, Mojtabai R, Alhusen JL. Contraceptive use by disability status: new national estimates from the national survey of family growth. Contraception. 2018;97(6):552–8.
108. Li H, Mitra M, Wu JP, Parish SL, Valentine A, Dembo RS. Female sterilization and cognitive disability in the United States, 2011–2015. Obstet Gynecol. 2018;132(3):559–64.
109. de Fiebre GY. Contraceptive use and sterilization among people with disabilities. 2022.
110. Namkung EH, Valentine A, Warner L, Mitra M. Contraceptive use at first sexual intercourse among adolescent and young adult women with disabilities: the role of formal sex education. Contraception. 2021;103(3):178–84.
111. Senders A, Horner-Johnson W. Contraceptive use among adolescents with and without disabilities. J Adolesc Health. 2022;70(1):120–6.
112. Ethics Committee of the American Society for Reproductive Medicine. Provision of fertility services for women at increased risk of complications during fertility treatment or pregnancy: an ethics committee opinion. Fertil Steril. 2022;117(4):713–9.
113. Agaronnik N, Pendo E, Lagu T, DeJong C, Perez-Caraballo A, Iezzoni LI. Ensuring the reproductive rights of women with intellectual disability. J Intellect Develop Disabil. 2020;45(4):365–76.
114. Baertschi B, Jouannet P, Bed'hom B, Dosquet C, Dubart-Kupperschmitt A, Lemaitre C, Nisand I, Jouet IR. Eugenics and medicalized reproduction conceptual, historical, medical, and ethical considerations. 2024.
115. Konečná H, Svatoš R. Alternative or nonstandard forms of parenthood in the context of reproductive technologies. Lawyer Quarterly. 2021;11(2).
116. Ono M, Kuji N, Ueno K, Kojima J, Nishi H. The long-term outcome of children conceived through assisted reproductive technology. Reprod Sci. 2023;1-8:583.

117. Velez MP, Dayan N, Shellenberger J, Pudwell J, Kapoor D, Vigod SN, Ray JG. Infertility and risk of autism spectrum disorder in children. JAMA Netw Open. 2023;6(11):e2343954.
118. Jenabi E, Bashirian S, Khazaei S, Farhadi Nasab A, Maleki A. The association between assisted reproductive technology and the risk of autism spectrum disorders among offspring: a meta-analysis. Curr Pediatr Rev. 2023;19(1):83–9.
119. Cynkar RJ. Buck v. bell: felt necessities v. fundamental values. Colum L Rev. 1981;81:1418.
120. Cohen A. Imbeciles: the supreme court, American eugenics, and the sterilization of Carrie buck. Penguin; 2017.
121. Lombardo PA. Three generations, no imbeciles: eugenics, the supreme court, and buck v. bell. JHU Press; 2022.

Chapter 5
Access to Care

Natasha Raj-Derouin

Introduction

According to the Centers for Disease Control and Prevention (CDC), it is estimated that 9.7 million women aged 15–49 years have impaired fecundity or impaired ability to get pregnant [1]. Among such women surveyed between 2015 and 2019, only 12.2% received any type of infertility services and 0.5% received assisted reproductive technologies (ART). The large gap between those seeking fertility care and those who receive it exists in large part due to numerous barriers to care. Access to care has been defined as the "timely use of personal health services to achieve the best possible health outcomes" [2]. The Agency for Healthcare Research and Quality breaks down access to care into four main components: coverage, services, timeliness, and workforce [3]. "Coverage" permits one's entry into the healthcare system; limited insurance coverage represents one of the largest obstacles to entering care. "Services" encompasses having a reliable source of care and "timeliness" ensures the ability to receive health care when a need is recognized. Finally, "workforce" involves having access to qualified and competent providers. Many of the barriers to equitable infertility care can be defined within this framework. Most patients do not have insurance coverage or the personal financial resources for assisted reproductive technologies (ART) or have a local ART center with an ample workforce to provide them with reliable and timely services. Numerous reviews in the literature have explored disparities in access to infertility care in depth and described the main causes of limited access to fertility care [4, 5]. This chapter provides a comprehensive and exhaustive review of the existing literature with the aim of categorizing and contextualizing the barriers to access to care. Using the

N. Raj-Derouin (✉)
Department of Obstetrics and Gynecology, Kaiser Permanente Los Angeles Medical Center, Los Angeles, CA, USA

D. A. Kaplan (ed.), *Cultural Responsiveness in Assisted Reproductive Technology*, https://doi.org/10.1007/978-3-031-76204-8_5

framework previously described, this chapter delineates the barriers to access to fertility care into three main categories: the limitations to the definition of infertility, the role of insurance mandates in reducing costs, and the impact of geographical factors.

The Definition of Infertility

In 1993, the American Society of Reproductive Medicine (ASRM) released a practice committee statement that "infertility is a disease" [6]. It quoted the Dorland's Medical Dictionary, which defined a disease as "any deviation from or interruption of the normal structure or function of any part, organ, or system…." Since infertility is a deviation from the normal functioning of the reproductive system, its presence is consistent with the recognized definition of a disease. ASRM was the first institution to recognize infertility as a disease; it took another 16 years before another international organization contributed to the dialogue [7]. In 2009, the World Health Organization (WHO) in conjunction with the International Committee for Monitoring Assisted Reproductive Technologies (ICMART) developed a glossary of infertility and ART terminology in the hopes of standardizing data collection internationally [8]. As part of this glossary, it released a new definition of infertility as "a disease of the reproductive system defined by the failure to achieve a clinical pregnancy after 12 months or more of regular unprotected sexual intercourse."

Around the same time, another powerful movement was blossoming under the Reproductive Justice framework. In 1994, a coalition of Black and Indigenous women congregated in Chicago in response to a US government proposal for healthcare reform that de-emphasized reproductive care and disproportionately adversely affected women of color [9]. This coalition, which began as the Women of African Descent for Reproductive Justice, further organized into a national group called SisterSong that pioneered the concept of reproductive justice [9]. The reproductive justice framework encompasses four main tenets: every human has a right to have children, to not have children, to parent children in a safe community, and to their bodily autonomy [10]. Though the movement was born in a time when abortion rights and the notion of "choice" were heavily debated, the reproductive justice framework emphasizes access rather than choice, arguing that many would not have functional access to abortion and contraception even if they were given the legal right to choose to use them. The reproductive justice movement emphasizes the need for increasing access to all reproductive healthcare, including abortion, contraception, comprehensive sex education, adequate prenatal care, and assisted reproductive technologies. Additionally, the framework underscores the importance of recognizing and addressing the intersecting issues of race, class, gender, and socioeconomic status and their impact on access to care.

The often overlooked tenet of the reproductive justice framework is the human right to have a child and the corresponding right to access ART for those who are unable to have biological children on their own [11]. Defining infertility as a disease was one small step toward acknowledging the desire to have a child as a human right, but further advocacy work remains to apply the reproductive justice framework to improve ART access for all communities, including marginalized ones such as BIPOC, LGBTQIA+, and individuals with disabilities.

Defining infertility as a disease state had profound effects on improving access to fertility care. First, it validated the emotional trauma suffered by millions of patients around the world, often silently and internally, by acknowledging the medical nature of their infertility. It also provided a clear timeframe as to when to refer patients to a Reproductive Endocrinology and Infertility (REI) specialist for further infertility work-up and treatment. Additionally, soon after the WHO released their definition of infertility, the International Classification of Diseases (ICD) released billing codes for female, male, and mixed infertility that further facilitated diagnostic classifications, disease monitoring, and reimbursement. Finally, the definition of infertility paved the road for insurance mandates to require coverage for fertility services. Health insurance companies often delineate which medical services are covered based on the concept of "medical necessity." A medically necessary service is one that "provides for the diagnosis, treatment, cure, or relief of a health condition, illness, injury, or disease." The classification of infertility as a disease deemed all the services required for its diagnosis and treatment as medically necessary and therefore eligible for insurance coverage.

Though the WHO definition of infertility was an important start in dispelling the notion that fertility care is elective, it excluded certain patient populations. Specifying infertility as the inability to achieve pregnancy after 12 months of regular unprotected sexual intercourse excludes patient populations such as LGBTQIA+ individuals and unpartnered individuals interested in family building. Since these institutional definitions are used as the basis for insurance coverage, using a definition of infertility that relies solely on the results of heterosexual intercourse further limits access to fertility care for these patient populations. In October 2023, the ASRM released a new, more inclusive definition of infertility as "a disease, condition, or status characterized by…the inability to achieve a successful pregnancy based on a patient's medical, sexual, and reproductive history, age, physical findings, diagnostic testing or any combination of those factors" ([12], p.1). The committee opinion also further specified that "nothing in this definition shall be used to deny or delay treatment to any individual regardless of relationship status or sexual orientation" ([12], p. 1). This updated language is not only more inclusive but also has the potential to increase access to fertility care if it is accepted by insurance plans as a guideline for determining what services and which patients qualify for coverage.

Costs of ART

The cost of ART is one of the most limiting factors in access to fertility care for patients. A single IVF cycle can cost an average of $15,000–$30,000 [13]. The cost increases when taking into account the costs of consultation, follow-up visits, medication co-pays, embryo storage fees, genetic testing fees, and increased visits throughout pregnancy before resulting in a live birth. According to an 18-month prospective cohort study examining the costs for infertility treatment, the median cost per live birth is $61,377 for IVF and $72,642 for IVF with donor egg [13]. Furthermore, many patients require multiple rounds of IVF in order to achieve a successful pregnancy and a single live birth. In comparison, the median disposable personal income in the United States in a year is estimated to be $16,751, only 27% of the median cost of a single IVF cycle and associated expenses [14]. This significant cost can be highly prohibitive for individuals seeking out infertility treatment.

The high costs of IVF are due to a combination of complex medical procedures, advanced laboratory techniques, and the intricate nature of fertility treatments. The process involves a series of highly specialized steps, including ovarian stimulation, egg retrieval, fertilization, and embryo transfer, all of which require advanced medical expertise and technology. One study showed that ovarian stimulation medication prices have risen by 50% between 2014 and 2020, mainly due to a lack of cheaper, generic alternatives [15]. In 2020, the average price of Gonal-F and Follistim, two commonly used medications that stimulate the ovaries during an IVF cycle, was $1463 and $1800, respectively [15]. In addition, the need for care by skilled professionals, such as reproductive endocrinologists, embryologists, and specialized nurses, adds to the overall cost. Furthermore, the use of cutting-edge technologies and equipment, stringent quality control measures, and the need for a controlled environment in IVF laboratories contributes significantly to the accumulating expenses. Hidden additional costs to patients can also accrue if patients decide to undergo preimplantation genetic testing (PGT), endometrial receptivity analysis (ERA), or sperm or oocyte cryopreservation that includes yearly storage fees.

Insurance coverage can significantly reduce the out-of-pocket expenditures for patients. Yet the main argument against mandated coverage for IVF is that it would be too costly to insurance companies to cover IVF and the associated pregnancy outcomes. This argument is majorly unfounded as shown by numerous studies demonstrating that the incremental cost to insurance companies of IVF coverage is minimal [16]. An analysis of cost expenditures in a state with comprehensive IVF coverage showed that infertility services accounted for only 0.41% of total expenditures within the insurance plan [17]. Other studies corroborate these statistics with similar findings, such as a case study examining the infertility insurance benefit provided by Southwest Airlines to its employees that showed that only 0.85% of insurance expenditures were for infertility-related costs [18]. One economic prediction model estimated that one IVF cycle would increase the *annual* premium for an insured employee by only $2.56 [19]. An additional benefit to insurers of covering IVF is the promotion of single-embryo transfer, which would reduce overall healthcare spending by reducing the rates of multiple gestation and associated maternal/neonatal morbidity and mortality [20, 21]. While the out-of-pocket costs of IVF and other ART procedures to the individual patient are high, it is comparatively miniscule to the insurer and would provide the benefit of reducing the costs associated with higher order gestation pregnancies, the cost burden of which is borne primarily by insurance companies.

Insurance Mandates

Historically, insurance companies did not provide coverage for most infertility treatments and patients paid for these services fully out of pocket. However, in 1984, a woman in Maryland who suffered from long-standing infertility secondary to endometriosis mounted a grassroots coalition to have the IVF she needed to achieve pregnancy covered by her health insurance. The work of her coalition resulted in the Maryland Senate Bill 793 and House Bill 1660, requiring that state-licensed payors "may not exclude benefits for all expenses arising from in vitro fertilization procedures" with the prerequisite that patients have "a history of infertility of at least 5 years' duration and all less costly available infertility treatment for which coverage is available have been exhausted" ([22], p. 824). Though the bill in its original form was restrictive in its eligibility criteria and itself likely deprived many patients of timely access to care, it set a monumental precedent for state-mandated insurance coverage for infertility treatments. An insurance mandate requires certain benefits to be included in a healthcare insurance policy by law. Federal and state governments use mandates to prevent insurance companies from excluding coverage for medically necessary procedures such as infertility treatment [23].

Since then, the Maryland Senate Bill has undergone several revisions to provide more inclusivity, such as reducing the duration of infertility to 2 years and including male infertility, same-sex couples, and medically necessary fertility preservation procedures. Several other states followed suit. As of July 2024, 23 states (Arkansas, California, Colorado, Connecticut, Delaware, Hawaii, Illinois, Kentucky, Louisiana, Maine, Maryland, Massachusetts, Montana, New Hampshire, New Jersey, New York, Ohio, Oklahoma, Rhode Island, Texas, Utah, Washington D.C., and West Virginia) have passed fertility insurance coverage laws [24]. Of these states, however, only fifteen have laws that include IVF coverage, and eighteen have laws that include fertility preservation for medically-induced infertility.

Research has demonstrated higher rates of ART utilization in states with insurance mandates as opposed to those without. Economic analyses have shown that a reduction in the cost of an IVF cycle by 1% of disposable income increases the utilization of IVF by 3.2% [25]. A study published in the *New England Journal of Medicine* that examined CDC and US Census data revealed a 277% increase in utilization of ART in states with complete coverage relative to states with no coverage [20]. Other studies have supported this association, including an analysis in 2018 from the CDC ART Fertility Clinic Success Rates Report that demonstrated that states with insurance mandates have double the IVF utilization of states without mandates [5]. This study additionally illustrated that an increase in utilization results in an increase in demand, as seen by the growing number of IVF clinics and cycles performed per clinic in states with insurance mandates.

In addition to the state-enforced insurance mandates, private employers and large corporations have separately started to offer broadened coverage for IVF and oocyte cryopreservation as an employee health benefit. In 2014, Facebook and Apple announced that they were including oocyte and sperm preservation in their employee health benefit package [26]. Since then, numerous other companies have followed suit. The rising popularity of fertility preservation created a new market for egg freezing start-ups that sell fertility benefits to employers. These companies have secured hundreds of millions in venture capital funding to provide fertility health benefits [27]. Despite this growing popularity of employer-provided coverage for fertility preservation, many employers were criticized for providing coverage that was viewed as self-serving to the companies themselves by promoting delayed childbearing in the interest of increased work productivity [28]. Regardless of employer intent, these policies provide choice and access to their employees on their reproductive health and reduce the barrier of cost in pursuing fertility services. Employer-sponsored fertility insurance coverage above that offered in general employer-sponsored health insurance plans has added to the expanding coverage provided by state mandates and further increased access to fertility services.

Limitations to Insurance Mandates

Despite the immense progress in passing insurance mandates since the first in 1984, there remain gaps in accessibility due to the inclusion criteria of the mandates and differences in breadth of coverage among states. Most insurance mandates have exemptions for religious employers, employers who self-insure, employers with fewer than a set number of employees, and publicly funded insurance such as Medicaid [24]. Patients who are covered by these forms of insurance, such as those with Medicaid, are often the ones who need financial support through insurance mandates the most. There also exists great variability among the services covered by each state mandate. For example, unlike other states, California and Texas only require that group insurance companies offer infertility services that employers can *choose* to include in their employee health plans, but do not require that employers provide that coverage. State mandates also vary in the caps they place on coverage [24]. Some states base their cap on expenditures: for example, Massachusetts covers a lifetime maximum of $100,000, whereas Arkansas has a lifetime maximum of only $15,000. Other states base their cap on the number of services, with Hawaii limiting coverage to one IVF cycle and Colorado limiting coverage to six egg retrievals and two IVF cycles [24]. Insurance mandates can be further restrictive on the prerequisite of duration of infertility, ranging from 1 year of inability to conceive in states such as Illinois to 5 years in Hawaii. These mandates additionally exclude patients such as unpartnered individuals, transgender patients, and same-sex couples by their inclusion criteria. For example, Arkansas defines infertility as the inability to achieve pregnancy between a patient and her spouse and specifies that the patient's egg must be fertilized with her spouse's sperm, therefore limiting coverage to married heterosexual couples and precluding the use of donor gametes [24].

Though the primary goal of insurance mandates is to decrease the costs and therefore barriers to accessing infertility services, the restrictions and variability among mandates may instead further exacerbate the disparities. As mentioned above, LGBTQIA+ individuals are often excluded from state mandates. One study demonstrated that LGBTQIA+ patients reported difficulties with insurance approval for treatment as the major barrier to accessing fertility care [29]. While progressive steps are being made toward providing more inclusivity to LGBTQIA+ patients with the broadening of ASRM's definition of infertility, more work and time are needed to see states adopt these new definitions in how they structure insurance mandates. Furthermore, many LGBTQIA+ patients require the use of third party collaborators such as gestational carriers or gamete donors, services for which a vast majority of the state mandates do not provide coverage. The cost of hiring a gestational carrier and its associated expenses can be as high as $100,000, not including the cost of an IVF cycle [30]. These additional expenses can accrue and deter LGBTQIA+ patients from pursuing fertility treatment, even if they reside in a state with comprehensive IVF coverage.

Additionally, racial and ethnic disparities in access to infertility services have been well documented in the literature. The 2002 National Survey of Family Growth demonstrated that married Black women were twice as likely to have infertility as married White women, even when adjusting for education, income, and history of pelvic inflammatory disease [31]. In addition, a 2007 population-based analysis from a large database found that Black women had a twofold increase in odds of infertility in comparison to White women after adjusting for socioeconomic status and infertility risk factors such as smoking, testosterone levels, fibroids, and ovarian volume [32]. Though minority racial groups such as Black and Hispanic patients are shown to have higher rates of infertility, they are less likely to seek or have access to infertility services. Kelley et al. studied approximately five million women who reported infertility using data from the National Health and Nutrition Examination Survey and found that Black and Hispanic women less frequently sought infertility care than White and non-Hispanic Asian women [33]. Several other studies have demonstrated similar findings of lower utilization of infertility services by Black and Hispanic patients in comparison to other racial groups [34, 35].

Though state insurance mandates aim to decrease barriers to accessing infertility care, they may not necessarily increase access equitably across all racial and ethnic groups. A retrospective analysis examining over 20,000 patients between 2010 and 2020 in a state with comprehensive, mandated coverage found that there was no significant increase in the number of consults among Black patients after implementation of the mandate, while White and Asian patients had an increase in consults and completion of infertility treatment [36]. Additionally, Correia et al. demonstrated that while utilization of ART was higher among all racial and ethnic groups in mandated states in comparison to non-mandated states, the rate of increase in utilization was still higher for non-Hispanic White and non-Hispanic Asian women [37]. These studies show that racial and ethnic disparities in access to infertility care persist even with state-mandated insurance coverage and greater efforts are needed to address these racial inequities.

Geographic Availability

Another major barrier to accessing adequate fertility services is geographic availability of fertility clinics. The 2016 Assisted Reproductive Technology Surveillance Report from the CDC found that 10 states, including Alaska, Arkansas, Idaho, Maine, Montana, New Hampshire, North Dakota, Rhode Island, South Dakota, and Wyoming, had 0–1 ART clinics in the entire state [38]. In contrast, some states were overserved with ART centers, such as California (69 clinics), Texas (43 clinics), and New York (37 clinics). The overarching issue is further elucidated by a recent population-based cross-sectional study that demonstrated that over 25 million reproductive-aged women lived in an area with either just a single ART clinic or no ART clinics [39]. This means that nearly 40% of the US population has limited access to ART services due to geographic constraints. Women are not the only patients with limited access to fertility care, as Nangia et al. demonstrated a scarcity of urologists and male infertility specialists in regions without ART centers [40].

Research has shown that ART clinics and specialists tend to concentrate in metropolitan urban regions with denser patient populations and higher median levels of income and in states with IVF insurance mandates [41]. Though rural areas encompass 75% of the US national landmass and almost 25% of the US population of reproductive-aged women, it is well documented that women in rural regions have limited access to healthcare providers, especially women's health providers [42]. Studies have also demonstrated that IVF availability is positively correlated with median state income, percentage of state residents holding a bachelor's degree, and percentage of urbanization [41]. Moreover, the variability of state-mandated insurance additionally exacerbates the geographic disparities in access to fertility care as a higher density of ART centers is found in states that have mandated insurance coverage for IVF. A study conducted by the CDC showed that the number of ART clinics in states with comprehensive IVF coverage was 1.31 per 100,000 reproductive-aged women in comparison to 1.00 per 100,000 in states without mandated coverage [5].

Patients with limited access to a local ART clinic face additional barriers to care that may result in delays in diagnosis and treatment. Not only do these patients endure increased travel time to a distant ART clinic, but they also bear other economic burdens such as work absenteeism and transportation costs. For some patients, the cost of overnight stays in locations far from home and childcare for any existing children in their family further compounds the burden. Receiving care at a geographically distant clinic may also reduce the availability of social support. One study evaluating the time costs of fertility care found that in an 18-month observation period, couples spent an average of 125 h dedicated to fertility care, with 73.3 h dedicated to provider visits and 43.4 h dedicated to travel time. During this time period, couples also reported an average of 17.7 days of work missed [43]. The time dedicated to fertility care had a positive correlation to distance from an ART center. In addition, IVF often requires multiple consultation visits, high frequency of imaging surveillance, phlebotomy-based tests, and cycle-dependent timing of appointments that can further worsen the time and travel burdens for patients who live far from an ART center.

Some progress has been made on improving the geographic accessibility of fertility care. The COVID-19 pandemic necessitated an expedited advancement in telehealth with numerous ART centers incorporating telehealth into their practices. A study performed by an ART center in central Georgia evaluated the efficacy of a novel telehealth program for their patients, who had to travel an average of 3 h to reach their clinic [44]. Their telehealth ART program included an initial consultation with an infertility specialist via a phone or video visit, subsequent procedures such as surveillance ultrasounds, hysterosalpingograms, saline-infusion sonohysterograms, and ovarian stimulation monitoring performed by a local gynecologist, and the final oocyte retrieval and embryo transfers performed at the ART center. In the study, they found there to be equivalent live birth rates between the telehealth and non-telehealth groups (44 vs. 47%), with 73% of patients reporting high satisfaction with the telehealth program. Another retrospective cohort study demonstrated that patients whose initial consultation was via telehealth were just as likely to pursue treatment as those who had in-person initial consultations [45]. The combination of advancing technology with telehealth and partnerships between ART centers and local gynecologists can reduce the travel and time cost burdens for patients with limited geographic access to fertility clinics.

Geographic disparities in fertility care access further deepened with the landmark overturning of *Roe v Wade* on June 24, 2022. In the *Dobbs v Jackson Women's Health* case, the US Supreme Court disbanded federal protections for abortion and gave individual states the authority to regulate abortion as they desired [46]. Almost immediately after the decision, 13 states enacted trigger laws that effectively banned abortion on the basis of "personhood" [47]. These states introduced legislation that defines personhood at the time of fertilization [48]. This not only has profound implications for abortion and reproductive rights but can also significantly influence the accessibility of IVF services across different geographical regions. Shortly afterward, in February 2024, the Alabama Supreme Court declared that embryos stored in a cryopreservation tank had the legal status of a "child" in the case of *LePage v Center for Reproductive Medicine* [49]. Thus, disposal or donation to research of unused embryos would fall under Alabama's Wrongful Death of a Minor Act. Following the court decision, IVF centers across Alabama temporarily paused cycles, making fertility services inaccessible to the entire state. Though a subsequent law was rapidly passed to protect IVF providers and their patients in order for cycles to resume, the consequences of these legal decisions still have the potential to affect ART practices such as the creation of multiple embryos per treatment cycle, pre-implantation genetic testing, storage of supernumerary embryos, and disposal of unused embryos or those with identified genetic abnormalities [50]. For example, an ART center in a state with personhood laws may fertilize fewer eggs per patient to avoid the creation of supernumerary embryos, which can reduce the overall successful live birth rate per IVF cycle for a patient. It may also increase costs for patients due to yearly storage fees for supernumerary embryos that patients may otherwise have discarded or donated to research. An REI physician in a state with personhood legislation could also be reluctant to perform an embryo transfer in a patient with a history of recurrent pregnancy loss due to the patient's inability to obtain a medical or surgical abortion locally in the event that the embryo transfer results in a missed spontaneous miscarriage, the conception of a fetus with a genetic anomaly incompatible with life, or an ectopic pregnancy. This reluctance could potentially require the patient to travel farther for reproductive care. Thus, patients in states with restrictive abortion or personhood laws may currently or potentially face a disproportionate lack of access to reproductive health care solely based on their geographic location.

Future Directions

Identifying barriers to fertility care can help inform the types of solutions needed to address these disparities. Understanding the importance of definitions of illness forces the scientific community to reevaluate our current standards for defining infertility, as illustrated by ASRM introducing a more inclusive definition for infertility that incorporates marginalized patient populations such as LGBTQIA+, single women, those requiring third-party collaborators, and male patients. Additionally, the influence insurance coverage has on reducing expenditures for patients and therefore accessibility of ART services has been extensively validated in the scientific literature. As the number of states that provide insurance mandates increases, more work needs to be done to standardize the coverage across states and enact federal guidelines for insurance mandates. An ideal future would include universal insurance coverage for ART services for all patients regardless of socioeconomic status, medical history, marital status, race, or sexual orientation. To further bridge the geographic gaps in accessibility to ART centers, federal funding incentives could be provided to REI physicians to open up practices in geographically underserved areas. The remainder of this chapter further delves into other developing solutions to improve access to fertility care.

One of the tenets of access to care discussed earlier in this chapter was "workforce." The workforce of fertility care consists of REI-trained physicians, advanced practice providers, nurses, embryologists, ultrasonographers, and affiliated care providers including professionals in the fields of law, mental health, and genetics. To provide adequate access to care, there needs to be a sufficient supply of professionals such as REI physicians to meet the demand for ART services. It is estimated that there were approximately 1500 board-certified REI physicians across the United States and 413,776 ART cycles performed in 2021 according to the CDC's Fertility Clinic Success Rates Report [51, 52]. This means that an individual REI physician would need to oversee an average of 275 cycles per year. With the increasing demand for ART services, this number will only continue to rise.

The main limiting factor to increasing the number of REI-trained physicians is the number of REI training programs. As of 2022, there were 49 REI fellowship programs in the United States with each program accepting 1–2 fellows per year

[53]. Strong arguments have been made to increase the number of REI fellowship programs, increase the number of fellows per year in each program, and shorten the training from 3 to 2 years to facilitate an increase in the number of qualified, board-certified REI physicians trained annually [54]. In conjunction, new fellowship programs should be established in geographic regions that are underserved in ART services. Studies have shown that a large proportion of the accredited REI fellowship programs are located in the Northeast with a dearth in the South and West [55]. The geographic location of REI fellowships is associated with the ultimate number of REI physicians in that region, as many trainees remain in the state in which they were trained to practice. Federal funding incentives should be enacted to promote the creation of new REI fellowships, specifically in underserved geographic regions, to increase the supply of workforce and address geographic disparities.

Novel IVF Technologies

Another important avenue for improving access to fertility care is to reduce the cost associated with ART procedures by developing novel and cutting-edge technology that can streamline the process [56]. Numerous protocols are under investigation for this purpose including mild ovarian stimulation, in vitro oocyte maturation, and intravaginal incubating devices. Mild stimulation utilizes the concept that "less is more" by focusing on optimizing competent oocytes and embryos with a lower dose of gonadotropins or combining gonadotropins with oral medications. Oral ovulation stimulation medications, such as letrozole and clomiphene citrate, in combination with gonadotropins, have been shown to decrease the overall amount of gonadotropins used and therefore the cost of medications, while maintaining pregnancy rates in patients characterized as poor responders to IVF treatment [57]. In addition, one retrospective study demonstrated that the addition of oral clomiphene citrate to gonadotropins for ovarian stimulation may reduce costs and lower the injection burden by removing the need for an injectable GnRH antagonist with no significant difference in mature oocyte yield [58]. In a similar vein, modified natural IVF cycles are being implemented that forego controlled ovarian stimulation prior to oocyte retrieval with only the administration of a GnRH antagonist for prevention of premature ovulation. These modifications appear to result in reduced cost without compromising pregnancy rates [59].

Another novel protocol under development is in vitro maturation of oocytes, wherein immature oocytes are cultured to maturity in the laboratory after minimal to no exposure to gonadotropins in vivo to lower the costs and medication burden to patients [60]. This would also lead to less waste as many practices currently discard immature oocytes that are deemed not viable for insemination.

Finally, researchers are evaluating new cutting-edge technology for incubation of embryos through intravaginal culture. With intravaginal culture, oocytes, sperm, and culture media are combined in a gas-permeable sealed device that is placed in the vaginal cavity during early embryo development. Early research has shown that this new vessel is safe and produces similar pregnancy outcomes to traditional embryo cultures and would reduce the costs associated with laboratory equipment and personnel [56, 61]. As ongoing research advances the field, emerging technological solutions will enhance not only the efficacy and success rates of IVF but also help to mitigate associated costs.

Conclusions

Since the first live birth from IVF in 1978, ART services have been an essential treatment for those experiencing infertility and the number of patients seeking these services has dramatically increased. As the demand for ART continues to rise, it becomes more important than ever to consider an individual's ability to access these services. This chapter explored various barriers to accessing fertility care such as the limitations of the definition of infertility, cost of services, insurance mandates, and the impact of geographical factors. Advocacy work is being done in each of these arenas as well as other avenues such as increasing the REI workforce and advancing IVF technology. A collaborative effort among healthcare providers, lawmakers, economic stakeholders, professional organizations, and insurance companies is needed to improve access to fertility care in the United States for all patients for whom assistance in having a longed-for child is required.

References

1. NSFG—Listing I—Key Statistics from the National Survey of Family Growth. 2022. https://www.cdc.gov/nchs/nsfg/key_statistics/i-keystat.htm. Accessed 21 Jun 2023.
2. Institute of Medicine (US) Committee on Monitoring Access to Personal Health Care Services (1993) Access to Health Care in America. Washington, DC: National Academies Press (US).
3. Access to Care. https://www.ahrq.gov/topics/access-care.html. Accessed 19 Dec 2023.
4. Disparities in access to effective treatment for infertility in the United States: an Ethics Committee opinion. Fertil Steril. 2021;116:54–63.
5. Impact of comprehensive state insurance mandates on in vitro fertilization utilization, embryo transfer practices, and outcomes in the United States. Am J Obstet Gynecol. https://www.ajog.org/article/S0002-9378(22)00175-2/fulltext. Accessed 30 Nov 2023.
6. Definition of "infertility". Fertil Steril. 2004;82:206.
7. Adashi EY. Infertility: a disease by any other name. JAMA Forum Arch. 2018; https://doi.org/10.1001/jamahealthforum.2018.0007.
8. Zegers-Hochschild F, Adamson GD, de Mouzon J, Ishihara O, Mansour R, Nygren K, Sullivan E, Vanderpoel S. International Committee for Monitoring Assisted Reproductive Technology (ICMART) and the World Health Organization (WHO) revised glossary of ART terminology. Fertil Steril. 2009;92:1520–4.
9. The Black history of reproductive justice | Progress Texas. 2021. https://progresstexas.org/blog/black-history-reproductive-justice. Accessed 29 Apr 2024.
10. Reproductive Justice. In: Sister song. https://www.sistersong.net/reproductive-justice. Accessed 4 Dec 2023.

11. Perritt J, Eugene N. Inequity and injustice: recognizing infertility as a reproductive justice issue. FS Rep. 2021;3:2–4.
12. Definition of infertility: a committee opinion. 2023. https://www.asrm.org/practice-guidance/practice-committee-documents/denitions-of-infertility/. Accessed 29 Apr 2024.
13. Katz P, Showstack J, Smith JF, Nachtigall RD, Millstein SG, Wing H, Eisenberg ML, Pasch LA, Croughan MS, Adler N. Costs of infertility treatment: results from an 18-month prospective cohort study. Fertil Steril. 2011;95:915–21.
14. U.S. Bureau of Economic Analysis. Real Disposable Personal Income. In: FRED Fed. Reserve Bank St Louis. 1959. https://fred.stlouisfed.org/series/DSPIC96. Accessed 20 Nov 2023.
15. IVF medication prices rose by 50% over the past 5 years. In: GoodRx. https://www.goodrx.com/conditions/fertility/ivf-in-vitro-fertilization-prices-rose-50-percent-over-5-years. Accessed 4 Dec 2023.
16. Omurtag KR, Styer AK, Session D, Toth TL. Economic implications of insurance coverage for in vitro fertilization in the United States. A review. J Reprod Med. 2009;54:661–8.
17. Griffin M, Panak WF. The economic cost of infertility-related services: an examination of the Massachusetts infertility insurance mandate. Fertil Steril. 1998;70:22–9.
18. Silverberg K, Meletiche D, Rosario GD. An employer's experience with infertility coverage: a case study. Fertil Steril. 2009;92:2103–5.
19. Collins JA, Bustillo M, Visscher RD, Lawrence LD. An estimate of the cost of in vitro fertilization services in the United States in 1995. Fertil Steril. 1995;64:538–45.
20. Jain T, Harlow BL, Hornstein MD. Insurance coverage and outcomes of in vitro fertilization. N Engl J Med. 2002;347:661–6.
21. Little SE, Ratcliffe J, Caughey AB. Cost of transferring one through five embryos per in vitro fertilization cycle from various payor perspectives. Obstet Gynecol. 2006;108:593–601.
22. Adashi EY, Schlaff WD. Against all odds: the first state infertility mandate (Maryland). Fertil Steril. 2018;110:824–5.
23. Mandated Benefit Laws.pdf.
24. Insurance Coverage by State | RESOLVE: The National Infertility Association. 2021.
25. Chambers GM, Hoang VP, Sullivan EA, Chapman MG, Ishihara O, Zegers-Hochschild F, Nygren KG, Adamson GD. The impact of consumer affordability on access to assisted reproductive technologies and embryo transfer practices: an international analysis. Fertil Steril. 2014;101:191–198.e4.
26. Perk up: facebook and apple now pay for women to freeze eggs. https://www.nbcnews.com/news/us-news/perk-facebook-apple-now-pay-women-freeze-eggs-n225011. Accessed 5 Dec 2023.
27. van de Wiel L. The speculative turn in IVF: egg freezing and the financialization of fertility. New Genet Soc. 2020;39:306–26.
28. Mertes H. Does company-sponsored egg freezing promote or confine women's reproductive autonomy? J Assist Reprod Genet. 2015;32:1205–9.
29. Bell AV. The margins of medicalization: diversity and context through the case of infertility. Soc Sci Med. 2016;156:39–46.
30. How Much Does IVF Cost In 2023? Forbes health. https://www.forbes.com/health/family/how-much-does-ivf-cost/. Accessed 30 Jun 2023.
31. Fertility, family planning, and reproductive health of U.S. women; data from the 2002 national survey of family growth. https://stacks.cdc.gov/view/cdc/6690. Accessed 27 Nov 2023.
32. Wellons MF, Lewis CE, Schwartz SM, Gunderson EP, Schreiner PJ, Sternfeld B, Richman J, Sites CK, Siscovick DS. Racial differences in self-reported infertility and risk factors for infertility in a cohort of black and white women: the CARDIA women's study. Fertil Steril. 2008;90:1640–8.
33. Kelley AS, Qin Y, Marsh EE, Dupree JM. Disparities in accessing infertility care in the United States: results from the National Health and Nutrition Examination Survey, 2013–16. Fertil Steril. 2019;112:562–8.

34. Greil AL, McQuillan J, Shreffler KM, Johnson KM, Slauson-Blevins KS. Race-ethnicity and medical services for infertility: stratified reproduction in a population-based sample of U.S. Women. J Health Soc Behav. 2011;52:493–509.
35. Kessler LM, Craig BM, Plosker SM, Reed DR, Quinn GP. Infertility evaluation and treatment among women in the United States. Fertil Steril. 2013;100:1025–1032.e2.
36. Korkidakis A, Thornton KL, Leung AQ, Shah JS, Amaral B, Penzias AS. Racial disparities in access to infertility care in a state with mandated infertility coverage. Fertil Steril. 2021;116:e46–7.
37. Correia KFB, Kraschel K, Seifer DB. State insurance mandates for in vitro fertilization are not associated with improving racial and ethnic disparities in utilization and treatment outcomes. Am J Obstet Gynecol. 2023;228:313.e1–8.
38. Sunderam S. Assisted reproductive technology surveillance—United States, 2016. MMWR Surveill Summ. 2019; https://doi.org/10.15585/mmwr.ss6804a1.
39. Harris JA, Menke MN, Haefner JK, Moniz MH, Perumalswami CR. Geographic access to assisted reproductive technology health care in the United States: a population-based cross-sectional study. Fertil Steril. 2017;107:1023–7.
40. Nangia AK, Likosky DS, Wang D. Distribution of male infertility specialists in relation to the male population and assisted reproductive technology centers in the United States. Fertil Steril. 2010;94:599–609.
41. Hammoud AO, Gibson M, Stanford J, White G, Carrell DT, Peterson M. In vitro fertilization availability and utilization in the United States: a study of demographic, social, and economic factors. Fertil Steril. 2009;91:1630–5.
42. Committee opinion no. 586: health disparities in rural women. Obstet Gynecol. 2014;123:384.
43. Wu AK, Elliott P, Katz PP, Smith JF. Time costs of fertility care: the hidden hardship of building a family. Fertil Steril. 2013;99:2025–30.
44. Mikhael S, Gaidis A, Gavrilova-Jordan L. Regional disparities in access to assisted reproductive technology: assessment of patient satisfaction when employing modern technology to close the gap. J Assist Reprod Genet. 2021;38:889–94.
45. Alexander VM, Schelble AP, Omurtag KR. Traits of patients seen via telemedicine versus in person for new-patient visits in a fertility practice. FS Rep. 2021;2:224–9.
46. Ranji U, Diep K, Published AS. Key facts on abortion in the United States. KFF; 2023.
47. Institute G Interactive Map: US abortion policies and access after Roe. https://states.guttmacher.org/policies/. Accessed 14 Dec 2023.
48. Feinberg EC, Kawwass JF, Cedars MI. Roe v Wade and the threat to fertility care. Obstet Gynecol. 2022;140:557.
49. LePage v. Center for Reproductive Medicine, P.C. In: Justia Law. 2024. https://law.justia.com/cases/alabama/supreme-court/2024/sc-2022-0579.html. Accessed 30 Apr 2024.
50. Bayefsky MJ, Caplan AL, Quinn GP. The real impact of the alabama supreme court decision in LePage v Center for Reproductive Medicine. JAMA. 2024;331:1085–6.
51. ART Success Rates | CDC. 2023. https://www.cdc.gov/art/artdata/index.html. Accessed 20 Dec 2023.
52. Stadtmauer L, Sadek S, Richter KS, Amato P, Hurst BS. Changing gender gap and practice patterns in reproductive endocrinology and infertility subspecialists in the United States: a Society for Reproductive Endocrinology and Infertility report. Fertil Steril. 2022;117:421–30.
53. 2023-SMS-Results-and-Data-Book.pdf.
54. Hariton E, Alvero R, Hill MJ, et al. Meeting the demand for fertility services: the present and future of reproductive endocrinology and infertility in the United States. Fertil Steril. 2023;120:755–66.
55. Diego D, Shandley LM, Feinberg EC, Cedars MI, Adashi EY, Kawwass JF, Hipp HS. REI clinics and fellowship training—a national snapshot to improve access to reproductive care. J Assist Reprod Genet. 2023;40:2101–8.
56. Davis OK, Sokol RZ. Introduction: access to fertility care. Fertil Steril. 2016;105:1111–2.

57. Haas J, Casper RF. In vitro fertilization treatments with the use of clomiphene citrate or letrozole. Fertil Steril. 2017;108:568–71.
58. Mandelbaum RS, Melville S, Masjedi A, Sriprasert I, Quinn MM, Paulson RJ, Wilcox JG, Guner JZ. Clomiphene citrate throughout the duration of ovarian stimulation: an approach to decrease costs, reduce injection burden, and prevent premature ovulation in patients with diminished ovarian reserve. Fertil Steril. 2023;120:e5.
59. Ho JR, Paulson RJ. Modified natural cycle in in vitro fertilization. Fertil Steril. 2017;108:572–6.
60. Yang Z-Y, Chian R-C. Development of in vitro maturation techniques for clinical applications. Fertil Steril. 2017;108:577–84.
61. Cooper AR. Intravaginal embryo culture: a successful alternative to standard IVF that may improve access to care. Curr Opin Obstet Gynecol. 2022;34:179–83.

Part II
Medical Considerations in ART with Diverse Populations

Chapter 6
ART Outcomes in Black Patients

David Boedeker, Charlene Echague, Katelyn Simpkins, and Torie C. Plowden

Background

Health disparities are differences in the quality of health, health care, and health outcomes experienced by socially disadvantaged populations. Racial and ethnic disparities have been consistently identified as significant drivers of inequity in access and utilization of healthcare, particularly reproductive healthcare [1]. Data indicate that Black women are more likely to suffer from infertility [2–5] yet seek infertility evaluation and treatment at significantly lower rates than their White counterparts [3, 6, 7]. These statistics require consideration and identification of concomitant barriers that affect access and pursuit of fertility care such as age, parity, marital status, education level, poverty level, and fertility diagnosis.

Reproductive health care cannot be discussed without addressing the historic manifestations of health disparities resulting from racial trauma experienced by African Americans dating back to slavery. Racial trauma, which refers to threats, prejudices, harm, shame, humiliation, and guilt associated with all types of racial discrimination, continues to affect individuals and shape cultures [8]. For instance, racial trauma experienced during slavery involved legalized sexual and reproductive exploitation of enslaved people. This trauma persisted beyond slavery through other reproductive practices such as forced sterilization. The collective weight of the historical manipulation of Black people's reproductive capacity heavily impacted the culture

D. Boedeker · K. Simpkins
Department of Gynecologic Surgery and Obstetrics, Walter Reed National Military Medical Center, Bethesda, MD, USA

C. Echague
Naval Medical Center San Diego, San Diego, CA, USA

T. C. Plowden (✉)
Walter Reed National Military Medical Center, Bethesda, MD, USA

D. A. Kaplan (ed.), *Cultural Responsiveness in Assisted Reproductive Technology*, https://doi.org/10.1007/978-3-031-76204-8_6

surrounding current reproductive health for many African American patients today [9, 10]. This history and the associated intergenerational and historical trauma that persist as a result are discussed at length throughout this volume. For the purposes of this chapter, the complex legacy of slavery and structural racism will be discussed as they relate specifically to access to reproductive healthcare and outcomes in treatment.

Due to the culturally inherent biases that have persisted for decades, limited or poor access to care remains a core barrier to medical care for racial and ethnic minority patients with fertility problems. The National Society of Family Growth (NSFG) found that patients who utilize fertility services are more likely to be non-Hispanic White, older, married and more highly educated than non-users [11]. This gap in access is further supported by data showing that non-Hispanic Black women are 1.8 times more likely to have infertility than their counterparts of other races yet are less likely to utilize fertility services at the same level [12].

Assisted reproductive technology (ART) includes in vitro fertilization (IVF), which is currently the most successful form of fertility treatment as measured by its high pregnancy rates when compared to other treatment options. We know that health inequities play a significant role in accessing care, but when Black patients do pursue fertility treatment, how do race and ethnicity impact their IVF outcomes [6]?

This chapter aims to address barriers to care and subsequent outcomes for Black patients in order to extend quality fertility care and mitigate inequities. By analyzing outcomes related to access, live birth rate, spontaneous abortions, and use of donor oocytes, we will better understand the lived experiences and barriers many Black patients face when pursuing IVF.

Access

There is a well-documented history of poor reproductive outcomes among Black individuals [4, 7, 13, 14]. Much of this research comes from large, national datasets, namely the Society for Assisted Reproductive Technologies Clinic Outcome Reporting System (SART CORS). Based on the Fertility Clinic Success Rate and Certification Act, IVF clinics are required to submit their data to the national government [15]. SART is a voluntary reporting organization that relays these data to the CDC for its members; SART member clinics are asked to provide detailed data on every cycle initiated in their clinic in a given reporting year. Given that the vast majority of clinics are SART members, much of our knowledge of ART outcomes and patient demographics relies on their data [16, 17].

When analyzing these national data, we see that Black women are noticeably underreported and underrepresented compared to their White counterparts [18]. In one SART CORS analysis published in 2016, Black patients only underwent 4.6% of the included IVF cycles, whereas cycles undergone by White individuals made up 85.4% of the total [19]. These data paint a stark difference in the patient makeup of ART users and suggest that Black patients are underrepresented among IVF users in these data. In an attempt to better understand the demographics of ART users,

SART now requires race to be reported [7]. However, this field is patient reported and even with this mandate, approximately 40% of cycles reported to SART have missing race variables [18]. Furthermore, reporting of race has not significantly increased over the past ten years [7], suggesting that SART's intention in mandating the change is not being met with corresponding changes in clinic procedures to more comprehensively capture this information. Accurate race reporting is paramount should we wish to better understand disparities affecting Black individuals and other minority groups pursuing infertility care. It is also critical to eliminating bias in research studies that aim to answer questions about why these disparities persist [14, 20].

The low percentage of Black patients completing ART cycles is of particular importance given that infertility rates among this group are increasing even as infertility rates are decreasing among White individuals [18]. There is a known discrepancy between the percentage of infertile women and those who ultimately pursue infertility care [18]. According to the CDC, approximately 19% of nulliparous individuals are infertile, but only 12% of them have sought fertility services [14]. However, this disparity is more pronounced among Black individuals, as evidenced by the fact that Black patients have an estimated twofold higher odds of infertility compared to their White peers [2]. Overall, only 25% of individuals with infertility in the United States are said to have their infertility care needs met. Criteria affecting whether their needs are met are not limited to race and ethnicity alone, as other factors including sexual orientation and geography affect access as well. However, race and ethnicity are consistently linked to barriers to accessing infertility services and ensuring that patients' needs are adequately met when marginalized patients do access care [20].

When Black women do seek reproductive care, they are more likely to do so at clinics with lower IVF volumes and poorer success rates than larger clinics frequented by White women [18, 19]. However, for many Black individuals, accessing a clinic in general presents challenges. Work constraints and distance from the location of the nearest clinic are routinely cited as barriers for Black patients seeking infertility care. Additionally, many cite the inability to find a physician they are comfortable with as a logistical constraint when initiating their reproductive care [20]. Minority patients are more likely to choose a physician of their own race when seeking any kind of healthcare [21, 22]. However, data from the 2019–2020 academic year indicate that only 0.3% of obstetrics and gynecology residents identify as Black. Training a diverse pool of residents and REI fellows that reflects the national population can improve access to care for minority and underserved populations, while also promoting more culturally responsive care. Addressing both the lack of Black physicians in the training pipeline and the dearth of opportunities for these physicians to be mentored by senior colleagues has direct implications for the reproductive care of Black patients, a concept explored more fully in the writings of Dr. Gloria Richard-Davis [21].

Once a Black patient decides to pursue infertility care, they are more likely to discontinue treatment prematurely than their White peers. Additionally, Black patients are slower to return to treatment than their peers after a failed cycle. These findings cannot be explained by the high cost of IVF care; the higher likelihood of premature treatment discontinuation among Black women exists independent of their insurance coverage. If they do proceed with treatment, Black individuals also face higher treatment failure rates [23]. However, experiences of infertility-specific care alone do not fully explain the racial disparities in IVF outcomes among Black patients and their peers. Rather, disparities are evident before Black patients are ever seen for infertility care.

When Black patients present to infertility clinics, they are more likely to be over the age of 35 and have a diagnosis of diminished ovarian reserve, which suggests they did not receive timely access to care [7, 18, 20, 24, 25]. In fact, Black patients seek infertility care on average 6–15 months later than White patients [20]. An observational study compared the number of Black patients seeking IVF care between 1999–2000 and 2004–2006. Over time, the number of Black patients under the age of 35 seeking care decreased, but the number of Black women over the age of 37 increased, a trend not mirrored among White patients [7]. When women present to clinics at a later age, they also run the risk of not meeting criteria for an elective single embryo transfer. This potentially puts them at an increased risk during pregnancy due to the gestation of multiples, should their transfer be successful [7]. The implications of these findings include an overall lower likelihood that Black patients' treatment and subsequent pregnancy and perinatal health outcomes will be favorable [20].

Some suggest that Black women presenting to clinics at a later age than their White counterparts can be linked to inconsistent referral patterns and adherence to guidelines for referral by their primary care physicians and gynecologists [20, 21]. The prohibitively high cost of IVF is also hypothesized to play a key role precluding many Black women and other patients from seeking infertility care [14, 26]. Since cost has been a key barrier, it was thought that mandating ART coverage would create more equity in accessing treatment [7, 18, 20]. Numerous studies have sought to answer whether IVF insurance mandates, or state laws that require insurers to cover a portion of ART, improve access to infertility treatments. Unfortunately, the studies evaluating these policies have shown that even though overall utilization increases, disparities in utilization persist [6, 14, 27]. For example, in Illinois, a state with mandated IVF coverage, Black individuals in Chicago represent only 5.3% of patients receiving IVF but comprise over 30% of the city's population [19]. Furthermore, in states with insurance mandates, utilization has actually increased the most among Asian and White women, groups that already demonstrated the highest rates of IVF use [14]. The intent of the mandates, therefore, appears to not be realized in many circumstances. A further discussion of the impact of these mandates on live birth can be found in a later section of this manuscript.

One notable flaw with these mandates includes the fact that no state mandate currently requires Medicaid programs to cover infertility treatment. Given that Black individuals are more likely to participate in this program than White individuals, Medicaid's omission of mandated coverage for infertility care may contribute to the persistent racial disparities seen in states with IVF insurance mandates [14]. Feinberg et al. shed insight into the effects of patients receiving care in an equal access-to-care setting in their 2006 paper [28]. The authors compared reproductive services utilization and outcomes between Black and White women seeking care in the military healthcare system. This healthcare system provides universal healthcare insurance to all active-duty service members, including subsidized IVF. The authors found that ART utilization among Black women was four times higher in the military population compared to the general U.S. population. However, Black patients had poorer ART outcomes, which the authors surmised may be related to a higher prevalence of fibroids [28].

Spontaneous Abortion

Once a Black patient does pursue IVF, their outcomes are significantly worse than those of their White peers [29–33]. In 2008, Seifer et al. conducted an analysis of the SART CORS database to examine the success rates of Black versus White IVF patients whose cycles were performed between 1999 and 2000. Of the patients seeking care at centers performing greater than 50 cycles per year, 80,309 patients met their inclusion criteria. Their primary outcome, live birth rate, was equivocal for cryopreserved embryos. However, even after controlling for pelvic pathologies, they found that Black race was an independent risk factor for pregnancy loss [34]. In fact, numerous studies demonstrate higher spontaneous abortion rates among Black women who conceive via IVF, which persist even when controlling for age [13, 34].

The authors continued to push forward our understanding of ART outcomes among Black women in a follow-up study published in 2010 [18]. In this paper, the authors compared live birth among patients seeking care at SART member clinics between 1999–2000 and 2004–2006. This retrospective cohort study included 158,693 IVF autologous embryo cycles. Despite the progression of time and advances in IVF technology, they demonstrated that the disparities they previously commented on persisted. For example, although the spontaneous abortion rate did not statistically change in the overall IVF patient population over this period, it continued to be more common among Black patients. The authors additionally performed a logistic regression to estimate the impact of race on treatment outcomes and compare relative risks between these two time cohorts (1999–2000 and 2004–2006). They then calculated relative risks to determine the effect race had on not achieving a live birth. Their comparison of the relative risks showed that the magnitude of these two numbers increased, suggesting worse outcomes for Black patients over time (31–33% in 2004–2006, 24–38% in 1999–2000). Additionally, although their initial study failed to identify any statistical significance in pregnancy loss rates among Black and White patients using cryopreserved embryos, this follow-up study did find a 10% increased risk of not achieving a live birth among Black patients pursuing this method of ART [18].

Another SART analysis performed by Baker et al. in 2010 [29] sought to further characterize predictive factors of live birth and pregnancy loss among users of ART. These researchers included 225,889 fresh embryo transfers from SART member clinics between the years 2004 and 2006. Again, they found that Black patients, in addition to Asians and Hispanics, had a significantly lower chance of achieving a live birth than their peers. Additionally, they note that Black patients had a higher rate of pregnancy loss in all trimesters [29].

Some surmise that this increased risk can be attributed to higher rates of pelvic pathologies in Black patients, such as hydrosalpinges and fibroids [28, 34]. Tubal factor infertility, for example, is up to three times more common in Black women compared with White women [20]. Given the well-known adverse effects hydrosalpinges have on embryo implantation, this subfertility diagnosis has detrimental effects on reproductive outcomes [31]. Additionally, fibroids are also more common in Black women, which can impair embryo implantation success and place the patient at increased obstetric risk should the transfer be successful [28]. In a secondary analysis of the Assessment of Multiple Gestations from Ovarian Stimulation (AMIGOS) clinical trial, the authors similarly found an increased prevalence of fibroids in their cohort. Although the authors acknowledge that the primary outcome of the AMIGOS trial was not related to spontaneous abortions, they report that patients who had a spontaneous abortion were more likely to be Black patients with fibroids, compared to non-Black patients with fibroids [25]. These data, therefore, suggest that the presence of pelvic pathology alone is not sufficient to explain the higher spontaneous abortion rates among Black women. Instead, it is important to keep in mind that when pathologies are more common in Black patients, a provider's implicit biases can result in missed or incorrect diagnoses or inadequate plans of care. This, in combination with already present racial disparities, has the potential to negatively influence aspects of these patients' reproductive care and their eventual pregnancy outcomes [20].

Live Birth

The ultimate goal and perhaps the most clinically meaningful measure of success in ART is the attainment of a live birth. It is important to recognize that, while all patients pursue ART in the hope of expanding their family, its benefits are not equally distributed across racial demographics. Numerous studies over the years have recognized that differences in race profoundly influence this outcome measure, particularly within the Black community [2]. The next several studies underscore the pervasive nature of racial disparities in reproductive healthcare and their impact on live birth.

Data accumulated in the SART CORS database have been used to determine the effect of race and ethnicity on ART outcomes. One such study, conducted by Shapiro et al., examined autologous ART cycles performed between 2004 and 2013. Of the 1,132,844 cycles analyzed, non-Hispanic Black women demonstrated a lower likelihood of achieving live birth as compared to their non-Hispanic White counterparts. Furthermore, after adjusting for age, this finding persisted throughout the duration of the study period [35].

An extrinsic factor potentially influencing suboptimal outcomes in ART across various races and ethnicities, particularly in Black women, is the financial accessibility of reproductive healthcare. Theoretically, the high out-of-pocket costs of infertility care for patients without insurance coverage for these services could lead patients and providers to pursue less costly but less effective methods of treatment. Relatedly, patients who assume the costs of infertility care without assistance from insurance could be forced to discontinue treatment prematurely on financial grounds alone, leading to decreased rates of success.[1] As fertility care can be cost-prohibitive, some states have implemented mandated insurance coverage of ART. To assess the impact of enhanced access on reproductive care, Correia et al. aimed to investigate the association between state insurance mandates and treatment outcomes [14]. Utilizing the SART CORS database, the authors conducted a retrospective analysis of autologous ART cycles performed between 2014 and 2019. Their study comprised 1,096,539 cycles from 487,191 unique individuals, the majority of whom obtained care from states without mandated insurance coverage for ART. After adjusting for patient demographics, Black patients were noted to have decreased odds of clinical pregnancy and an overall reduced cumulative live birth rate as compared to White patients, irrespective of the status of mandated insurance coverage. Moreover, Black patients experienced higher odds of both spontaneous abortion per pregnancy and cycle cancellation, regardless of mandated coverage. Thus, the authors concluded that, while state insurance mandates might mitigate the financial burden associated with reproductive healthcare, they do not seem to be enough to improve live birth outcomes [14].

Similarly, McQueen et al. evaluated the effect of racial disparities on ART outcomes through a retrospective analysis of 4045 patients receiving care at a single infertility practice in a state with mandated insurance coverage for IVF [33]. Their study examined the initial autologous retrieval cycle and subsequent fresh embryo transfers spanning the years of 2010 to 2012. Among individuals self-identifying as Black, there was a notable reduction in the number of mature oocytes (MIIs), normally fertilized oocytes (2PNs), day 5 blastocysts, and supernumerary blastocysts as compared to White patients. Additionally, this demographic demonstrated a higher rate of cycle cancellation. Regarding reproductive outcomes, Black patients experienced a significantly lower clinical pregnancy rate and a higher rate of spontaneous abortion. Live birth in Black patients was significantly reduced by nearly 50% compared to their White counterparts. Multivariable regression analysis adjusting for age, body mass index (BMI), day 3 follicle stimulating hormone (FSH) levels, smoking status, and infertility diagnoses again exhibited the finding of a significantly lower likelihood of live birth in Black patients [33]. This study further underscores the reality that, despite strides made in rectifying inequities in access to reproductive healthcare, there are still underlying factors that portend a poorer prognosis in Black patients undergoing ART.

[1] As discussed in the chapter on adverse pregnancy outcomes, disparities in insurance coverage can also lead to decreased rates of live births due to the quality of prenatal care and that of the hospitals in which underinsured patients give birth.

Shifting focus from the observed reduction in live birth among Black individuals, it is important to explore methods of predicting cycle outcome success. Various predictive methodologies have been utilized over the years, including assessment of baseline anti-Müllerian hormone (AMH) levels and oocyte yield. A more recent addition to this array of techniques is the ovarian sensitivity index (OSI), which is calculated as the number of oocytes retrieved divided by the total gonadotropin dose, multiplied by 1000. Normal OSI is defined as 1.697–10.07, with higher values indicative of greater ovarian responsiveness to stimulation. Since its integration into ART in 2013, the current body of literature does not describe any variations in levels among different races or ethnicities. As it has been studied primarily in White populations, however, true information about interracial differences in the OSI has been difficult to obtain [36].

Considering this, researchers sought to determine if race or ethnicity influenced the ovarian responsiveness to gonadotropin stimulation, as measured by the OSI. In one study, the authors investigated whether differences in OSI levels predicted live birth outcomes across diverse racial and ethnic groups. Their retrospective cohort study included a total of 4875 cycles, 553 of which involved patients who self-identified as Black. Following adjustment for multiple retrievals in the same patient, age, BMI, infertility diagnosis, and cycle number, Black patients were found to have a higher OSI level as compared to White patients. Despite this predicted greater response to gonadotropin stimulation, the likelihood of live birth was lower in the same demographic [36]. This discordant finding underscores the multifaceted factors contributing to the racial disparities impacting reproductive success within the Black population.

Donor Oocyte Cycles

Since its evolution from an experimental procedure to an established method of fertility preservation, there has been an increase in the utilization of oocyte cryopreservation. This has both made it possible for women to cryopreserve their own oocytes for use in later autologous cycles and for patients in need of third-party collaborators to access a larger pool of donor oocytes from egg banks rather than through coordinated cycles with a specific donor. As a result, ART with the use of donor oocytes has become more common as a means of achieving pregnancy among individuals with a history of diminished ovarian reserve, poor response to ovarian stimulation, advanced reproductive age, or an absence of oocytes, particularly for those without a biologic female partner [27]. While there is an innumerable amount of literature regarding reproductive outcomes in ART using autologous oocytes across various races and ethnicities, a significant gap exists in understanding the impact of race on outcomes of oocyte donation cycles.

One of the earliest studies to investigate this was a retrospective, matched cohort study conducted by Bodri et al. at a single, private infertility center between 2003 and 2008. The authors sought to compare ongoing pregnancy rates between Black donor oocyte recipients and matched Caucasian controls undergoing fresh day 2–3 embryo transfers. Although there was a significantly higher number of oocytes retrieved, mature oocytes (MIIs), and normally fertilized oocytes (2PNs) in Black recipients, rates of implantation, clinical pregnancy, and ongoing pregnancy were significantly lower than those of their matched Caucasian counterparts. Additionally, the miscarriage rate was observed to be higher in Black recipients as compared to Caucasian recipients. When a multiple regression analysis was performed, accounting for variables determined to influence the attainment of an ongoing pregnancy, Black race emerged as an independent risk factor associated with a diminished likelihood of achieving an ongoing pregnancy after oocyte donation [13].

Perhaps one of the largest studies evaluating the impact of Black race on ART cycles using donor oocytes was conducted by Shapiro et al. [35]. Using data reported to the Society for Assisted Reproductive Technologies Clinic Outcome Reporting System (SART CORS) between 2004 and 2013, the authors found that among the 217,030 cycles using third-party methods of ART, individuals of non-Hispanic Black race demonstrated lower live birth overall. While this study did not distinguish among reproductive outcomes resulting from donor gametes, donor embryos, gestational carrier, or a combination of methods, the trend remained consistent over the span of the study [35].

Finally, investigating the effect of Black race on frozen embryo transfer (FET) cycles involving donor oocytes, Liu et al. aimed to determine whether race had any bearing on the outcome of live birth. Their retrospective cohort study used data from a national oocyte bank spanning the years of 2008 to 2015. They included 327 oocyte donors and 899 oocyte recipients who underwent a total of 1601 programmed FETs, using embryos at either the cleavage or blastocyst stage. While the number of surviving and fertilized oocytes was similar between self-reported Black and White donors, there was a higher number of usable embryos in Black donors. However, FET initiated in a Black recipient resulted in a lower probability of live birth as compared to White recipients after adjusting for infertility attributable to tubal or uterine factors and body mass index (BMI). Although there were a limited number of cases in which the donor and recipient were of discordant races, live birth was found to be significantly lower in Black recipients, irrespective of the donor's race [32].

Collectively, the aforementioned studies underscore the impact of Black race on reproductive outcomes in the setting of ART involving donor oocytes. While some studies were limited by their small sample sizes, they highlight the fact that Black race reduces the likelihood of achieving both an ongoing pregnancy and live birth. As donor oocytes are presumed to be an option to optimize the chance of achieving pregnancy, this raises the question of whether there are other factors that might contribute to the diminished chance of ART success, such as an impaired uterine milieu or other environmental, behavioral, or genetic factors.

Inequities in donor-assisted conception are not limited to pregnancy outcomes for those pursuing reproduction with the aid of third-party collaborators. A recent cross-sectional study published in 2022 evaluated whether the racial and ethnic distribution of oocyte donors is representative of the demographics of reproductive-aged women in the United States. Analyzing data from 12 donor oocyte banks, Tsai et al. [37] found that the proportion of donors who self-identified as either Black or African American was notably lower than the overall population of Black or African-American women in the United States. Moreover, there were fewer Black or African American donors relative to the number of recipients from the same racial group, indicating an imbalance in representation [37].

Similar challenges exist for patients seeking to conceive with donor sperm. In a recent study of 20 sperm banks with a total of 1647 available donors, self-identified Black donors were significantly underrepresented compared to the U.S. population of Black men, at 3.2% vs 11.3%, respectively [38]. Perhaps unsurprisingly, then, patients seeking to conceive with gametes from a non-Hispanic Black donor report lower rates of satisfaction with donor selection and ultimately have lower utilization rates of donor gametes [39]. These studies shed light on the concerning discrepancy between the racial and ethnic makeup of gamete donors and that of the general population. They emphasize the pressing need for equitable representation and access within all aspects of ART care, including the recruitment of gamete donors that more closely mirror the characteristics of patients in need of their collaboration.

Conclusion

There is a long-standing history of poor reproductive outcomes among Black patients compared to their White counterparts, which extends to IVF. Despite efforts to improve access, Black patients face unique barriers to establishing care with a clinic and finding providers with whom they identify. Additionally, although insurance mandates for the inclusion of fertility benefits are intended to increase ART utilization among minority groups, they appear to primarily benefit groups who already have access to these services. Once pregnant, Black patients have higher miscarriage rates than their White peers, even when controlling for pelvic pathologies or the use of donor oocytes. This suggests that other factors, such as physician implicit biases and structural inequities, may be playing a role in these poorer outcomes.

The remedies to these inequities in access and outcomes are multifaceted, involving change at individual, systemic, and structural levels. It is our hope that the information provided in this chapter serves as a reminder of the urgency of enacting these changes. Working toward equity in infertility care for Black patients furthers the goal of increasing pregnancy and healthy live birth rates for all those whose family-building efforts we are ethically charged to support.

References

1. Beroukhim G, Mahabamunuge J, Pal L. Racial disparities in access to reproductive health and fertility care in the United States. Curr Opin Obstet Gynecol. 2022;34(3):138–46.
2. Beroukhim G, Seifer DB. Racial and ethnic disparities in access to and outcomes of infertility treatment and assisted reproductive technology in the United States. Endocrinol Metab Clin. 2023;52(4):659–75.
3. Janitz AE, Peck JD, Craig LB. Racial/ethnic differences in the utilization of infertility services: a focus on American Indian/Alaska Natives. Matern Child Health J. 2019;23:10–8.
4. Humphries LA, Chang O, Humm K, Sakkas D, Hacker MR. Influence of race and ethnicity on in vitro fertilization outcomes: systematic review. Am J Obstet Gynecol. 2016;214(2):212–e1.
5. Snow M, Vranich TM, Perin J, Trent M. Estimates of infertility in the United States: 1995–2019. Fertil Steril. 2022;118(3):560–7.
6. Dieke AC, Zhang Y, Kissin DM, Barfield WD, Boulet SL. Disparities in assisted reproductive technology utilization by race and ethnicity, United States, 2014: a commentary. J Women's Health. 2017;26(6):605–8.
7. Seifer DB, Simsek B, Wantman E, Kotlyar AM. Status of racial disparities between black and white women undergoing assisted reproductive technology in the US. Reprod Biol Endocrinol. 2020;18:1–3.
8. Cénat JM. Complex racial trauma: evidence, theory, assessment, and treatment. Perspect Psychol Sci. 2023;18(3):675–87.
9. Miller F, Miller P. Transgenerational trauma and trust restoration. AMA J Ethics. 2021;23(6):480–6.
10. Owens DC, Fett SM. Black maternal and infant health: historical legacies of slavery. Am J Public Health. 2019;109(10):1342–5.
11. Chandra A, Copen CE, Stephen EH. Infertility service use in the United States: data from the National Survey of Family Growth, 1982–2010. US Department of Health and Human Services, Centers for Disease Control and Prevention, National Center for Health Statistics; 2014.
12. Chandra A, Copen CE, Stephen EH. Infertility and impaired fecundity in the United States, 1982–2010: data from the National Survey of Family Growth. US Department of Health and Human Services, Centers for Disease Control and Prevention, National Center for Health Statistics; 2013.
13. Bodri D, Guillen JJ, Lopez M, Vernaeve V, Coll O. Racial disparity in oocyte donation outcome: a multiethnic, matched cohort study. Hum Reprod. 2010;25(2):436–42.
14. Correia KF, Kraschel K, Seifer DB. State insurance mandates for in vitro fertilization are not associated with improving racial and ethnic disparities in utilization and treatment outcomes. Am J Obstet Gynecol. 2023;228(3):313–e1.
15. Lawrence DL, Rosenwaks Z. Implications of the fertility clinic success rate and certification act of 1992. Fertil Steril. 1993;59(2):288–90.
16. Curchoe CL, Tarafdar O, Aquilina MC, Seifer DB. SART CORS IVF registry: looking to the past to shape future perspectives. J Assist Reprod Genet. 2022;39(11):2607–16.
17. Wellons MF, Fujimoto VY, Baker VL, Barrington DS, Broomfield D, Catherino WH, Richard-Davis G, Ryan M, Thornton K, Armstrong AY. Race matters: a systematic review of racial/ethnic disparity in Society for Assisted Reproductive Technology reported outcomes. Fertil Steril. 2012;98(2):406–9.
18. Seifer DB, Zackula R, Grainger DA, Society for Assisted Reproductive Technology Writing Group Report. Trends of racial disparities in assisted reproductive technology outcomes in black women compared with white women: Society for Assisted Reproductive Technology 1999 and 2000 vs. 2004–2006. Fertil Steril. 2010;93(2):626–35.
19. Eichelberger KY, Doll K, Ekpo GE, Zerden ML. Black lives matter: claiming a space for evidence-based outrage in obstetrics and gynecology. Am J Public Health. 2016;106(10):1771–2.

20. Butts SF. Health disparities of African Americans in reproductive medicine. Fertil Steril. 2021;116(2):287–91.
21. Richard-Davis G. The pipeline problem: barriers to access of Black patients and providers in reproductive medicine. Fertil Steril. 2021;116(2):292–5.
22. Saha S, Taggart SH, Komaromy M, Bindman AB. Do patients choose physicians of their own race? To provide the kind of care consumers want, medical schools might be able to justify using race as an admissions criterion. Health Aff. 2000;19(4):76–83.
23. Bedrick BS, Anderson K, Broughton DE, Hamilton B, Jungheim ES. Factors associated with early in vitro fertilization treatment discontinuation. Fertil Steril. 2019;112(1):105–11.
24. Dimitriadis I, Batsis M, Petrozza JC, Souter I. Racial disparities in fertility care: an analysis of 4537 intrauterine insemination cycles. J Racial Ethn Health Disparities. 2017;4:169–77.
25. Styer AK, Jin S, Liu D, Wang B, Polotsky AJ, Christianson MS, Vitek W, Engmann L, Hansen K, Wild R, Legro RS. Association of uterine fibroids and pregnancy outcomes after ovarian stimulation–intrauterine insemination for unexplained infertility. Fertil Steril. 2017;107(3):756–62.
26. McCarthy-Keith DM, Schisterman EF, Robinson RD, O'Leary K, Lucidi RS, Armstrong AY. Will decreasing assisted reproduction technology costs improve utilization and outcomes among minority women? Fertil Steril. 2010;94(7):2587–9.
27. Liao C, Kotlyar AM, Seifer DB. Effect of state insurance mandates on racial/ethnic disparities in the utilization and outcomes of donor oocyte–assisted reproductive technologies. Fertil Steril. 2023;120(1):111–22.
28. Feinberg EC, Larsen FW, Catherino WH, Zhang J, Armstrong AY. Comparison of assisted reproductive technology utilization and outcomes between Caucasian and African American patients in an equal-access-to-care setting. Fertil Steril. 2006;85(4):888–94.
29. Baker VL, Luke B, Brown MB, Alvero R, Frattarelli JL, Usadi R, Grainger DA, Armstrong AY. Multivariate analysis of factors affecting probability of pregnancy and live birth with in vitro fertilization: an analysis of the Society for Assisted Reproductive Technology Clinic Outcomes Reporting System. Fertil Steril. 2010;94(4):1410–6.
30. Dhillon RK, McLernon DJ, Smith PP, Fishel S, Dowell K, Deeks JJ, Bhattacharya S, Coomarasamy A. Predicting the chance of live birth for women undergoing IVF: a novel pretreatment counselling tool. Hum Reprod. 2016;31(1):84–92.
31. Fujimoto VY, Luke B, Brown MB, Jain T, Armstrong A, Grainger DA, Hornstein MD, Society for Assisted Reproductive Technology Writing Group. Racial and ethnic disparities in assisted reproductive technology outcomes in the United States. Fertil Steril. 2010;93(2):382–90.
32. Liu Y, Hipp HS, Nagy ZP, Capelouto SM, Shapiro DB, Spencer JB, Gaskins AJ. The effect of donor and recipient race on outcomes of assisted reproduction. Am J Obstet 8pGynecol. 2021;224(4):374–e1.
33. McQueen DB, Schufreider A, Lee SM, Feinberg EC, Uhler ML. Racial disparities in in vitro fertilization outcomes. Fertil Steril. 2015;104(2):398–402.
34. Seifer DB, Frazier LM, Grainger DA. Disparity in assisted reproductive technologies outcomes in black women compared with white women. Fertil Steril. 2008;90(5):1701–10.
35. Shapiro AJ, Darmon SK, Barad DH, Albertini DF, Gleicher N, Kushnir VA. Effect of race and ethnicity on utilization and outcomes of assisted reproductive technology in the USA. Reprod Biol Endocrinol. 2017;15:1–1.
36. Lee IT, Berger DS, Koelper N, Senapati S, Mainigi M. Race, ovarian responsiveness, and live birth after in vitro fertilization. Fertil Steril. 2023;120(5):1023–32.
37. Tsai S, Chung EH, Truong T, Farrell AS, Wu J, Ohamadike O, Eaton JL. Racial and ethnic disparities among donor oocyte banks in the United States. Fertil Steril. 2022;117(3):622–8.
38. Hobbs C, Gadson A, Raker C, Eaton JL. Racial and ethnic disparities among donor sperm banks in the United States. Fertil Steril. 2022;118(5):e25–6.
39. Mebane S, Harris BS, Woodward J, Brucker A, Erkanli A, Nagle C, Steele D, Neal S. A survey study evaluating donor gamete utilization rates, patient satisfaction and fertility treatment outcomes according to desired race and ethnicity. Fertil Steril. 2024;

Chapter 7
ART Outcomes in Latinx Patients

Anita Pershad and Arielle Yeshua

Introduction

In the United States, approximately 7.4 million women suffer from infertility, constituting about 12% of women of reproductive age [1]. While the 2022 United States Census indicates that 18.5% of the US female population identifies as Latinx, Latinx patients make up a mere 5.4% of the US population accessing assisted reproductive technology [2–4]. Overall, Latinx patients are significantly underrepresented in infertility treatment and use infertility services at a lower rate than non-Latinx patients. According to a 2022 report, 15% of White women between ages 25 and 44 years old in the United States have accessed infertility care, in contrast to 7.6% of Hispanic women [2]. A 2014 survey echoed these disparities, reporting that Latinx women had lower than average assisted reproductive technology (ART) utilization rates compared to non-Hispanic women in the United States [5]. Understanding the demographic landscape and medical outcomes of the Latinx community utilizing ART will help to promote increased access to care and reproductive health equity for Latinx patients.

A. Pershad (✉)
Department of Obstetrics and Gynecology, Eastern Virginia Medical School,
Norfolk, VA, USA
e-mail: pershaa@evms.edu

A. Yeshua
Department of Reproductive Endocrinology and Infertility, Eastern Virginia Medical School,
Shady Grove Fertility, Norfolk, VA, USA

D. A. Kaplan (ed.), *Cultural Responsiveness in Assisted Reproductive Technology*, https://doi.org/10.1007/978-3-031-76204-8_7

Background of ART in the Latinx Community

There are several historical, cultural, and social factors that impact ART outcomes in the Latinx population. These factors influence ART access, treatment decisions, rates of treatment uptake, and outcomes in care for Latinx patients.

Socioeconomic Factors

Socioeconomic disparities directly impact ART access and treatment success rates. Treatment cost and limited insurance coverage of fertility treatment is a known barrier to care, leading to decreased access to ART for patients with lower incomes. The average cost of an in vitro fertilization (IVF) cycle with medications is about $19,200 in the United States according to the American Society for Reproductive Medicine (ASRM). Socioeconomic barriers to care disproportionately impact Latinx patients. The median household income in 2021 for non-Hispanic White families was $74,932, compared to $60,566 for Hispanic families, suggesting that Latinx patient have less disposable income to put towards infertility care [6]. Further, although racial and ethnic disparities in overall insurance coverage were reduced by the passage of the Affordable Care Act in 2014, Hispanic adults remain disproportionately more likely to be uninsured or to be covered by public rather than private insurance and consequently less likely to have insurance coverage for infertility care than non-Hispanic White or Asian patients [1].

However, it is important to acknowledge that cost and insurance coverage is not the only factor that impedes Latinx patients from accessing ART. This is demonstrated by the persistent disparity seen in Massachusetts, which mandates insurance coverage for infertility. Massachusetts has the most comprehensive infertility insurance coverage in the United States. However, the use of IVF services by Latinx patients is notably less than projected based on population demographics: while 6.8% of the state population identifies as Latinx, only 3.9% of infertility patients identify as Latinx [7].

This effect is also seen in the military healthcare system. Healthcare in the military is often considered a surrogate for an equal access to care model, due to the equality in insurance coverage among military service members and the low cost of infertility care at military-affiliated medical facilities such as Walter Reed Army Hospital. In addition, active-duty military personnel have passed English proficiency testing and graduated from high school, which helps to correct for variables that may influence treatment seeking for infertility care including language barriers and health literacy. Despite these potentially equalizing factors, while 9% of people in the Department of Defense (DoD) are Hispanic, only 4% of patients seeking infertility treatment within the DoD system are Hispanic [8].

Reproductive Health Literacy

Health literacy and awareness of ART also shape medical outcomes for Latinx populations. Generally, among reproductive aged people, fertility literacy is low. There is limited understanding of age-related changes in fertility, male risk factors, spontaneous pregnancy rates, and fertility treatments among adults in the United States [9]. Low fertility literacy is especially prominent among patients with low socioeconomic status and levels of education [10]. In a 2021 study of 500 women, the authors investigated the impact of racial or ethnic disparities in fertility awareness. The study found that Black and Hispanic women had lower fertility awareness than non-Hispanic White women [11]. An additional study found that Hispanic women were less likely than non-Hispanic White women to recognize that smoking negatively impacts fertility [12, 13].

Having decreased fertility knowledge is a significant risk factor for poor reproductive outcomes, as fertility knowledge is positively associated with shorter time to seeking fertility evaluation and treatment [14, 15]. Latinx patients have been shown to have significant delays in accessing and presenting for fertility treatment due to lower rates of reproductive health literacy. After one year of trying to conceive without success, 78% of White women, compared to 65% of Latinx women, sought infertility treatment [14, 15]. Additionally, a 2013 study found that after an infertility evaluation, Hispanic women are less likely to receive treatment for their infertility [16], with one study indicating that Latinx patients were 27% less likely to have ever used fertility services compared to White patients and less likely to receive more intensive ART interventions such as IVF and intrauterine insemination (IUI) [3].

Cultural Factors

Cultural beliefs and attitudes toward fertility, parenthood, and medical interventions may also impact ART utilization and outcomes for Latinx patients. In one study, authors interviewed Hispanic women to understand the cultural factors surrounding infertility beliefs and uptake of treatment. These interviews were conducted with 88 women and 30 men in California. Hispanic women generally reported a cultural belief that children were the basis of the marital relationship and that childless marriages were considered a failure. Another prevalent belief reported among Latinx patients was that couples should engage in persistent efforts to try to conceive naturally without medical intervention until menopause. The researchers concluded that infertility is a culturally devastating experience for Latinx patients that has a profound impact on individuals and on the couple's relationship [12, 13]. The study also noted a difference in approaches to infertility treatment between women raised in the United States and those raised in Latin American countries. Latinx patients raised in the United States advocated for their healthcare needs more assertively and were more likely to see providers who practice Western medicine rather than alternative, homeopathic approaches. As a result of social and cultural stigma, Latinx women may be hesitant to seek help or talk about their experiences, making it difficult for them to access information about fertility options and find support from friends and family. This stigmatization may cause couples to avoid or delay seeking treatment, ultimately leading to poorer fertility outcomes.

Latinx patients may also experience religious-based stigmas related to the use of fertility treatments. In one study, Latinx patients were twice as likely as non-Hispanic White patients to report being very worried about using science and technology to conceive due to religious reasons, reporting discomfort around manipulating a perceived natural process [17].

Language Barriers

Language barriers and limited access to culturally competent care profoundly impact access and utilization of ART. A 2008 study examined the experiences of low-income Latinx patients from Mexico and Central America who suffered from infertility and their ability to access medical treatment. This study found that these patients had difficulty understanding their diagnoses and treatment options, and expressing their questions, concerns, and experiences to physicians [14, 15]. There were also notable difficulties in communicating with the fertility clinic staff, as patients reported difficulty with appointment scheduling, follow-up visits, and timed laboratory procedures due to language barriers [14, 15].

Disparities in Medical Care:

Barriers in accessing ART care directly manifest in disparities in reproductive health outcomes for Latinx patients. Infertility is a multifactorial disease, with many possible causes including ovulatory dysfunction, tubal disease, uterine factors, endocrinopathies, genetic disorders, and male factor infertility. Obesity is linked to ovulatory dysfunction, which increases the risk of infertility. Obesity and ovulatory dysfunction also decrease the effectiveness of ART [18]. Latinx patients are more likely to be affected by obesity than White women, as obesity effects 43% of Hispanic women in the United States in 2017–2018 [19]. Additionally, Latinx patients have higher rates of tubal factor infertility compared to their White counterparts [20, 21]. Tubal factor infertility usually requires IVF to achieve pregnancy [22]. The prevalence of uterine fibroids is also higher among Latina women than their White counterparts, with some studies suggesting a greater disease burden among Latina women with fibroids than among either White or Black women [23]. Finally, Latinx patients have decreased access to reproductive healthcare in general, with findings from a recent study reporting a 35% decrease in Latina women aged 21–65 years old who received a pap smear in the last 3 years when compared to non-Hispanic White patients [24].

Limitations to Research Findings

Accurate information about treatment outcomes for Latinx patients in ART care is limited by a dearth of empirical research that includes substantial representation of Latinx patients in the study population. There is essentially no reliable data comparing the efficacy of ART treatments, such as clomid, letrozole, and IUI, for Latinx and non-Latinx populations. Information about outcomes for Latinx patients in infertility care is based on limited data that is difficult to interpret; studies are characterized by small sample sizes and present conflicting results. There is a similar problem with the research on factors that impact infertility, such as endometriosis [25].

It is also important to note that much of the data available does not include consistent race and ethnicity reporting. About 39% of the data reported in the Society for Assisted Reproductive Technology Clinic Outcome Reporting System (SART-CORS) national database is missing information on patient race and ethnicity. For cycles where race and ethnicity are reported, there is inconsistency in whether the data are based on patient self-report or clinician judgment. Further, SART CORS does not allow users to input data on patient socioeconomic status, a relevant social determinant of health for many minoritized patients [26]. This further reduces the number of patients able to be studied when examining medical outcomes in ART for Latinx patients and increases the likelihood of significant bias and inaccuracies in any study conclusions. While the results of these initial pilot studies are described below, there is an overwhelming need for additional research on IVF outcomes in Latinx patients.

ART Outcomes

The two main studies that compare IVF success rates between Latinx and Caucasian populations report the following findings. Fujimoto et al. examined data from 2004 to 2006, using a large dataset from 95% of US ART clinics. The authors found 13% lower rates of clinical pregnancy among Latinx women relative to non-Hispanic White women undergoing IVF [22]. This study was limited by differences among clinic treatment protocols and general demographic variations in clinic populations. In contrast, a single site study of IVF patients who received treatment between 2010 and 2012 found no statistically significant difference in IVF success rates between Latinx and non-Hispanic White patients [27]. This study involved more similar comparison groups with fewer confounding variables in treatment and population. However, the use of data from a single clinic with a small sample size raises questions on its generalizability. It should also be noted that both studies used data gathered over a decade ago, before the advent of improvements in stimulation protocols, egg vitrification, and techniques to improve endometrial receptivity [28]. Updated research that includes representative samples is needed to determine what, if any, impact these advances have had on disparities in ART outcomes for Latinx patients.

The early data from smaller studies regarding IVF success and Latinx patients are complex and yield unclear conclusions. However, clearer data exist on the disparities in maternal and fetal health outcomes following infertility treatment. A study of the SART CORS database examined racial and ethnic disparities in ART outcomes [29]. The data set, comprising cycles initiated between 2014 and 2016, included over 140,000 IVF cycles using autologous oocytes, partner sperm, and fresh embryo transfers. Of these, about 9000 of the cycles included Hispanic women. This study found that compared to non-Hispanic White women, the odds of live birth were significantly reduced for Hispanic women as well as Asian and Black women. Latinx patients were 13% less likely than non-Hispanic White women to have a live birth as their pregnancy outcome. This decreased live birth rate was evident for patients both with and without a prior history of ART care [29]. Additionally, Latinx patients are significantly more likely than non-Hispanic White patients to have preterm deliveries and infants with lower birth weights [30]. Similarly, a recent study highlighted racial disparities in the success of ART. Overall the study found that ART cycles in Hispanic and Asian women resulted in lower rates of live birth per cycle compared to cycles in non-Hispanic women, after correcting for age, parity, body mass index, etiology of infertility, use of intracytoplasmic sperm injection, or number of embryos transferred [31].

A handful of smaller, older studies have presented contradictory evidence to the above ART outcomes. These earlier studies report similar IVF outcomes for both Latinx and non-Latinx patients. A study of about 4000 Latinx patients reported no difference in clinical intrauterine gestation rates or live birth rates in Latinx women compared to White women [27]. Similarly, a study of about 1400 patients found no significant difference between Hispanic and White patients for IVF outcomes including clinical pregnancy rates, live birth rates, implantation rates, or spontaneous abortion rates [27, 32]. This study specifically examined patients undergoing ART within the military health system, attempting to control for socioeconomic and insurance factors. A study in Texas conducted from 1998 to 2008 collected IVF cycle data from about 130 Latinx women and 300 non-Latinx women and reported no significant differences in clinical pregnancy rates or live birth rates [33]. Finally, a Chicago study conducted from 2010 to 2012 of about 4000 patients undergoing their first fresh autologous IVF cycle found that Latinx patients had similar pregnancy outcomes to White patients with similar clinical pregnancy rates, spontaneous abortion rates, and live birth rates [8]. However, this study also reported that Latinx patients were also more likely to have their IVF cycle canceled compared to White patients.

It has also been observed that Hispanic women have higher odds of adverse pregnancy outcomes such as fetal growth restriction and preterm delivery when compared with non-Hispanic White patients [34–36]. A 2012 systematic review showed that non-Hispanic White women consistently had higher live birth rates when compared with Black and Hispanic women, suggesting significant racial disparities in pregnancy outcomes in the United States regardless of the method of conception [37]. Further analysis suggests that a significant proportion of the disparities in outcomes can be explained by inequitable access to high-quality prenatal care and to the quality of the hospitals where patients deliver, pointing to systemic inequities that go far beyond those related to infertility care [34, 35]. Overall, compared to non-Hispanic White patients, Latinx patients are less likely to receive needed infertility treatment and have lower clinical intrauterine pregnancy rates, lower live birth rates, and higher rates of spontaneous abortions [37]. An additional study examined rates of adverse birth outcomes in singleton pregnancies conceived via ovulation induction and intrauterine insemination (IUI). While the incidence of adverse birth outcomes for all patients was less than 10%, the authors found that Hispanic patients had higher rates of fetal demise, neonatal death, perinatal death, and preterm birth defined as before 34 weeks gestation, compared to non-Hispanic White patients [36].

More recent research points to the fact that fertility outcomes are more likely to be compromised for Hispanic men as well. A 2024 study of clinically subfertile men in Utah suggests that the Hispanic men have a 40% lower likelihood of live birth than do their non-Hispanic counterparts when sociodemographic factors are controlled. This resulted in 14 fewer live births per 100 men per year among the Hispanic population. The authors suggest that some of this difference could be ameliorated by the uptake of infertility care but indicate that subfertile Hispanic men in this sample were significantly less likely to have ever accessed fertility treatment [38].

Finally, disparities are noted for Latinx patients regarding the frequency of multiple embryo transfer. Studies have shown that Latinx patients are more likely to have multiple embryos transferred in each transfer cycle. A study examining single transfers from 2004 to 2006 found that approximately 20% of Latinx patients received 4 or more embryos per transfer, compared to 16% of White patients [39]. It is established that multiple gestation pregnancies have significantly increased health risks to the mother and fetuses, including increased rates of postpartum hemorrhage, preeclampsia, preterm birth, and infant mortality [40]. While this study was conducted at a time when the transfer of multiple embryos was a more common practice, this racial disparity is still notable. It is unclear why this disparity exists; however, several factors are hypothesized to contribute. The discrepancy may have resulted from financial pressure to transfer multiple embryos per cycle due to limited insurance coverage or inability to afford multiple transfers. Other factors may have included poorer physician–patient communication, or late presentation to infertility care. It is important to note that a limitation of this study is that we do not know the quality of the embryos transferred, causing us to consider once again disparities in the effectiveness of ART caused by delays in treatment seeking and other factors impacting embryo quality [40].

Given the overall limited and inconsistent data, any conclusions regarding ART outcomes in Latinx patients are tentative at best. Conceptual arguments can be made that the widely differing findings result from the lack of uniformity among patients who are categorized as Latinx with regard to socioeconomic factors, language fluency, or nationality of heritage, and whether they self-identify as Latinx or are categorized as such by their providers. Regardless of the reasons for the inconsistency, additional and updated research with consistent race and ethnicity reporting is needed to examine and address disparities in ART outcomes for the Latinx population.

Ethnic disparities in fertility care are not limited to those impacting intended parents. An additional disparity was noted in the demographics of gestational carriers involved in international gestational surrogacy arrangements. A recent study of 40,177 embryo transfers to a gestational carrier from 2014 to 2020 noted that gestational carriers for international intended parents were more commonly younger than 30 years (42.8% vs. 29.1%) and identified as Hispanic (28.6% vs. 11.7%) compared with gestational carriers for US intended parents [41]. Cross-border surrogacy arrangements differ from those within the United States in legal and regulatory aspects, and screening of gestational carriers and counseling of intended parents can vary widely. Additionally, the psychosocial circumstances of these gestational carriers were not specified by the researchers [42]. Taken in combination, however, these findings raise the possibility that Latinx gestational carriers in international surrogacy arrangements may experience different levels of both need and psychological screening and may therefore be more vulnerable to adverse effects from participating in the surrogacy relationship.

Healthcare Policies and Recommendations

Multiple opportunities exist for healthcare providers and policymakers to improve fertility care and ART outcomes for Latinx patients. These involve improving access and affordability and providing culturally sensitive care for Latinx individuals seeking ART. Below are outlined best practice guidelines related to fertility care to decrease reproductive health disparities in the Latinx community.

Given that low fertility literacy and limited English language fluency are often barriers to accessing and participating in ART care, there is a need for readily available qualified medical Spanish interpreters. It is established that healthcare providers with limited Spanish fluency cannot elicit and address patients' concerns and improve their understanding of ART as well as professional interpreters or fluent Spanish-speaking providers [43, 44]. The ad hoc use of clinic staff or patients' family members and friends as interpreters risks both inaccurate communication of sensitive medical information and a violation of patient confidentiality; it has both been shown to worsen patient care outcomes and is not in accordance with federal statutes on the medical care of patients with limited English proficiency [45].

Professional interpreting is most helpful on initial intake visits, to help obtain a comprehensive medical history, when discussing a specific diagnosis, and when discussing poor prognoses, such as premature ovarian failure and azoospermia.

Studies have found that the use of qualified interpreters, increasing the number of Spanish speaking providers, and the use of visual aids can increase patient understanding of ART and their treatment options [46]. There have been two recent studies that found that participation in an 8-h to 2-week Spanish language immersion and cultural competency course improved provider knowledge, skills, and communication with Latinx patients [47–49]. Enhanced understanding between provider and patient can ultimately improve patient satisfaction and medical outcomes for patients.

Diversity in the Infertility Workforce

Increasing diversity among infertility care providers and clinic staff is an important component to providing culturally competent fertility care and ultimately improving medical outcomes for Latinx patients. Currently, there is limited diversity in the field of reproductive endocrinology and infertility (REI). The infertility workforce is overwhelmingly White and does not reflect the patient population of the United States. Compared to 18.9% of the US population identifying as Latinx, only 3% of REI trainees identify as Latinx [50]. It is important to actively train and promote individuals from diverse backgrounds. There should be a focus on creating pipelines for physicians from underrepresented groups such as the Latinx community to enter the field and to avail themselves of mentorship and opportunities for collaboration with senior clinicians.

Infertility clinics should also aim to have a diverse workforce of staff and affiliated providers that represents the patients they serve. Practice managers should focus on creating an inclusive and welcoming work environment for Latinx staff and those from other marginalized populations. Increasing diversity and Latinx representation in REI clinics is likely to improve patient satisfaction and engagement. There is no existing data on the outcomes of racially concordant infertility care, but comparisons can be drawn from other medical specialties. In a telephone survey of patients with appointments at multiple primary care practices, patients in race–concordant relationships with their physicians rated their visits as significantly more participatory and were more satisfied with their care than patients in race–discordant relationships [51]. Additionally, studies have shown that providers from minority backgrounds are more likely to focus on providing care to their minority communities, improving access to care and healthcare outcomes for members of these communities [52]. Minoritized providers are also more likely to express a desire to mentor more junior providers from marginalized groups, creating a virtuous cycle that increases diverse representation in healthcare [53]. Increasing the diversity of infertility staff and providers could therefore increase both the satisfaction of staff from marginalized groups and that of Latinx patients in infertility care. It may also reduce disparities in fertility care by increasing the pool of providers with a heightened interest in serving patients with similar cultural and ethnic backgrounds.

Advocacy and Education

Advocating for the specific needs of Latinx patients is an important aspect of improving medical outcomes and decreasing health disparities. Socioeconomic factors and insurance coverage are important barriers to accessing fertility care. As of September 2023, 21 states and Washington DC have passed fertility insurance coverage laws. Fifteen of those laws include IVF coverage, and 17 cover fertility preservation for iatrogenic infertility [54]. Describing infertility as a disease may increase insurance coverage and reduce the social and cultural stigma surrounding infertility in the Latinx community. REI providers can promote the fact that infertility is defined as a disease by the World Health Organization, the American Medical Association, and the American Society for Reproductive Medicine [55].

Establishing fertility clinics in low- and middle-income communities can also increase access to fertility care for minority populations. Minority women more frequently live in neighborhoods with fewer resources overall, including fewer medical facilities such as reproductive health clinics [56]. Greater accessibility via telemedicine and online resources may increase access to care [57]. To address the lack of fertility knowledge and increase awareness of available options among Hispanic populations, REI providers should increase education and outreach initiatives to promote fertility health literacy. Fertility clinics should provide multilingual pamphlets with easily accessible information, multilingual short videos, and illustrations on fertility to reduce the language barrier and improve fertility care for Latinx patients. Providers should focus on providing clear, thorough explanations using a vocabulary that the patients can understand.

To help all patients increase fertility awareness, it is important that all primary care providers—including advanced practice nurses, physician assistants, family practice and internal medicine physicians, and obstetrics and gynecology specialists—improve their knowledge of infertility. Patients with limited access to specialized fertility care often turn to their primary care providers and general obstetrician-gynecologists first for their infertility needs. These first-line providers should be familiar with the treatment options and initial workup to help improve patient understanding of infertility, access to care, and treatment options [58].

Conclusion

There are significant gaps in the current research and a profound need for greater understanding of ART outcomes in the Latinx community. Future studies should address these gaps with larger studies with consistent race and ethnicity reporting to enhance knowledge in this area. Engagement and collaboration with the Latinx community is important to advance research and improve medical outcomes. We emphasize a need for understanding and addressing disparate ART outcomes within the Latinx community. This is a call to action for continued efforts to improve access, equity, and quality of care in fertility treatments for all individuals, regardless of ethnicity or cultural background.

References

1. Ethics Committee of the American Society for Reproductive Medicine. Disparities in access to effective treatment for infertility in the United States: an Ethics Committee opinion. Fertil Steril. 2021;116(1):54–63. https://doi.org/10.1016/j.fertnstert.2021.02.019.
2. Genadek K, Sanders J, Stevenson A. Measuring US fertility using administrative data from the Census Bureau. Demogr Res. 2022;47:37–58. https://doi.org/10.4054/demres.2022.47.2.
3. Chandra A, Copen CE, Stephen EH. Infertility service use in the United States: data from the National Survey of Family Growth, 1982–2010. Natl Health Stat Rep. 2014;73:1–21.
4. Chandra A, Martinez GM, Mosher WD, Abma JC, Jones J. Fertility, family planning, and reproductive health of U.S. women: data from the 2002 National Survey of Family Growth. Vital Health Stat 23. 2005;(25):1–160.
5. Dieke AC, Zhang Y, Kissin DM, Barfield WD, Boulet SL. Disparities in assisted reproductive technology utilization by race and ethnicity, United States, 2014: a commentary. J Womens Health (Larchmt). 2017;26(6):605–8. https://doi.org/10.1089/jwh.2017.6467.
6. Guzman G. Household income: 2021. American Community Survey Briefs; 2022.
7. Jain T, Hornstein MD. Disparities in access to infertility services in a state with mandated insurance coverage. Fertil Steril. 2005;84:221–3.
8. Feinberg EC, Larsen FW, Wah RM, Alvero RJ, Armstrong AY. Economics may not explain Hispanic underutilization of assisted reproductive technology services. Fertil Steril. 2007;88(5):1439–41. https://doi.org/10.1016/j.fertnstert.2007.01.031.
9. Pedro J, Brandão T, Schmidt L, Costa ME, Martins MV. What do people know about fertility? A systematic review on fertility awareness and its associated factors. Ups J Med Sci. 2018;123(2):71–81. https://doi.org/10.1080/03009734.2018.1480186.
10. Hoffman JR, Delaney MA, Valdes CT, Herrera D, Washington SL, Aghajanova L, Smith JF, Herndon CN. Disparities in fertility knowledge among women from low and high resource settings presenting for fertility care in two United States metropolitan centers. Fertil Res Pract. 2020;6:15. https://doi.org/10.1186/s40738-020-00084-1.
11. Siegel DR, Sheeder J, Polotsky AJ. Racial and ethnic disparities in fertility awareness among reproductive-aged women. Womens Health Rep (New Rochelle). 2021;2(1):347–54. https://doi.org/10.1089/whr.2021.0034.
12. Maher JY, Pal L, Illuzzi JL, Achong N, Lundsberg LS. Racial and ethnic differences in reproductive knowledge and awareness among women in the United States. F S Rep. 2022;3(Suppl. 2):46–54. https://doi.org/10.1016/j.xfre.2022.03.006.
13. Becker G, Castrillo M, Jackson R, Nachtigall RD. Infertility among low-income Latinos. Fertil Steril. 2006;85(4):882–7. https://doi.org/10.1016/j.fertnstert.2005.09.052.
14. Swift BE, Liu KE. The effect of age, ethnicity, and level of education on fertility awareness and duration of infertility. J Obstet Gynaecol Can. 2014;36(11):990–6. https://doi.org/10.1016/S1701-2163(15)30412-6.
15. Nachtigall RD, Castrillo M, Shah N, Turner D, Harrington J, Jackson R. The challenge of providing infertility services to a low-income immigrant Latino population. Fertil Steril. 2009;92(1):116–23. https://doi.org/10.1016/j.fertnstert.2008.05.037.
16. Kessler LM, Craig BM, Plosker SM, Reed DR, Quinn GP. Infertility evaluation and treatment among women in the United States. Fertil Steril. 2013;100(4):1025–32. https://doi.org/10.1016/j.fertnstert.2013.05.040.

17. Galic I, Swanson A, Warren C, Negris O, Bozen A, Brown D, Lawson A, Jain T. Infertility in the Midwest: perceptions and attitudes of current treatment. Am J Obstet Gynecol. 2021;225(1):61–e1.
18. Pasquali R, Patton L, Gambineri A. Obesity and infertility. Curr Opin Endocrinol Diabetes Obes. 2007;14(6):482–7. https://doi.org/10.1097/MED.0b013e3282f1d6cb.
19. Hales CM, Carroll MD, Fryar CD, Ogden CL. Prevalence of obesity and severe obesity among adults: United States, 2017–2018 NCHS Data Brief, no 360. Hyattsville: National Center for Health Statistics; 2020.
20. Komorowski AS, Jain T. A review of disparities in access to infertility care and treatment outcomes among Hispanic women. Reprod Biol Endocrinol. 2022;20(1):1. https://doi.org/10.1186/s12958-021-00875-1.
21. Huddleston HG, Cedars MI, Sohn SH, Giudice LC, Fujimoto VY. Racial and ethnic disparities in reproductive endocrinology and infertility. Am J Obstet Gynecol. 2010;202(5):413–9.
22. Fujimoto VY, Luke B, Brown MB, Jain T, Armstrong A, Grainger DA, et al. Racial and ethnic disparities in assisted reproductive technology outcomes in the United States. Fertil Steril. 2010;93(2):382–90. https://doi.org/10.1016/j.fertnstert.2008.10.061.
23. Orellana M, Riggan KA, DSouza K, Stewart EA, Venable S, Balls-Berry JE, Allyse MA. Perceptions of ethnoracial factors in the management and treatment of uterine fibroids. J Racial Ethn Health Disparities. 2022;9(4):1184–91.
24. Spencer JC, Kim JJ, Tiro JA, Feldman SJ, Kobrin SC, Skinner CS, Wang L, McCarthy AM, Atlas SJ, Pruitt SL, Silver MI. Racial and ethnic disparities in cervical cancer screening from three US healthcare settings. Am J Prev Med. 2023;65(4):667–77.
25. Cox K, Sriprasert I, Nguyen B. Endometriosis management patterns among women in the national survey of family growth (2017–2019) [A98]. Obstet Gynecol. 2022;139:29S.
26. Curchoe CL, Tarafdar O, Aquilina MC, Seifer DB. SART CORS IVF registry: looking to the past to shape future perspectives. J Assist Reprod Genet. 2022;39(11):2607–16.
27. McQueen DB, Schufreider A, Lee SM, Feinberg EC, Uhler ML. Racial disparities in in vitro fertilization outcomes. Fertil Steril. 2015;104(2):398–402.e1. https://doi.org/10.1016/j.fertnstert.2015.05.012.
28. Singh K, Dewani D. Recent advancements in in vitro fertilisation. Cureus. 2022;14(10)
29. Kotlyar AM, Simsek B, Seifer DB. Disparities in ART live birth and cumulative live birth outcomes for hispanic and asian women compared to white non-hispanic women. J Clin Med. 2021;10(12):2615. https://doi.org/10.3390/jcm10122615.
30. Crawford S, Joshi N, Boulet SL, Bailey MA, Hood ME, Manning SE, McKane P, Kirby RS, Kissin DM, Jamieson DJ. Maternal racial and ethnic disparities in neonatal birth outcomes with and without assisted reproduction. Obstet Gynecol. 2017;129(6):1022–30.
31. Beroukhim G, Seifer DB. Racial and ethnic disparities in access to and outcomes of infertility treatment and assisted reproductive technology in the United States. Endocrinol Metab Clin N Am. 2023;52(4):659–75. https://doi.org/10.1016/j.ecl.2023.05.005.
32. Grainger DA, Seifer DB, Frazier LM, Rall MJ, Tjaden BL, Merrill JC. Racial disparity in clinical outcomes from women using advanced reproductive technologies (ART): analysis of 80,196 ART cycles from the SART database 1999 and 2000. Fertil Steril. 2004;82:S37–8. https://doi.org/10.1016/j.fertnstert.2004.07.098.
33. Shuler A, Rodgers AK, Budrys NM, Holden A, Schenken RS, Brzyski RG. In vitro fertilization outcomes in Hispanics versus non-Hispanic whites. Fertil Steril. 2011;95(8):2735–7. https://doi.org/10.1016/j.fertnstert.2011.04.031.
34. Nasiri K, Moodie EE, Abenhaim HA. To what extent is the association between race/ethnicity and fetal growth restriction explained by adequacy of prenatal care? A mediation analysis of a retrospectively selected cohort. Am J Epidemiol. 2020;189(11):1360–8.
35. Dongarwar D, Garcia BY, Booker A, Sankhavaram M, Salihu HM. Implications of social determinants of health characteristics on fetal growth restriction among various racial/ethnic groups. Matern Child Health J. 2023 Apr;27(4):650–8.

36. Lisonkova S, Ukah UV, John S, Yearwood L, Muraca GM, Razaz N, Sabr Y, Yong PJ, Bedaiwy MA. Racial and ethnic disparities in the perinatal health of infants conceived by ART. Pediatrics. 2022;150(5):e2021055855.
37. Wellons MF, Fujimoto VY, Baker VL, Barrington DS, Broomfield D, Catherino WH, Richard-Davis G, Ryan M, Thornton K, Armstrong AY. Race matters: a systematic review of racial/ethnic disparity in Society for Assisted Reproductive Technology reported outcomes. Fertil Steril. 2012;98(2):406–9. https://doi.org/10.1016/j.fertnstert.2012.05.012.
38. Langston DM, Fendereski K, Halpern JA, Iko IN, Aston KI, Emery BE, Ferlic EA, Ramsay JM, Horns JJ, Hotaling JM. Hispanic ethnicity and fertility outcomes. Urology. 2024;
39. Luke B, Brown MB, Grainger DA, Cedars M, Klein N, Stern JE, Society for Assisted Reproductive Technology Writing Group. Practice patterns and outcomes with the use of single embryo transfer in the United States. Fertil Steril. 2010;93(2):490–8.
40. Day MC, Barton JR, O'Brien JM, Istwan NB, Sibai BM. The effect of fetal number on the development of hypertensive conditions of pregnancy. Obstet Gynecol. 2005;106:927–31.
41. Herweck A, DeSantis C, Shandley LM, Kawwass JF, Hipp HS. International gestational surrogacy in the United States, 2014–2020. Fertil Steril. 2024;121(4):622–30. https://doi.org/10.1016/j.fertnstert.2023.12.039.
42. González NI. Legal and ethical issues in cross-border gestational surrogacy. Fertil Steril. 2020;113(5):916–9.
43. Fernandez A, Schillinger D, Grumbach K, Rosenthal A, Stewart AL, Wang F, et al. Physician language ability and cultural competence an exploratory study of communication with Spanish-speaking patients. J Gen Intern Med. 2004;19:167–74.
44. Baker DW, Hayes R, Fortier JP. Interpreter use and satisfaction with interpersonal aspects of care for Spanish-speaking patients. Med Care. 1998;36:1461–70.
45. Karliner LS, Jacobs EA, Chen AH, Mutha S. Do professional interpreters improve clinical care for patients with limited English proficiency? A systematic review of the literature. Health Serv Res. 2007;42(2):727–54.
46. Khoong EC, Fernandez A. Addressing gaps in interpreter use: time for implementation science informed multi-level interventions. J Gen Internal Med. 2021;36(11):3532–6.
47. Rivadeneyra R, Eldlerkin-Thompson V, Silver RC, Waitzkin H. Patient centeredness in medical encounters requiring an interpreter. Am J Med. 2000;108:470–4.
48. Barkin SR, Balkrishnan R, Manuel J, Hall MA. Effect of language immersion on communication with Latino patients. N C Med J. 2003;64:258–62.
49. Assemi MC, Cullander C, Hudmon KS. Implementation and evaluation of cultural competency training for pharmacy students. Ann Pharmacother. 2004;38:781–6.
50. Portugal A, Kosturakis AK, Onyewuenyi TL, Rivera-Cruz G, Jimenez PT. Breaking down barriers: advancing toward health equity in fertility care for black and hispanic patients. Obstet Gynecol Clin N Am. 2023;50(4):735–46. https://doi.org/10.1016/j.ogc.2023.08.007.
51. Cooper-Patrick L, Gallo JJ, Gonzales JJ, Vu HT, Powe NR, Nelson C, Ford DE. Race, gender, and partnership in the patient-physician relationship. JAMA. 1999;282(6):583–9. https://doi.org/10.1001/jama.282.6.583.
52. Mabeza RM, Christophers B, Ederaine SA, Glenn EJ, Benton-Slocum ZP, Marcelin JR. Interventions associated with racial and ethnic diversity in US Graduate Medical Education: a scoping review. JAMA Netw Open. 2023;6(1):e2249335. https://doi.org/10.1001/jamanetworkopen.2022.49335.
53. Wyatt TR, Rockich-Winston N, Crandall S, Wooten R, Gillette C. A comparison of professional identity experiences among minoritized medical professionals. J Natl Med Assoc. 2022;114(4):456–64.
54. Korkidakis A, DeSantis C, Kissin D, Hacker M, Koniares K, Yartel A, Adashi E, Penzias A, Collaborative for Assisted Reproductive Technology Epidemiologic Research. State insurance mandates and racial and ethnic inequities in assisted reproductive technology utilization. Fertil Steril. 2024;121(1):54–62. https://doi.org/10.1016/j.fertnstert.2023.09.015.

55. Practice Committee of the American Society for Reproductive Medicine. Definitions of infertility and recurrent pregnancy loss: a committee opinion. Fertil Steril. 2020;113(3):533–5. https://doi.org/10.1016/j.fertnstert.2019.11.025. Epub 2020 Feb 27
56. Crear-Perry J, Correa-de-Araujo R, Lewis Johnson T, McLemore MR, Neilson E, Wallace M. Social and structural determinants of health inequities in maternal health. J Women's Health. 2021;30(2):230–5.
57. Brodeur TY, Grow D, Esfandiari N. Access to fertility care in geographically underserved populations, a second look. Reprod Sci. 2022;29(7):1983–7.
58. Harper JC, Hammarberg K, Simopoulou M, Koert E, Pedro J, Massin N, Fincham A, Balen A. The International Fertility Education Initiative: research and action to improve fertility awareness. Human Reprod Open. 2021;2021(4):hoab031.

Chapter 8
Cultural and Clinical Considerations in Assisted Reproductive Therapy in Asia

Wanxuan Wang and Tat Xin Ee

Case Study

Catherine Smith is a 33-year-old American business manager working at a fintech start-up company. She was recruited and hired on lucrative terms to head a team in Singapore. Catherine has been in Singapore for a year and has done very well for the company. She is currently without a partner and has not yet met a person with whom she would consider having children. However, it is also Catherine's dream to have a child of her own in her early thirties before she reaches advanced maternal age. She is well informed and worries about pregnancy in advanced maternal age giving rise to problems such as increasing risks of birth and genetic defects and pregnancy issues such as miscarriage, pre-eclampsia and gestational diabetes.

Prior to leaving her home country, she was scheduled to undergo fertility treatment with donor sperm to achieve her dream of becoming a parent. However, due to the move to Singapore, that plan was put on hold. When she had finally settled into her new job and a new country of residence, Catherine went to a reputable fertility clinic in Singapore, hoping to restart the process of going through fertility treatment with donor sperm. However, to her horror, she was informed by the fertility specialist that she was not allowed to undergo assisted reproductive treatment as she was not married. She was also told that she was not eligible for the sperm donation programme due to the social and non-medical indication of her request. Whilst Catherine was shocked and disappointed with the situation, she did some research on her own and

W. Wang · T. X. Ee (✉)
Department of Reproductive Medicine, KK Women's and Children's Hospital, Singapore, Singapore
e-mail: wang.wanxuan@singhealth.com.sg; ee.tat.xin@singhealth.com.sg

D. A. Kaplan (ed.), *Cultural Responsiveness in Assisted Reproductive Technology*, https://doi.org/10.1007/978-3-031-76204-8_8

understood the intentions of the Singaporean government's strict regulatory framework on fertility treatment.

Catherine will be exploring her options for her quest for a child in the neighbouring countries in Southeast Asia, after understanding the clinical and cultural considerations in each country.

Introduction

Assisted reproductive therapy (ART) has become increasingly prevalent worldwide, including in Asia. As Asia catches up with the rest of the world industrially and economically, many Asian countries are faced with a concomitant decline in birth rates. The total fertility rate in Singapore declined from 1.04 to 0.97 between 2022 and 2023 alone [1]. A similar trend showed fertility rates of 0.87 in Taiwan for 2022 and 0.72 for South Korea in 2023 [2, 3]. Across the world, the practice of ART is shaped by differing geographical, demographical, political, economic and social influences. Understanding the cultural and clinical factors that influence ART practices in this diverse region is essential for providing effective and ethical care to patients. In this chapter, we explore the cultural influences, ethical and regulatory considerations and clinical practices that shape ART in an ethnically heterogenous Asian country like Singapore.

Singapore in Perspective

Singapore is a small island country located at the southern tip of the Malay Peninsula in Southeast Asia, with a total land area of approximately 720 square kilometers. Despite its small size, Singapore has a population of around 5.92 million people, making it one of the most densely populated countries in the world [4]. The main industry driving Singapore's economy is manufacturing, particularly in the electronics and biomedical sectors, which accounts for about 20% of the country's GDP. Singapore is also a major financial hub, with a thriving services sector [5]. One of the defining characteristics of Singapore is its heterogeneous population, comprising people of different ethnicities, including Chinese, Malays, Indians and Eurasians. This diversity is reflected in the country's four official languages: English, Malay, Mandarin Chinese and Tamil [4]. Despite its economic success, Singapore faces challenges such as falling birth rates, with a total fertility rate of 0.97 children per woman in 2023, which is one of the lowest in the world [1]. This has led to the Singaporean Government implementing various measures to boost the birth rate, an initiative that has influenced both financial and clinical aspects of ART practice in Singapore over the last few years.

Cultural Beliefs and Stigma

Asian cultures often place a strong emphasis on family and fertility, leading to significant stigma surrounding infertility and the use of ART [6]. For example, in some societies, infertility may be viewed as a personal failure, leading to social ostracism and marital discord [7]. Older Singaporean residents, regardless of ethnicity, are used to couples marrying young and having bigger families [8]. However, Singapore faces the same situation as the rest of the world; rising inflation and increasing competition for employment are key factors in young people's choice to delay marriage and family building across all ethnic groups. In 2021 and 2022, about 21% of all first births in Singapore and Japan were to women ages 35 and older; the percentages of first births to older mothers in South Korea, Hong Kong and Taiwan were even higher [9]. This will naturally have an effect on how ART is conducted, as treatment is increasingly conducted with a population for whom fertility concerns related to aging will need to be considered.

Religious Perspectives

Case Study
Mary Lee, a 39-year-old devout Singaporean Catholic woman who works as a teacher, has been trying to conceive with her husband for the past 3 years. She has been diagnosed with polycystic ovarian syndrome (PCOS) and tried one year of ovulation induction before going on to six failed cycles of IUI. She has been advised to give IVF a go by her fertility specialist, but she is reluctant due to the likelihood of creating more embryos than needed in view of her high ovarian reserves. This possibility makes Mary concerned about the dilemma of needing to dispose of supernumerary embryos when her family is complete. Her husband, who is also a Catholic but has differing views and interpretations of the religious laws, is very keen to start IVF. He worries about their advancing ages and the likely diminishing returns of continuing to attempt to conceive via IUI. The couple has had many disagreements about how to proceed and has not been able to come to an agreement on this issue. Mary is currently thinking of starting her 7th IUI cycle.

Religious beliefs play a significant role in shaping attitudes towards infertility and ART in Asia [10]. As Singapore is a multi-ethnic, multicultural melting pot of a cosmopolitan city, there are many religious considerations of which ART practitioners must take note. For instance, Muslim patients may find different ART procedures to be more or less permissible [11–14], depending on their practice and interpretation of Islamic laws in Singapore. Most Muslim patients are able to undergo ART with their own gametes but some draw the line at the use of donor gametes as it contravenes their religious beliefs, even if they have little to no chance of conceiving with their own gametes [12–14]. Catholics in Singapore, on the other hand, generally adhere to stringent teachings that do not support the use of most assisted reproductive therapy to conceive. Catholics believe in the beginning of life after fertilization such that the zygote, pre-embryo, embryo and foetus are viewed as persons. The prospect of needing to dispose of unused embryos therefore becomes a problem [15]. Many Catholic patients in Singapore may choose to undergo repeated IUIs even with a low chance of success rather than embarking on a single cycle of IVF due to the boundaries of what is acceptable in their religious framework.

Social Norms and Gender Roles

Case Study

Sam Wong and Nora Binte Roslan are a Singaporean couple who got married last year when Sam legally changed his gender from female to male. They went to a public hospital IVF centre to enquire about going through IVF with donor sperm. The couple was evaluated clinically and psychologically and underwent a thorough counselling process with a trained psychologist to understand the implications of donor conception for themselves and their future children. After they had adequate time to discuss and consider, they decided to proceed with IVF with donor sperm to achieve their dream of having a child. They were then directed to a certified sperm bank to obtain a suitable donor sperm specimen and started the IVF process.

Gender preferences and traditional gender roles can influence decisions regarding infertility treatment in Asia [16]. Especially in some cultures, there may be a preference for male children, leading to pressure on women to undergo ART procedures until a male offspring is conceived [17]. In some Asian countries, there is the option to determine the sex of the embryo prior to transfer, enabling couples to use genetic testing for sex selection. In Singapore, however, embryo selection is done without regard for the sex of the embryo; when PGS is performed in Singapore, the results for the sex chromosomes are concealed. Whilst not currently prevalent, gender selection may still be on the minds of some patients in Singapore. These patients may then seek treatment elsewhere in the region where gender selection through PGS may be possible.

In Singapore, a marriage is legally recognised only when it is between a man and a woman and IVF is only able to be performed for married couples. In a partnership between two natal females, IVF with donor sperm is only possible if one partner undergoes a legal change of gender to male. This process is closely audited by the Ministry of Health and the couple must fulfill all the criteria for the use of donor gametes, including being assessed for psychosocial fitness to have a child, before they are allowed into the IVF programme. The general mindset surrounding sexual orientation and gender identity in Singapore is also more traditional, with the older generation frowning upon non-heterosexual relationships and identification as LGBTQ+ [18]. This is in contrast with Thailand, where gender roles have always been more fluid, making it a regionally recognised destination for gender confirmation surgeries. As Thailand has legalised same-sex marriage, it will likely mean that more Asian LGBTQ+ couples looking to start a family will eventually be able to achieve this via IVF and gestational surrogacy through cross-border medical travel. Surrogacy arrangements, however, are currently restricted to legally married Thai residents and Thailand is not open for commercial surrogacy arrangements for foreigners [19].

Accessibility and Affordability

Disparities in access to ART exist across Asia, with wealthier countries and urban areas generally having better access to facilities than poorer countries and rural regions [20]. The high cost of ART procedures can be prohibitive for many individuals and couples, particularly in low- and middle-income countries [21]. The birth rate of the country may also determine the affordability and accessibility of ART, with some governments motivated to provide financial support for ART as a means of increasing fertility rates. In Singapore, the cost of a single cycle of IVF ranges from 7000 to 23,000 USD and a single cycle of IUI costs 1500–2300 USD. While the costs of ART are prohibitive, there is a co-funding system for ART available in Singapore. This is a government program that provides financial support to eligible citizens. The program covers up to 75% of the costs for assisted reproductive treatments, including in vitro fertilization (IVF) and intra uterine insemination (IUI), with varying levels of co-funding based on the couple's citizenship status. MediSave, a national savings program, is also available in Singapore; the program lets individuals set aside part of their income for use in the payment of inpatient and outpatient bills, including ART treatment. Couples may use 3000–4500 USD from their MediSave accounts to pay for their cycles [22]. As private insurance plans do not provide coverage for fertility treatment in Singapore, these measures by the government greatly lower the financial barrier to entry for many couples to receive fertility treatment.

Regulatory Framework

The regulatory landscape for ART varies widely across Asian countries, with some nations having comprehensive laws governing ART practices, and others having minimal regulation [23]. In Singapore, ART is tightly regulated by the Healthcare

Services (Assisted Reproduction Service) Regulations (HCSAR) framework, which is a regulatory framework governing ART in Singapore. The HCSAR framework is administered by the Singapore Ministry of Health (MOH) and sets standards for the provision of ART, including in vitro fertilization (IVF), in Singapore. This framework is stipulated in the Healthcare Services Act 2020—Healthcare Services (Assisted Reproduction Service) Regulations 2023 [24]. The framework aims to ensure that ART is provided in a safe, ethical and responsible manner.

The HCSAR framework includes the following key elements:

1. IVF procedures (oocyte retrieval and embryo transfer) may only be performed by ART practitioners who are licensed to perform IVF and have at least 6 months of independent practical hands-on experience after obtaining their license.
2. All providers of ART service must adhere to established clinical guidelines which will be audited regularly.
3. Suitability for ART will be assessed on a case-by-case basis for each individual patient seeking such treatment and only patients who fulfill medical criteria will receive such treatment. Patients must be above 35 years old or have medical indications for the performance of ART, and they have to be legally married to a man who also consents to the procedure. For patients above the age of 45 years old, they must be assessed to be fit to carry a pregnancy and to adequately care for a child as he or she grows.
4. In the assessment of each patient's eligibility for ART, providers will disclose information on the centre's success rates, risks and costs of treatment for patients with similar characteristics.
5. Before the initiation of ART cycles, informed consent is obtained from the couple after extensive counselling regarding the process, risks, benefits and alternatives. Counselling is performed by trained doctors. This consent is captured and documented in the patient's case notes.
6. There are strict guidelines concerning embryo storage and disposal, with patients required to pay an annual fee to continue storage of embryos. This allows annual recurring assessment by the IVF centre regarding the couple's status and well-being pertaining to continued storage of their embryos [24].

The HCSAR framework serves to ensure that all patients undergoing ART in Singapore receive high-quality care and are protected from unethical practises. Although the age limit on the provision of ART services has been lifted in recognition of shifting social norms that have led to more women getting married after age 35, emphasis is still placed on assessment of these older women's medical fitness for pregnancy and ability to care for their children. The increased age limit on eligibility for treatment indicates the Singaporean government's supportive stance towards helping couples who wish to have a family do so.

The practice of elective egg freezing was also allowed in Singapore in July 2023. Prior to this, egg freezing was only allowed where medically indicated, such as before initiation of chemotherapy for cancer treatment. Women between the age of 21 and 38, regardless of marital status, are eligible for elective egg freezing in any public or private fertility centre in Singapore but must assume the associated expenses themselves. This change in policy was made after careful consideration by the Singaporean government regarding the desires of many women who wished to preserve their fertility but who were not married yet because of personal circumstances. Many women and related groups had lobbied for years for this to happen while the Singaporean government took time to deliberate the risks and benefits of such a change, even though elective egg freezing had been popularised in many other countries since the start of the last decade [25]. It can be seen from the various amendments to the legal framework governing the provision of ART services in Singapore made in the past few years that it is necessary for the services provided to move with the times in order to cater to the social circumstances and fertility needs of a changing patient population.

Counselling and Support Services

In many Asian cultures, people may experience a reluctance to seek professional psychological support for mental health issues as compared to their Western counterparts [26]. Pursuing ART is an emotionally and physically demanding endeavour, and the emotional rollercoaster that often results from both infertility and its treatment is frequently associated with higher rates of anxiety and depression [27]. Integrating counselling services within ART clinics and providing support groups can help address the emotional sequelae of infertility and help people to better navigate the stresses associated with treatment [28]. Whilst it is not mandatory to send patients for counselling, many IVF centres in Singapore include an in-house counselling service and will readily refer couples for counselling if the practitioners sense that couples are not prepared for the intensity of fertility treatment or are discordant with respect to treatment decisions. Patients who are undergoing IVF at very advanced maternal ages above 45 years are also referred for counselling to ensure that the couple understands the very poor prognosis, the physical and social impact of delayed parenthood and the inherently high-risk nature and possible complications of pregnancy at this stage. For those involved in third-party reproduction, both donors and recipients are often referred for counselling to allow them time and space to understand the gamete donation process and the implications of participating in a donor programme for all parties. There are many more patient support groups for couples with infertility now ever than before due to the emergence of social media and the diminishing stigma around infertility and fertility treatment in Asia. Patients now find themselves armed with much more knowledge and support from people who previously went through infertility treatment before embarking on their own treatment journey. Fertility counselling and support services are crucial services for couples undergoing ART. In 2021, there were 263 registered psychiatrists and 551 registered psychologists in Singapore [29]. In contrast, New York City, with a population less than twice as large as that of Singapore, had a total of 3,121 registered psychologists as of 2024 [30]. Although there is no consensus on what constitutes the optimal concentration of mental health professionals, the availability of mental health services and specialized training in infertility counselling can be further strengthened to improve the Singaporean patient's journey and experience in infertility care.

Surrogacy and Third-Party Reproduction

Case Study

Nicole Davids was a 35-year-old single Singaporean Eurasian woman with a known history of obesity and well controlled diabetes. She was unfortunately diagnosed with early-stage endometrial cancer with more than 50% myoinvasion and the grade of the cancer was reported to be aggressive. She was thus advised to undergo a hysterectomy as a definitive treatment. However, she still had hopes of having children of her own progeny with a partner in the future. Hence, she asked about her fertility preservation options should she agree to the proposed treatment plan. She was informed that she could still cryopreserve her eggs, but there would be no guarantee of a chance of using a gestational carrier in Singapore in the future, and she might have to export her eggs to other regions in which gestational surrogacy would be possible. Nicole decided to pursue egg cryopreservation and froze 20 mature oocytes, keeping the faith that when the time to utilize those eggs came, she would be able to do so legally in Singapore.

Surrogacy laws vary across Asia, with some countries prohibiting or restricting the practice and others having more permissive regulations [31]. Across the region, the legality and availability of gestational surrogacy are influenced by multiple factors. In Malaysia and Myanmar, for example, its legality depends on the religion of the parties involved. In other countries, legality hinges on whether the surrogacy arrangement is altruistic or compensated. Regulation can also exist at the level of the law, as it does in South Korea, or the individual practitioner, as is the case in Japan [31]. Ethical concerns surrounding the exploitation of gestational carriers and the commodification of children have led to ongoing debates about the ethics of surrogacy in Asia [32]. In Singapore, surrogacy is strictly prohibited by the Ministry of Health. Even for conditions such as Mullerian anomalies or cancer, patients who are unable to carry a pregnancy have no options to seek surrogacy in Singapore. There have been various groups lobbying for the lifting of restrictions on surrogacy for medical conditions; as of this writing, it remains to be seen if the Singaporean Government will change their stance on this practice.

In contrast to the prohibition on gestational surrogacy, the use of donor gametes is legal in Singapore. The use of donor sperm to conceive a pregnancy is currently an option available only to married couples; single women are not legally allowed to conceive using donor sperm. Sperm donors are required to comply with Ministry of Health guidelines for donation and undergo both medical and psychological screening. Although several public hospitals have their own sperm banks, donors can only be registered with one bank at a time. There are strict limits on the number of donations, with a maximum of three live births allowed per donor to decrease the likelihood of consanguinity. Under MOH guidelines, all sperm donors in Singapore remain deidentified, as do recipient parents [33].

In contrast, patients requiring egg donors are more typically advised to use a directed donor such as a friend or relative of the female partner. With the recent change in laws to allow for elective egg freezing, however, it is anticipated that there will be an increase in the number of unused frozen eggs that could potentially be made available for local donation. With this possibility comes the need for clear policies on the criteria for egg donation and clinic regulations that avoid conflicts of interest [34]. It is illegal for both egg and sperm donors to be paid for their donation, though they can be compensated for expenses associated with donation such as transportation costs.

Clinical Considerations in ART

The practice of ART in Singapore differs minimally from other countries. It is governed by international guidelines, clinical best practices and well-evidenced research outcomes. Depending on the fertility centre, a bespoke stimulation protocol is decided on by the fertility specialist based on the patient's parameters and conditions. The aim is to achieve a reasonable number of eggs without the complications of ovarian hyperstimulation syndrome (OHSS). Fresh and frozen transfers are performed according to patients' clinical condition or according to the physicians' preference. Blastocyst culture is the most commonly performed and single embryo transfer is highly encouraged. Physicians may choose to transfer up to 3 cleavage stage embryos or 2 blastocysts maximally as mandated by the Ministry of Health.

Preimplantation genetic testing (PGT) was first started in Singapore in 2004 starting with aneuploidy testing (PGT-A); structural and monogenic testing were subsequently introduced. Some researchers posit that many Singaporean patients may be averse to abortion based on their religious beliefs. They assert that this fact, in combination with traditional cultural stigmas associated with raising a child with aneuploidies, might make PGT-A a particularly useful option for older Singaporean patients who are willing to assume the cost of the testing [35]. However, PGT-A has been considered under an experimental framework until as recently as 2023 as policy makers continue to grapple with the controversies associated with it.

The use of other adjunctive therapies, such as immunotherapy, may also be performed depending on the fertility specialists' preferences and beliefs. However, some of these therapies need prior approval from the Health Sciences Authority (HSA) of Singapore before they can be performed for patients. Strict regulation of healthcare services has always been the hallmark of the Singaporean governance of ART as the policy makers of Singapore ensure that its people receive healthcare of the highest standards of safety and efficacy. The paradoxical consequence is that newer advancements such as PGS and the practice of elective egg freezing tend to reach our shores a few years later than other countries.

IVF Success Rates

According to statistics collated by the Singaporean government, the overall ART success rates for patients receiving care from 2017 to 2021 are 24.0%, 22.7%, 17.2% and 6.4% for patients below the age of 30, from 30 to 34, from 35 to 39 and 40 and above, respectively [36]. The success rates for public and private clinics are comparable. Despite the multiethnic nature of Singapore's population, data on success rates for specific subgroups are not generally reported, making it difficult to assess for differences in treatment outcomes by race or ethnicity [37].

Conclusion

Cultural and clinical considerations play a significant role in shaping ART practices in Asia. By understanding the cultural beliefs, clinical practices and ethical dilemmas inherent in ART, healthcare providers can deliver more culturally sensitive and ethical care to patients in the region. Singapore, with its blend of modern medical advancements and traditional Asian values, provides a wonderful microcosm of the complex and evolving landscape of reproductive healthcare and cultural attitudes towards fertility treatment in the larger Asian region.

References

1. Singstat.gov.sg. Department of Statistics Singapore Feb 2024, Births and Fertility Rates Government of Singapore. Available from: https://tablebuilder.singstat.gov.sg/table/TS/M810091.
2. National Development Council. Low Birth Rate. Government of Taiwan; 2023. Available from: https://www.ndc.gov.tw/en/Content_List.aspx?n=6F69D4E5D624660A.
3. The Chosun Daily. S. Korea's fertility rate hits another record low of 0.65, raising the concern of extinction. The Chosen Daily; 2024. The Chosun Daily. Available from: https://www.chosun.com/english/national-en/2024/02/29/57XIL6EB6VF6LNEHBUGQMZUTUI/.
4. National Population and Talent Division. Overview. www.population.gov.sg; 2022. Available from: https://www.population.gov.sg/our-population/population-trends/overview/.
5. World Bank. The World Bank in Signapore. The World Bank; 2019. Available from: https://www.worldbank.org/en/country/singapore/overview.
6. Vu MH, Nguyen AT, Alur-Gupta S. Asian Americans and infertility: genetic susceptibilities, sociocultural stigma, and access to care. F&S Rep. 2022;3(2):40–5.

7. Adamson GD. Global cultural and socioeconomic factors that influence access to assisted reproductive technologies. Women's Health. 2009;5(4):351–8. https://doi.org/10.2217/WHE.09.28.
8. Jones GW. Changing marriage patterns in Asia. In: Routledge handbook of Asian demography. Routledge; 2017. p. 351–69.
9. Chen M. Late transition to parenthood in high-income and low-fertility East Asian societies. Asian Popul Studies. 2024:1–4.
10. Serour GI, Serour AG. The Impact of religion and culture on medically assisted reproduction in the Middle East and Europe. Reprod Biomed Online. 2021;43(3):P421–33.
11. Inhorn MC. Religion and assisted reproductive technology: new pathways of engagement. J Religion Health. 2018;57(2):469–85.
12. Butt MQ, Shah MS. An overview of Islamic teachings on infertility. Jurnal Al-Adwa. 2012;48:32.
13. Nordin MM. An Islamic perspective of assisted reproductive technologies. Bangladesh J Med Sci. 2012;11(4):252.
14. Sallam HN, Sallam NH. Religious aspects of assisted reproduction. Facts Views Vision ObGyn. 2016;8(1):33.
15. Alvare HM. Catholic teaching and the law concerning the new reproductive technologies. Fordham Urb LJ. 2002;30:107.
16. Inhorn MC, Patrizio P. Infertility around the globe: new thinking on gender, reproductive technologies and global movements in the 21st century. Hum Reprod Update. 2015;21(4):411–26.
17. Dyer SJ, Abrahams N, Mokoena NE, van der Spuy ZM. 'You are a man because you have children': experiences, reproductive health knowledge and treatment-seeking behaviour among men suffering from couple infertility in South Africa. Hum Reprod. 2004;19(4):960–7.
18. Zhou M, Hu T. Social tolerance of homosexuality: a quantitative comparison of Mainland China, Singapore, and Taiwan. Chinese Soc Rev. 2020;52(1):27–55.
19. Chung E. Surrogate coverage under Thailand's health insurance on standby. Pacific Prime Thailand's Blog; 2024 [cited 2024 August 23]. Available from: https://www.pacificprime.co.th/blog/surrogate-coverage-under-health-insurance-in-thailand-on-standby.
20. Kumar D, Hessini L. Cultural and ethical issues in reproductive health: a focus on developing countries. Fertil Steril. 2009;92(4):1174–81.
21. Ombelet W, Cooke I, Dyer S, Serour G, Devroey P. Infertility and the provision of infertility medical services in developing countries. Hum Reprod Update. 2008;14(6):605–21.
22. MOH: Medisave. www.moh.gov.sg. Available from: https://www.moh.gov.sg/healthcare-schemes-subsidies/medisave.
23. Pennings G. The rough guide to insemination: cross-border travelling for donor semen due to different regulations. FVV Obgyn. 2010:55–60. (Monograph)
24. Healthcare Services (Assisted Reproduction Service) Regulations 2023—Singapore Statutes Online. Agc.gov.sg; 2023 [cited 2024 August 25]. Available from: https://sso.agc.gov.sg/SL/HSA2020-S429-2023?DocDate=20230623&WholeDoc=1.
25. Lee GJ. Reconciling moral discourses on choice, risk and pronatalism: the politics of elective egg freezing in Singapore. Cult Health Sex. 2024:1–5.
26. Javed A, Lee C, Zakaria H, Buenaventura RD, Cetkovich-Bakmas M, Duailibi K, Ng B, Ramy H, Saha G, Arifeen S, Elorza PM. Reducing the stigma of mental health disorders with a focus on low-and middle-income countries. Asian J Psychiatry. 2021;58:102601.
27. Kiani Z, Simbar M, Hajian S, Zayeri F. The prevalence of depression symptoms among infertile women: a systematic review and meta-analysis. Fertil Res Pract. 2021;7(1):6. https://doi.org/10.1186/s40738-021-00098-3.
28. Ying L, Wu LH, Loke AY. The effects of psychosocial interventions on the mental health, pregnancy rates, and marital function of infertile couples undergoing in vitro fertilization: a systematic review. J Assist Reprod Genet. 2016;33:689–701.
29. MOH, News Highlights. www.moh.gov.sg. Available from: https://www.moh.gov.sg/news-highlights/details/sufficiency-of-number-of-practising-psychiatrists-and-psychologists-

in-singapore#:~:text=There%20are%20263%20psychiatrists%20registered,9.7%20psychologists%20per%20100k%20population.
30. NYS Psychology: License Statistics. Nysed.gov 2024. Available from: https://www.op.nysed.gov/professions/psychology/license-statistics.
31. Aguiling-Pangalangan EH. Surrogacy in Asia. In: Research handbook on surrogacy and the law. Edward Elgar Publishing; 2024. p. 395–435.
32. Spar D. For love and money: the political economy of commercial surrogacy. Rev Int Polit Econ. 2005;12(2):287–309.
33. How To Be A Sperm Donor—HealthXchange. Healthxchange.sg 2019. Available from: https://www.healthxchange.sg/men/prostate-health/how-to-be-sperm-donor.
34. Chin AH. Singapore needs to update regulation of frozen egg donation after permitting social egg freezing. J Assist Reprod Genet. 2022;39(7):1497–500.
35. Chin AH, Sun N. Sociocultural imperatives for Singapore to permit preimplantation genetic testing-aneuploidy (PGT-A) despite uncertain results and ongoing controversy. J Assist Reprod Genet. 2023;40(6):1377–9.
36. Statistics of Assisted Reproductive Technology Success Rates for Public and Private Centres. Ministry of Health; 2023. Available from: https://www.moh.gov.sg/news-highlights/details/statistics-of-assisted-reproductive-technology-success-rate-for-public-and-private-centre.
37. Mee HL, Ni LS, Ling YS. Live birth rates of assisted reproductive technology treatment and spontaneous conception among subfertile couples in Singapore: a follow-up study. Asian Pacific J Reprod. 2018;7(5):206–13.

Chapter 9
Racial Disparities in Adverse Pregnancy Outcomes

Ashley L. Parker

Introduction

Bringing life into this world is a milestone and an event many people live their lives anticipating. Childbirth is one of the most miraculous and joyous occasions in life. Unfortunately, for some it may also be the most dangerous. Often, we think of maternal mortality in the context of under-resourced countries. After all, Western society has made strides in the development of medications, surgical techniques, devices, and protocols intended to save lives during and after childbirth [1–3].

Concerningly, non-Hispanic Black women in the United States are as likely to die during childbirth and in the postpartum period as are women in some developing countries [4]. Disparities exist for cardiovascular disease, hypertensive disorders of pregnancy, diabetes, infection, hemorrhage, preterm birth, and other pregnancy related morbidity. Racial and ethnic minority women develop these conditions at earlier ages, are less likely to have their conditions adequately managed, and are more likely to have complications and mortality from these conditions, with non-Hispanic Black women representing the population most impacted [5]. This burden is not only carried by non-Hispanic Black women experiencing poverty. Even Serena Williams, one of the greatest tennis players of all time, and Allyson Felix, a 6-time Olympic track gold medalist, came near death with the birth of their children [6]. Being elite athletes with financial security did not protect them from preventable complications of pregnancy. When controlling for education and socioeconomic status [7], non-Hispanic Black women are still 3–5 times more likely to die in childbirth. The disparities in outcomes exist for other racial minorities as well. Native Americans/Native Alaskans, Asians/Pacific Islanders, and some subgroups

A. L. Parker (✉)
Massachusetts General Hospital, Boston, MA, USA
e-mail: aparker18@mgh.harvard.edu

D. A. Kaplan (ed.), *Cultural Responsiveness in Assisted Reproductive Technology*, https://doi.org/10.1007/978-3-031-76204-8_9

of Hispanic women experience complications related to pregnancy at variably higher rates compared to their non-Hispanic White counterparts [8–10].

In recent years, there has been a focus on racial disparities in obstetric outcomes in the United States. Approximately half of the severe maternal morbidity events and mortalities are preventable, which means there are identifiable targets for improvement in how care is executed [11, 12]. Research has been done to look at the multifactorial nature of the disparities in patient outcomes, including economics, psychosocial variables, and education. Racial bias, framed by systemic racism in the United States, is the factor that remains the same across educational and socioeconomic subgroups. Racism is deeply ingrained in the history and training of Obstetrics and Gynecology. The American Congress of Obstetrics and Gynecology (ACOG), the governing body for practicing OBGYNs in the United States, agrees that racism is an issue that needs to be addressed directly, recently stating that they are "committed to eliminating racism and racial inequities that lead to disparate health outcomes through deep reflection, listening, accountability, collaboration, and direct action" [13].

The research on racial disparities has used various terms for racial groups. For the purposes of this chapter, women from the African Diaspora will be referred to as non-Hispanic Black. People of European ancestry will be referred to as non-Hispanic White.

Disparities in Maternal Health Outcomes in the United States

The disparity in maternal deaths in the United States has grown in the last century with non-Hispanic Black women representing the demographic with a persistent surplus of maternal death [4]. According to the CDC, a total of 6765 pregnancy-related deaths occurred in the United States between 2007 and 2016. The pregnancy-related mortality ratios were highest among non-Hispanic Black (40.8) and non-Hispanic American Indian/Alaska Native (29.7) women. These rates were 3.2 and 2.3 times the pregnancy-related mortality ratios for non-Hispanic White women (12.7) [14]. A study by Berg et al. showed that between the years 1991 and 1997 Black women had a greater risk of pregnancy-related death regardless of age, live-birth order, marital status, or trimester of onset of prenatal care [7] (Fig. 9.1).

Cesarean Delivery

Cesarean section rates have been used as a quality indicator for hospitals because of the associated morbidity. Cesarean deliveries are associated with risk of surgical complications, increased obstetrical related costs, greater likelihood of delivery by cesarean in subsequent births, and risk of abnormal placentation and hysterectomy

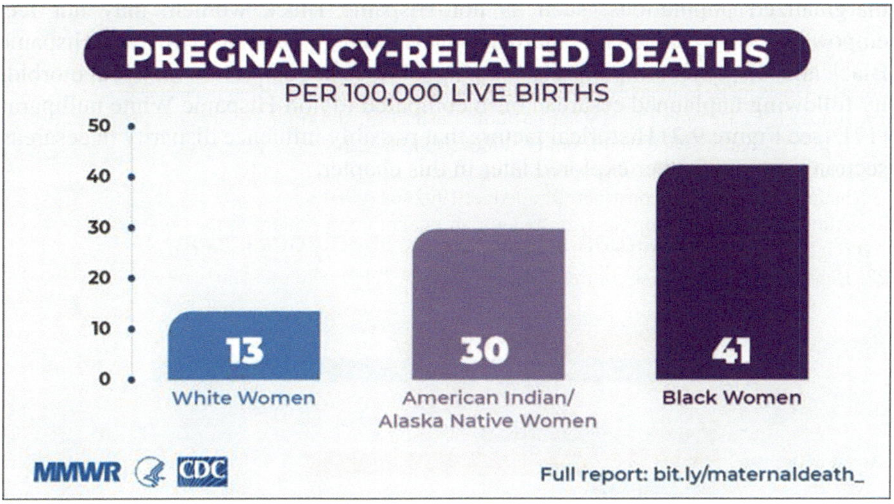

Fig. 9.1 U.S. overall PRMR was 16.7 pregnancy-related deaths per 100,000 births. Non-Hispanic Black (Black) and non-Hispanic American Indian/Alaska Native women experienced higher PRMRs than did all other racial/ethnic groups. Source: Petersen et al.

[15]. Studies have shown differences in primary cesarean section rates for racial minorities compared to non-Hispanic White women, with non-Hispanic Black women having the highest rates of cesarean. Non-Hispanic Black women were most likely to have cesarean section for fetal intolerance to labor and Asian and Hispanic women were more likely to be diagnosed with failure to progress. These disparities in cesarean delivery rates were not accounted for by facility, maternal, or neonatal factors [16]. A recent retrospective cohort study supported those findings. The study evaluated associations between maternal race/ethnicity and unplanned cesarean birth among nulliparous pregnant people. It found that rates of unplanned cesarean birth were significantly higher among non-Hispanic Black (24.1%) and Hispanic (24.7%) birthing patients compared to non-Hispanic White participants (17.4%) [17]. After adjusting for maternal age, BMI, gestational age at birth, development of hypertensive complications during pregnancy, and mode of labor onset, non-Hispanic White participants had 0.57 lower odds of unplanned cesarean birth compared to non-Hispanic Black participants. The odds were similar between Hispanic and Non-Hispanic Black participants with the primary indication for cesarean birth compared to non-Hispanic White people being non-reassuring fetal heart rate in the setting of spontaneous labor onset [17]. This reproduced a similar pattern noted in a 2012 study [18]. Potential causes for this outcome have been theorized as differences in fetal tolerance in labor based on maternal and fetal factors (stress, small for gestational age) versus differences in how fetal resuscitation is rendered to non-Hispanic Black, non-Hispanic White, and Hispanic women [16, 17]. Fear influencing the shared decision-making process for non-Hispanic Black women could also contribute to the disparity in primary cesarean section [16, 17]. Members of

marginalized populations, such as non-Hispanic Black women, may not feel empowered to advocate for alternatives to cesarean section [18]. Non-Hispanic Black and Hispanic nulliparas also had higher rates of postpartum maternal morbidity following unplanned cesarean birth compared to non-Hispanic White nulliparas [17]. (see Figure 9.2) Historical factors that possibly influence disparity in cesarean section rates are further explored later in this chapter.

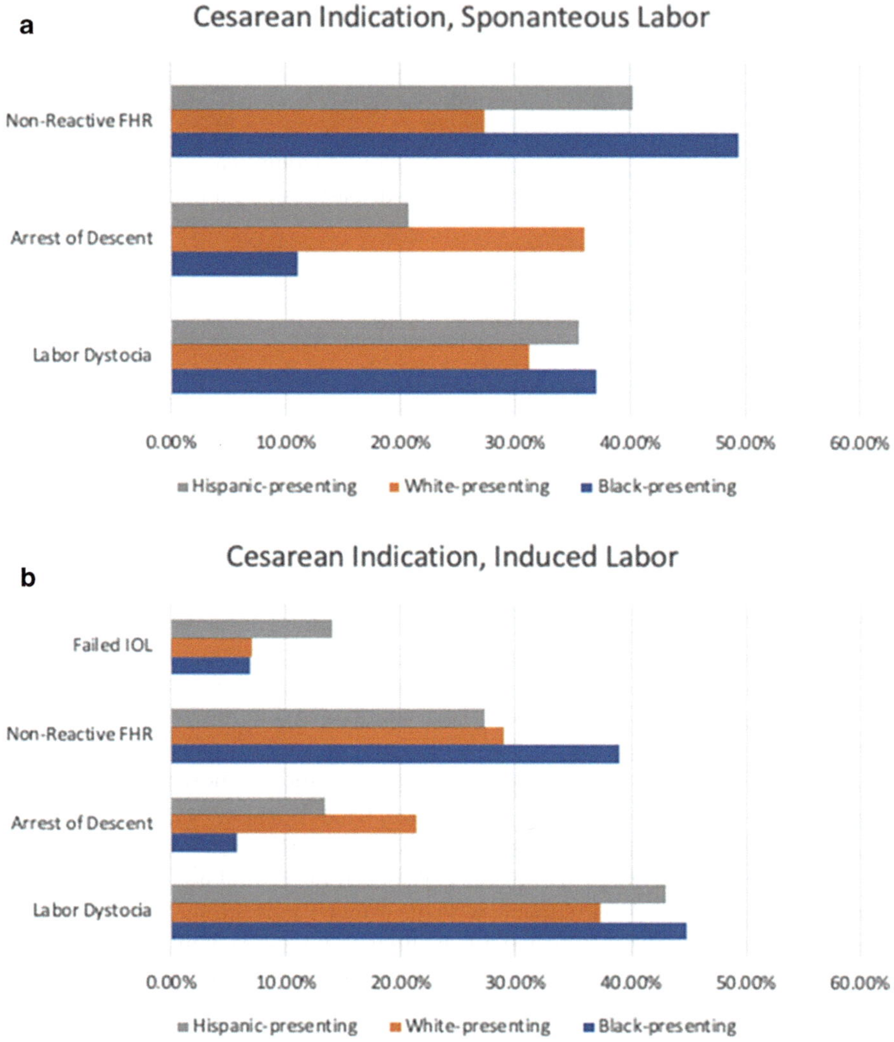

Fig. 9.2 Primary indication for unplanned cesarean birth by presenting race/ethnicity and mode of labor onset (n = 1001). Abbreviations: FHR, fetal heart rate; IOL, induction of labor. Panel (**a**) Primary indication of unplanned cesarean in laboring people with spontaneous labor onset ($p < 0.05$ difference between presenting race/ethnicity groups in non-reassuring FHR and arrest of descent), and (**b**) Induced labor onset ($p < 0.05$ difference between presenting race/ethnicity groups in arrest of descent. Source: Carslon et al. [17]

Hypertensive Disorders of Pregnancy

Hypertensive disorders of pregnancy are the leading cause of pregnancy-related death in the United States. These include chronic hypertension, gestational hypertension, preeclampsia, and eclampsia [19]. Non-Hispanic Black women experience more mortality from hypertensive disease than non-Hispanic White women. Hispanic women also have increased mortality related to hypertensive diseases of pregnancy with up to a three times higher risk of death compared to non-Hispanic White women [20].

A population-based study by Leonard et al. demonstrated that people with chronic hypertension were more likely to be non-Hispanic Black and age 35 years or older [21]. Comorbidities such as obesity, chronic renal disease, preexisting diabetes, preexisting cardiac disease, and thyroid disorder were notably higher in people with chronic hypertension than in those without chronic hypertension [21]. The highest rates of chronic hypertension were 5.1% in non-Hispanic Black people, 2.9% in Native Hawaiian or Other Pacific Islander people, and 2.5% in American Indian or Alaska Native people. Chronic hypertension was associated with increased risk of preeclampsia with severe features or eclampsia, acute renal failure, and pulmonary edema [21]. Additional studies have also shown an associated elevated risk of stillbirth, small for gestational age, gestational diabetes, iatrogenic preterm birth, and elective cesarean section associated with chronic hypertension [22]. Comparison among ethnic groups showed evidence that chronic hypertension contributes to more severe obstetric morbidity and acute renal failure among non-Hispanic Black and Native Hawaiian or Other Pacific Islander people than among other racial–ethnic groups while risk for cerebrovascular accident and pulmonary edema was highest in Non-Hispanic Black people [21].

Preeclampsia, separate from chronic hypertension, is also associated with increased pregnancy morbidity. Severely elevated systolic blood pressures have been associated with hemorrhagic strokes and a retrospective cohort study demonstrated that non-Hispanic Black women are at higher risk for stroke compared to women of any other racial or ethnic group [23, 24]. The same was shown for eclampsia and in-hospital death. Resemblant to studies of chronic hypertension, non-Hispanic Black women were at highest risk for pulmonary edema, acute heart failure, and renal failure compared to non-Hispanic White women and all other racial and ethnic groups [23]. Mortality related to preeclampsia is preventable with the development of antihypertensive medication administration, magnesium seizure prophylaxis, and aspirin prophylaxis [23]. It is unclear if these measures are implemented in a disparate manner, but potential causes for the disparities in mortality due to preeclampsia are evaluated later in the chapter.

Cardiovascular Complications

In addition to cerebrovascular accidents, other cardiovascular complications in pregnancy include cardiomyopathy and venous thromboembolism. Cerebrovascular accidents, or stroke, were previously discussed as a consequence of hypertensive disease. Hypertensive disease also increases risk of cardiomyopathy [25]. Non-Hispanic Black women experience higher mortality related to cardiomyopathy [10]. There are multiple factors that influence cardiometabolic risk postpartum, including race/ethnicity, poverty status, and prenatal cardiometabolic diseases. Studies show that non-Hispanic Black women who experienced pregnancy complications often have the greatest postpartum cardio-metabolic risk compared to non-Hispanic White and Hispanic women even when earning higher income [26]. This finding is duplicated in other studies including a nationwide retrospective study that found acute myocardial infarction, pulmonary embolism, and cardiovascular related mortality were substantially higher for non-Hispanic Black women compared to non-Hispanic White women [27]. Socioeconomic differences contributed to racial disparities, but the disparities persisted after adjustment for socioeconomic factors, with worse pregnancy-related cardiovascular events among high socioeconomic status non-Hispanic Black women when compared with low socioeconomic status non-Hispanic White women [27]. Risk factors that were more common for non-Hispanic Black women included prior history of cardiovascular disease, obesity, depression, smoking, and poor dietary habits. Hispanic women also have a persistent pattern of poor cardiovascular outcomes compared to non-Hispanic White women. Risk factors for this population include Type 2 diabetes, obesity, and food insecurity with resultant imbalanced diet [27].

As previously mentioned, peripartum cardiomyopathy is a major cause of postpartum mortality. Historical data show a sixfold increased risk of death for non-Hispanic Black women compared to non-Hispanic White women [28]. A recent retrospective cohort study found that though the ejection fraction at time of diagnosis of peripartum cardiomyopathy was not significantly different between non-Hispanic Black and non-Hispanic White women, non-Hispanic Black women had more severe persistent left ventricular systolic dysfunction [29]. This led to worse outcomes including the need for ICD placement and increased resource utilization. The persistent ventricular systolic dysfunction also resulted in poorer cardiac function entering a subsequent pregnancy which leads to poorer outcomes in subsequent pregnancies [29].

Preterm Birth and Small for Gestational Age

Preterm birth is known to be associated with neonatal morbidity, but it is also associated with increased maternal morbidity such as stroke and cardiovascular disease [30]. The United States has made efforts to reduce the preterm birth rate through

March of Dimes [31], but the rates of preterm birth have continued to be elevated for non-Hispanic Black women in the United States [32] (see Fig. 9.3). In a review of 30 studies, non-Hispanic Black women were found to have twice the risk of preterm birth compared to non-Hispanic White women. The same study found Hispanic and Asian ethnicity had a less consistent association with preterm birth rates [33]. The disparity remains in the most recent CDC data from 2023, which suggests a 1.5 times higher preterm birth rate for non-Hispanic Black women compared to non-Hispanic White women [34]. (see Figure 9.4) Risk is not only higher for non-Hispanic Black women to have an isolated preterm birth but recurrent preterm birth as well as preterm premature rupture of membranes [35, 36]. Compared to other causal factors, cervical insufficiency and chronic maternal stress are significantly higher among non-Hispanic Black women compared to non-Hispanic White women [37]. When considering neonatal outcomes, there is a similar pattern of disparity for ethnic/racial minorities. Spontaneous previable preterm birth rates are higher for non-Hispanic Black women and neonatal death rates are higher for non-Hispanic Black infants [38]. These outcomes are partially influenced by sociodemographic differences, such as neighborhood deprivation, but the effects are most significant for non-Hispanic Black mothers [39].

Much like maternal mortality, the disparity in preterm birth is not fully accounted for by differences in education level [40]. Psychosocial stress, smoking, and illicit drug use are risk factors traditionally associated with an elevated risk for preterm birth. In a study by Goldenberg, these risk factors were more common among non-Hispanic White women compared to non-Hispanic Black women, but 16.7% of

Table 18. Selected medical and health characteristics of births, by race of mother: United States, 2015

Characteristic	All races	White	Black	American Indian or Alaska Native	Asian or Pacific Islander
Mother			Percent		
Diabetes during pregancy	6.5	6.2	5.8	9.9	11.1
Weight gain of less than 11 lbs.	9.1	8.3	13.1	13.1	7.1
Weight gain of more than 40 lbs.	21.0	21.6	21.4	22.2	14.3
Induction of labor	23.8	24.5	22.9	24.2	18.5
CNM delivery[1]	8.5	8.7	7.4	17.8	7.2
Cesarean delivery	32.0	31.3	35.3	28.3	33.0
Infant					
Gestational age:					
Preterm[2]	9.6	9.0	13.2	10.5	8.6
Early preterm[3]	2.8	2.4	4.7	2.8	2.2
Late preterm[4]	6.9	6.6	8.4	7.7	6.4
Birthweight[5]:					
Very low birthweight[6]	1.4	1.1	2.8	1.3	1.1
Low birthweight[7]	8.1	7.0	13.0	7.5	8.4
4,000 grams or more	8.0	9.0	4.6	10.1	4.8
Twin birth[8]	33.5	32.8	38.7	25.1	29.9
Triplet or higher-order birth[9]	103.6	107.1	101.7	38.4	81.4

[1]Births delivered by certified nurse midwives (CNMs).
[2]Born before 37 completed weeks of gestation based on the obstetric estimate; see Technical Notes.
[3]Born before 34 completed weeks of gestation based on the obstetric estimate; see Technical Notes.
[4]Born between 34 and 36 completed weeks of gestation based on the obstetric estimate; see Technical Notes.
[5]Equivalents of gram weights in pounds are shown in Technical Notes.
[6]Less than 1,500 grams.
[7]Less than 2,500 grams.
[8]Live births in twin deliveries per 1,000 live births.
[9]Live births in triplet and other higher-order multiple deliveries per 100,000 live births.

NOTES: Race and Hispanic origin are reported separately on birth certificates. Race categories are consistent with 1977 Office of Management and Budget standards. Forty-nine states and the District of Columbia reported multiple-race data for 2015 that were bridged to single-race categories for comparability with other states; see Technical Notes. In this table, all women, including Hispanic women, are classified only according to their race; see Technical Notes.

Fig. 9.3 Proportion of preterm births, stratified by gestational age at delivery and maternal race, 2015. Sources: Martin et al. Final birth data 2015 [32]

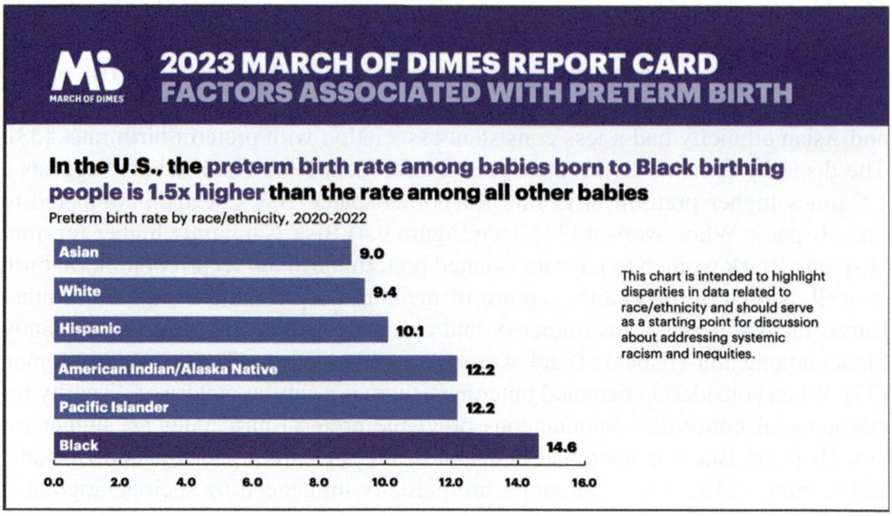

Fig. 9.4 Preterm birth rate by race/ethnicity, 2020–2022. Source: [44]

non-Hispanic Black women delivered preterm compared to 11.3% of non-Hispanic White women [41]. Short interval pregnancy, as defined by <6 months between delivery of one pregnancy and the conception of the next, is also a known risk factor for preterm birth [42]. Historically, demographic data suggest that short interval pregnancy is more common among non- Hispanic Black women compared to non-Hispanic White women. This was supported by a study conducted in California which showed non-Hispanic Black women had higher prevalence of short interval pregnancy at 7.6%, compared to 4.4% for non-Hispanic White women. The same study concluded that short interval pregnancy alone does not account for the magnitude of the disparity between non-Hispanic Black and non-Hispanic White women for preterm births [43]. Other studies suggest differences in epigenetics, microbiome, and inflammatory biomarkers as potential cause for the differences in preterm birth rates between non-Hispanic White women and non-Hispanic Black women, but the phenomenon is likely due to a complex interplay among all the above [40].

Hemorrhage

Postpartum hemorrhage (PPH) is the number one cause of maternal deaths in the developing world and is considered preventable [45]. Causes of postpartum hemorrhage include uterine atony, genital tract lacerations, retained placenta or products of conception, uterine inversion, abnormal placentation, inherited or acquired disorders of coagulation, and infection [46]. A meta-analysis performed by Okunlola et al. found that non-Hispanic White women had the lowest risk of PPH while non-Hispanic Black women had higher risk of PPH [47]. Some of this difference was attributed to higher prevalence of anemia, fibroids, and preeclampsia. As mentioned previously, the non-Hispanic Black women in a separate study were noted to have higher rates of cesarean delivery, which increases risk of blood loss [48]. Per Tucker et al., placental abruption and placenta previa were 2.4–3.3 times higher in non-Hispanic Black women than non-Hispanic White women [49]. Hemorrhage in non-Hispanic Black women was less likely related to atony, but more likely to require transfusion or hysterectomy [47]. Recent research showed that non-Hispanic White women undergoing peripartum hysterectomy were more likely to have an elective/anticipated peripartum hysterectomy than non-Hispanic Black women, while the non-Hispanic Black women were more likely to have an unscheduled or emergent hysterectomy and require reoperation after peripartum hysterectomy [50]. Suggested reasons for the disparity in indication for peripartum hysterectomy included disparate management of atony/postpartum hemorrhage versus inequitable referral patterns for suspected abnormal placentation by race/ethnicity [50].

It was also found that Hispanic, Asian, Native American, and Pacific Islanders had an increased risk of atonic PPH compared to non-Hispanic White women [47]. These findings were supported in studies that found that *quantitative* blood loss was higher in deliveries of non-Hispanic Black women and Hispanic women compared to non-Hispanic White women [48]. These same women were not noted to have significant differences in *estimated* blood loss, which suggested bias in reporting [48]. Consistent use of quantitative blood loss versus estimated blood loss also could be a target for eliminating bias and improving outcomes.

Diabetes

Gestational diabetes has health consequences in pregnancy and after delivery with increased lifetime cardiovascular risk and a ten-fold increased risk of developing type 2 diabetes in one's lifetime [51]. Compared to non-Hispanic White women, the risk of development of type 2 diabetes is fourfold for non-Hispanic Black women and threefold for Hispanic and South and Southeast Asian women [52]. These findings are consistent with earlier studies where Hispanic women had higher rates of diabetes than non-Hispanic White women [9]. Education level, insurance status, and WIC participation had less influence on later development of type 2 diabetes in non-Hispanic Black, Hispanic, and South and Southeast Asian individuals than in non-Hispanic White individuals, suggesting that other factors may influence the disparity [52]. The same was found in a separate study in addition to persistent racial/ethnic differences in risk for diagnosed type 2 diabetes after adjustment for age and BMI [53]. In addition to increased risk of type 2 diabetes, gestational diabetes-related adverse outcomes including preeclampsia, preterm delivery and neonatal hypoglycemia are highest among non-Hispanic Black women [54]. Other studies have also found lower birth weight and higher rates of Apgar scores under 7 for the neonates born to non-Hispanic Black women [55].

It has been hypothesized that "weathering" and chronic high levels of stress can contribute to accelerated aging and cardiometabolic and glucose dysregulation. The concept of "weathering" was originally hypothesized by Arline Geronimus and proposes that "the health of African-American women may begin to deteriorate in early adulthood as a physical consequence of cumulative socioeconomic disadvantage" [56]. Weathering can be credited to the cumulative effects of structural racism, discrimination, and psychological distress [57]. Differences in management of elevated glucose and diagnosis of type 2 diabetes after pregnancy may also play a role in the disparities in outcomes. A retrospective cohort study demonstrated that non-Hispanic White women with gestational diabetes received pharmacotherapy at a lower percent of abnormal blood glucose values than women of other races and ethnicities and non-Hispanic Black women had the highest percentage of abnormal values before initiation of treatment [55]. A separate study showed non-Hispanic Black and Hispanic women had significantly higher mean HbA1c levels after pregnancy, regardless of current diagnosed diabetes status, which suggests delay in diagnosis. Though they were screened more frequently and met criteria more often, non-Hispanic Black women were less likely to be formally diagnosed and henceforth less likely to receive treatment, resulting in more advanced stage disease [53]. Though the burden of disease is higher for Hispanic women than non-Hispanic White women, they were less likely to be screened for type 2 diabetes in the years after delivery. Some possible reasons included insurance status and access to care [53].

Pain Management

Despite a complete absence of factual evidence to support this claim, a longstanding belief dating back to the enslavement of African women is that women of African descent feel less pain. This belief was further perpetuated by Caldwell and Moloy's now-disputed 1933 categorization of pelvic typology into four distinct groups and the theory that Black women experienced easier childbirth with less pain than White women because of a more spacious pelvis that was more similar to that of apes [58]. Research demonstrates the common perception that non-Hispanic White women are thought to have significantly more labor pain than women of color [59]. Differential treatment of pain, however, is not solely because of perceived differences in experience of pain. A retrospective cohort study showed that during postpartum hospitalization non-Hispanic White women were less likely to report a higher pain score at discharge than both Hispanic and non-Hispanic Black women but received significantly greater morphine milligram equivalents per day as inpatients than Hispanic and non-Hispanic Black women [60]. Opiate pain prescriptions were also more likely to be provided to non-Hispanic White women at discharge compared to Hispanic and non-Hispanic Black women [60]. This finding was replicated in other studies including a meta-analysis in an anesthesia journal which showed that

Hispanic and non-Hispanic Black patients are more likely to undergo general anesthesia for cesarean deliveries, receive fewer postpartum pain assessments, and are less likely to receive postpartum opioid analgesia or opioid prescription at the time of discharge compared to non-Hispanic White women [61]. Similar discrepancies were found in a study by Thomas et al. where they found that non-Hispanic Black patients were twice as likely to receive general anesthesia for intrapartum cesarean section, and non-Hispanic White patients were more likely to receive neuraxial analgesia than non-Hispanic Black and Hispanic patients [62]. Use of general anesthesia in this study was associated with higher rates of composite severe maternal morbidity, intensive care unit admissions, fetal demise, and blood transfusions [62]. This suggests a disregard for the labor pain of women of color [59]. A contrasting belief that is equally detrimental is the idea that non-Hispanic Black women have superhuman qualities and resiliency that makes them more capable of coping with pain [63]. The belief that there is value in women's experiencing labor pain and that pain should not be treated is commonly held by those who also believe that women who are not non-Hispanic White experience less pain, and this also influences disparities in management of pain [59].

Perinatal Mood Disorders

Postpartum depression is increasing in prevalence and suicide because of perinatal mood disorders is one of the leading causes of death for women peri- and postpartum in the United States [64]. A retrospective cohort study showed that women most likely to have a positive depression screen or a diagnosis of depression were young, single, covered by public insurance, and multiracial or non-Hispanic Native American. It also demonstrated than non-Hispanic Black women with a positive depression screen during pregnancy were about half as likely to receive a formal diagnosis of depression as non-Hispanic White women, a finding with significant implications for timely referral to psychiatric care and subsequent treatment outcomes [65]. One longitudinal retrospective study in Baltimore found that a diagnosis of postpartum depression was made for non-Hispanic White women more than any other race, which was contrary to previous studies [66]. Proposed causes include stigma and lack of reporting or sampling bias based on access to care among racial and ethnic minority women [66]. They also found that non-Hispanic Black patients and Asian and Pacific Islander patients were more likely to be diagnosed with postpartum depression >8 weeks post-delivery [66]. It is unclear if this is the result of delay in diagnosis or later patient presentation to care. Similar results were found in another study that evaluated barriers to care. In this study, women from racial/ethnic minority backgrounds faced more challenges posed by lack of social support, trauma history, and difficulty getting time off work for treatment. Family disapproval, stigma, and clinician mistrust were barriers to care across ethnicities [67].

Impact of COVID-19

The COVID-19 pandemic disproportionately affected racial and ethnic minorities with non-Hispanic Black and Hispanic pregnant women being twice as likely to be infected with and/or die from COVID-19 as non-Hispanic White pregnant women [68]. There are also state and national data that suggest that people of racial and ethnic minorities experience more severe COVID-19-associated illness, are more likely to require hospitalization, and have higher risk for death from COVID-19 [69]. Hispanic/Latino followed by non-Hispanic Black, American Indian/Alaska Native, Asian, and Native Hawaiian/other Pacific Islander people were more likely to live in areas with the highest disease burden [69]. In a Boston hospital during the early pandemic, Hispanic women accounted for more than 60% of all pregnant women hospitalized for COVID-19 infection despite only accounting for 18% of the population [70]. In contrast with other populations, the rate of infections among Hispanic pregnant women continued to rise despite statewide distancing guidelines. This difference was possibly influenced by families living in multigenerational or multifamily homes, being employed in essential or low-wage jobs without insurance or paid time off, language barriers, and fear of deportation if presenting to medical care [70]. Additional influences may have been underlying medical conditions and higher levels of exposure to pollution and environmental hazards [69].

Possible Contributing Factors to Differences in Outcomes

Why is there a difference in these outcomes? Some proposed causal factors have been considered at the level of the system, patient, and provider [4]. In addition to these factors is the idea that race-based care, rather than race-conscious care, can be harmful and contributes more to disparities in outcomes [71]. The use of racialized medicine in clinical predictive models perpetuates a biological construct of race that is based in colonialism and eugenics [71]. This obscures the true causes of health disparities, such as structural racism as a chronic stressor [72]. Identifying these causal factors hopefully provide targets for improving outcomes for racial minority women.

System Factors

Historical Background

Though there are disparities in the prevalence of many of the medical complications of pregnancy, research in the management of those disease processes does not include representative samples of racial and ethnic minorities. The number of studies that include racial minorities has not improved much in over 30 years [73]. Some portion of this lack of representation in research is likely the result of the distrust of minorities in the ethics of research. As discussed in greater detail elsewhere in this volume, this distrust exists within the context of the Tuskegee experiment, in which impoverished Black men were purposely infected with syphilis and left untreated under the guise of receiving free health care from the United States government [74], and the work of J. Marion Sims, who performed unanesthetized gynecologic procedures on enslaved Black women without their consent [75]. Additional unethical practices were used in the case of Henrietta Lacks, whose cells were cultured to form the HeLa cell line, the first immortalized cell line. The handling of Lacks' genetic material raises issues regarding consent and privacy. Her cells were acquired from a tumor biopsied during treatment for cervical cancer at Johns Hopkins Hospital in 1951 without her consent. Her family was never compensated for their extraction or use, and the family's medical records were published without family consent [76]. Mistrust in the research process and in the adherence of researchers to ethical guidelines leads to limited sample sizes of minority populations in research. This, in turn, creates a paucity of reliable data to guide management of these disease processes in minority women.

We have discussed the disparities in rates of primary and repeat cesarean sections in the United States. These differences are likely partially due to the tools used by physicians to make these decisions; some of which are rooted in racism [18, 77]. For example, clinical pelvimetry and concern for risk of cephalopelvic disproportion have been used to counsel non-Hispanic Black women toward primary cesarean section [58]. The previously mentioned pelvic typology was used to support the theory that labor was easier for Black women and that duration of labor should be shorter, which influenced later suggestion of alternate labor curves and increased likelihood for surgical intervention during childbirth [58].

The use of race in our evaluation of risk in obstetric care has also influenced counseling for trial of labor after cesarean section. The vaginal birth after cesarean section (VBAC) calculator designed by The Maternal Fetal Medine Units Network provides individualized estimate of the probability for a VBAC using six factors including age, body mass index (BMI), race, and ethnicity [77, 78]. The original calculation estimated the probability of a successful vaginal birth after cesarean section as 5 to 15 percent lower for non-Hispanic Black and Hispanic patients compared to non-Hispanic White patients with identical risk factors [77]. It is unclear if the data used to create the calculator truly reflected racial or ethnic demographic differences that decreased the likelihood of success or if their influence on outcomes were the result of health inequities and racism [79]. This tool, which was intended to encourage shared decision-making using evidence-based medicine, became more of a deterrent for minority women from having a vaginal delivery [80]. Some studies found that non-Hispanic White women benefited both from having a higher prediction for a successful vaginal birth and from having the ability to use experiential knowledge to ultimately choose to have a VBAC despite the calculator's prediction [81]. Racialized assessments of risk in the context of perinatal care can lead to discrimination, tension between patients and care providers, and poor communication of information [82].

As previously detailed, hypertension and its consequences is one of the largest contributors to maternal mortality, and its management has also been dictated by race-based medicine. Examples include the salt sensitivity hypotheses as a cause of higher rates of high blood pressure in non-Hispanic Black people due to the differing genetic makeup of people of African descent and influence of slavery [71]. Variance in response to antihypertensives has been suggested by historical research. A combination pill of hydralazine and isosorbide dinitrate became the first drug to receive approval from the US Food and Drug Administration to treat specifically African Americans, and calcium channel blockers or thiazide diuretics were used preferentially in monotherapy for non-Hispanic Black patients based on flawed data [71, 83]. The evidence documenting racial disparities in drug responses has not resulted in elimination of the racial disparity in outcomes for non-Hispanic Black patients and in fact, use of standard medical therapy recommendations across races results in better outcomes [83]. Calculation of glomerular filtration rate used in the evaluation of kidney disease also erroneously uses race, which underestimates disease severity and ultimately leads to lack of management and progression to more advanced disease [71].

Potential Areas of Intervention within the Continuum of Care

Planning pregnancy and receipt of preconception care helps expectant mothers optimize health in anticipation of a future pregnancy [84]. Women in racial minority groups have been shown to have higher rates of medical comorbidities such as diabetes, hypertension, and obesity [85]. A study by Denny et al. demonstrated that tobacco dependence, alcohol misuse and diabetes were higher for American Indian/Alaskan Native women while obesity was more common in non-Hispanic Black women [85]. These factors individually confer risk in pregnancy; therefore, intervention prior to conception should influence racial and ethnic disparities in pregnancy morbidity [4]. Avoidance of pregnancy through access to adequate reversible contraception can allow time for appropriate management of these medical comorbidities [84].

Receipt of prenatal care is an important contributor to maternal morbidity and mortality. Rates of maternal death and severe morbidity are higher in patients who have received limited prenatal care [20]. Non-Hispanic White and Asian women are more likely to initiate prenatal care in the first trimester while the lowest initiation rates have been reported for non-Hispanic Black, American Indian/Alaskan Native and Native Hawaiian/Pacific Islanders [86]. Access to medical subspecialists and Maternal Fetal Medicine physicians improves maternal mortality [87] and many women are not referred despite having complex medical conditions in pregnancy [88]. Insufficient prenatal care among minority populations may be influenced by insurance status, availability of transportation, and hesitancy to initiate care secondary to medical trauma and experiences of racism in healthcare [89, 90].

Research shows that the quality of care rendered to non-Hispanic Black women differs in hospitals that serve predominantly Black communities compared to those that are outside of those communities [4]. At these hospitals, severe maternal morbidity occurs more frequently among non-Hispanic Black than non-Hispanic White women even after adjustment for confounders. These hospitals also have more poor outcomes across populations [91]. Howell et al. used simulation to show how delivery hospital in New York impacted disparities in severe morbidity and demonstrated that if non-Hispanic Black women delivered at the hospitals serving primarily non-Hispanic White women, severe morbidity would be reduced from 4.2% to 2.9%. Similarly, for Hispanic women the severe morbidity would be reduced from 2.7% to 2.3% [89].

Adherence to postpartum care has been an area of focus to improve maternal outcomes [92]. Women with poor maternal outcomes are at increased risk for recurrence in their next pregnancy and are at increased risk of chronic illness in later life [93]. The impact of limited prenatal care was previously addressed and is correlated with not attending postpartum visits [94]. A cross-sectional survey of patients with births from 2016 to 2019 found that postpartum visit attendance was lower among Medicaid-insured and racially minoritized patients [95]. This disparity was reinforced by the COVID-19 pandemic. A retrospective cohort study performed in the greater Boston area evaluated the differences in attended postpartum visits during the COVID-19 pandemic and found that overall visits decreased for all demographic groups during the pandemic. However, the decrease persisted during the late pandemic for non-Hispanic Black and Hispanic women, with non-Hispanic White women more likely to reengage in care after the COVID-19 peak [96]. Some reported reasons for lack of attendance at postpartum visits were concerns around childcare issues, availability of personal protective equipment at the healthcare facilities, and the feeling of being isolated [97, 98].

Patient Factors

Socioeconomics has been historically linked to poorer obstetric outcomes with non-Hispanic Black women thought to have lower income and access to care [99]. However, previous discussion of cardiovascular morbidity in pregnancy demonstrated that even affluent non-Hispanic Black women fare worse than non-Hispanic White women. Insurance status does not contribute as substantially as previously thought. A study showed an increase in myocardial infarction and stroke in non-Hispanic Black women with private insurance compared with non-Hispanic White women without insurance, suggesting that access to financial resources alone does not eradicate racial disparities [27].

Education and health care literacy are also thought to improve outcomes for patients across specialties [100, 101]. Evaluation of causal factors for racial and ethnic disparities has not found education to be protective for some groups of racial and ethnic minorities including non-Hispanic Black women. One study showed the pregnancy-related mortality ratios among non-Hispanic Black women with a completed college education or higher were 1.6 times that of non-Hispanic White women with less than a high school diploma. Among women with a college education or higher, the pregnancy-related mortality ratio for non-Hispanic Black women was 5.2 times than non-Hispanic White women [14]. Therefore, while education may be a contributor to these disparities, they are unfortunately not eliminated by the acquisition of higher education.

Advanced maternal age is an isolated risk factor for pregnancy-related morbidity with increased association with preeclampsia, diabetes, and cardiovascular complications [21, 53]. However, the pregnancy-related mortality ratio for non-Hispanic Black and American Indian/Alaskan Native women aged ≥30 years was approximately four to five times that for their non-Hispanic White counterparts [14]. Apart from increasing maternal age, the relative risk of pregnancy-related death for non-Hispanic Black women compared with non-Hispanic White women was greatest among those groups whose absolute risk of death was lowest [11, 102].

A proposed reason for racial disparities despite correction for income, education and other risk factors is the unique psychosocial experiences of non-Hispanic Black people in the United States such as chronic stress, racism, depression, and lack of social support [103]. This hypothesis has not yet been substantiated by research findings; differences in self-reported psychosocial factors in a large prospective observational study were not significantly associated with higher odds of the adverse pregnancy outcomes. The exception was perceived lack of social support, which was associated with preterm birth and small-for-gestational-age birth [103]. Separate from the external stressor of structural racism, internalized racism may manifest in low self-worth, low self-confidence, and depression, which may create behaviors that compromise both minoritized patients' health and their ability to access care [104].

The ethical issues and poor quality and limited research involving non-Hispanic Black people have downstream effects. This is represented by possibly limited data applicable to minority patients and cultural mistrust of research findings and care that is based on these findings [105]. This manifests as mistrust of White physicians, dissatisfaction with healthcare, and delayed medical treatment [105]. The racial disparities previously addressed regarding the COVID-19 pandemic are partially influenced by patient skepticism of the U.S healthcare system among minority populations and have resulted in poor vaccination uptake [106]. Work by both individual physicians and larger systems of care must be put forward to establish a strong physician–patient relationship and regain patients' trust in medical care.

Provider Factors

Racial disparities in maternal outcomes may be a consequence of communication failures and policies or procedures that are not in place or not followed [4]. For example, a study at a North Carolina hospital showed that half of the maternal deaths were among non-Hispanic Black women, of which 14% were due to hemorrhage. Ninety percent of the cases of hemorrhage were determined to be preventable and the result of medical care felt to be below the standard expected for the facility [3].

Overt and covert racism by the provider have known impacts on patient care. Non-Hispanic Black women have reported stigmatizing stereotyping from providers, including assumptions that they were single parents, had low incomes, and had multiple children, regardless of marital status, socioeconomic status, or parity [107]. Provider bias has an established influence on disparities in maternal outcomes and is discussed in depth elsewhere, but unconscious attitudes and stereotypes have been associated with disparities in treatment recommendations for non-Hispanic Black patients [108]. Differing treatment recommendations based on negative stereotypes can have detrimental effects on the patient as discussed above.

Solutions and Best Practices

Finding viable solutions to the long-standing problem of racial disparities in adverse pregnancy outcomes is a work in progress and requires resources that address each area of weakness within our healthcare system. Protocols, checklists, triggers (such as maternal early warning criteria), and the promotion of a safety culture have all been recommended in recent reviews [109]. A culture of safety includes implementation of national bundles for patient safety and team-based training practices aimed at improving care for racially diverse mothers [110]. For example, The Council on Patient Safety in Women's Health Care and the Alliance for Innovation in Maternal Health (AIM Program) published the "Reduction of Peripartum Racial/Ethnic Disparities Patient Safety Bundle" [111]. This bundle provides a blueprint for institutions and clinicians to implement to reduce disparities in maternal morbidity and mortality. Safety bundles can address system and provider issues through improving accurate and respectful data collection on linking identity to outcomes and applying coaching and education to raise awareness throughout a hospital system [110]. Examples of previously used safety bundles include those for hemorrhage, venous thrombotic disease, and hypertension, all of which improve care across racial and ethnic identities [109].

Another system target is improving access to quality care in the preconception, pregnancy, and postpartum periods, which can be implemented through coordination at the level of the community, health facility, patient and family, and health care provider [14]. Examples include use of group prenatal care and doulas as labor support to encourage shared decision making with patients [110]. Use of doulas for patient advocacy can lower rates of cesarean delivery, lower rates of forceps or vacuum deliveries, improve birth experiences, decrease maternal stress, and improve breastfeeding rates [112–114]. Doula services are not usually covered under available health insurance plans including Medicaid, which generates a barrier to care, but more recent legislation has been directed towards expanding coverage [115]. The benefit of doula care is amplified when the caregiver is community-based or of shared experiences; therefore, efforts to recruit individuals from racial minority groups is a focus for improving maternal outcomes [115].

Group prenatal care has been suggested to improve the care experience and outcomes for women from racial minority groups. The model consists of ten scheduled prenatal visits in groups of people with similar gestational ages and estimated due dates [79]. This model of care delivery is thought to make patients feel socially supported by their group and more comfortable asking questions of their providers and has been associated with improved perinatal outcomes [116, 117]. Patients receiving group care perceive themselves as receiving better communication and culturally sensitive care for their pregnancy and health. Most research on this model shows more improvement in neonatal outcomes but not necessarily maternal outcomes [117]. Neonatal outcomes of reduced preterm delivery and decreased short interval pregnancies have been noted in previous research [79].

Cultural competency training can help clinicians acknowledge cultural influences and biases that influence the health and experiences of racial minorities and "deprogram" clinicians' automatic responses instead of perpetuating racialized medicine and the false concept that there are biologic differences between races [59, 71]. Such training also acknowledges the systems and cultural structures that produce health inequities and promotes learning and advocacy to repair enduring harm from these systems [118]. Cultural competence describes attitudes, behaviors and policies that allow medical providers to properly serve clients of diverse racial/ethnic backgrounds [119]. Using cultural competence in the rendering of care can improve the systemic and provider issues that contribute to current racial disparities in maternal outcomes.

An additional goal is implicit bias recognition and elimination. This can be achieved by addressing implicit biases through a combination of cognitive and behavioral interventions and uncovering local or system-based biases through the routine use of quality assurance tools [110]. Unfortunately, techniques such as debiasing have not been shown to change attitudes or behaviors of physicians [110]. Small studies have suggested that exposure to counterstereotypes or positive representations of racial minority group members can change the attitudes towards members of that group, but the impact of these interventions tends to be short lived [120]. Though challenging, intensive behavior change techniques have been shown to be effective in altering the impact of implicit racial biases on the experiences of racialized patients in medical care. This involves dedicated time, financial, and personnel resources [121].

Race- concordant care has been shown to improve outcomes regarding the disparities in infant mortality [122] but there is less research on the maternal outcomes.

Non-Hispanic Black, Hispanic, and Native American physicians are underrepresented in medicine [123]. Increasing the likelihood of race-concordant care requires pipelines that make health care jobs more accessible and more representative of our diverse population [110, 122]. Moreover, studies have shown that members of racial minorities in the health professions are more likely to serve minority populations and to work with publicly insured and minority populations [124]. A publicly available list of the race/ethnicity of maternal health providers in the area has been suggested to improve access to race-concordant care [125].

A list of recommendations presented for caring for racial and ethnic minority women was proposed by the Black Mamas Matter Alliance; "(1) Listen to Black women; (2) recognize the historical experiences and expertise of Black women and families; (3) provide care through a reproductive justice framework; (4) disentangle care practices from the racist beliefs in modern medicine; (5) replace white supremacy and patriarchy with a new care model; (6) empower all patients with health literacy and autonomy; (7) empower and invest in paraprofessionals; and (8) recognize that access does not equal quality care" [126]. There is certainly more work to be done, but this wonderfully crafted list covers the core of how efforts should be directed. If consistent effort is placed into addressing the issues at the system, provider and patient level while keeping these recommendations in mind, maternal outcomes can improve.

References

1. American College of Obstetricians and Gynecologists. Committee opinion no. 464: patient safety in the surgical environment. Obstet Gynecol. 2010;116(3):786–90.
2. Nunes I, Nicholson W, Theron G, FIGO Childbirth and Postpartum Hemorrhage Committee. FIGO good practice recommendations on surgical techniques to improve safety and reduce complications during cesarean delivery. Int J Gynaecol Obstet Off Organ Int Fed Gynaecol Obstet. 2023;163(Suppl. 2):21–33.
3. Pahlavan P, Nezhat C, Nezhat C. Hemorrhage in obstetrics and gynecology. Curr Opin Obstet Gynecol. 2001;13(4):419–24.
4. Howell EA. Reducing disparities in severe maternal morbidity and mortality. Clin Obstet Gynecol. 2018;61(2):387–99.
5. Beckie TM. Ethnic and racial disparities in hypertension management among women. Semin Perinatol. 2017;41(5):278–86.
6. Mackenzie M, Felix A. Allyson Felix risked everything by speaking out. She's not finished. 2020 Jun 16 [cited 2024 May 11]; Available from: https://www.glamour.com/story/game-changer-allyson-felix
7. Berg CJ, Chang J, Callaghan WM, Whitehead SJ. Pregnancy-related mortality in the United States, 1991–1997. Obstet Gynecol. 2003;101(2):289–96.
8. Creanga AA, Bateman BT, Kuklina EV, Callaghan WM. Racial and ethnic disparities in severe maternal morbidity: a multistate analysis, 2008–2010. Am J Obstet Gynecol. 2014;210(5):435–8.
9. Guendelman S, Thornton D, Gould J, Hosang N. Obstetric complications during labor and delivery: assessing ethnic differences in California. Womens Health Issues Off Publ Jacobs Inst Womens Health. 2006;16(4):189–97.

10. Hopkins FW, MacKay AP, Koonin LM, Berg CJ, Irwin M, Atrash HK. Pregnancy-related mortality in Hispanic women in the United States. Obstet Gynecol. 1999;94(5 Pt 1):747–52.
11. Berg CJ, Harper MA, Atkinson SM, Bell EA, Brown HL, Hage ML, et al. Preventability of pregnancy-related deaths: results of a state-wide review. Obstet Gynecol. 2005;106(6):1228–34.
12. Braveman P. What are health disparities and health equity? We need to be clear. Public Health Rep Wash DC 1974. 2014;129(Suppl. 2):5–8.
13. Anon. Committee opinion no. 649 summary: racial and ethnic disparities in obstetrics and gynecology. Obstet Gynecol. 2015;126(6):1325.
14. Petersen EE, Davis NL, Goodman D, Cox S, Syverson C, Seed K, et al. Racial/ethnic disparities in pregnancy-related deaths—United States, 2007–2016. MMWR Morb Mortal Wkly Rep. 2019;68(35):762–5.
15. ACOG. Committee opinion no. 761: cesarean delivery on maternal request. Obstet Gynecol. 2019;133(1):e73–7.
16. Okwandu IC, Anderson M, Postlethwaite D, Shirazi A, Torrente S. Racial and ethnic disparities in cesarean delivery and indications among Nulliparous, term, singleton, vertex women. J Racial Ethn Health Disparities. 2022;9(4):1161–71.
17. Carlson NS, Carlson MS, Erickson EN, Higgins M, Britt AJ, Amore AD. Disparities by race/ethnicity in unplanned cesarean birth among healthy nulliparas: a secondary analysis of the nuMoM2b dataset. BMC Pregnancy Childbirth. 2023;23(1):342.
18. Washington S, Caughey AB, Cheng YW, Bryant AS. Racial and ethnic differences in indication for primary cesarean delivery at term: experience at one U.S. Inst Birth Berkeley Calif. 2012;39(2):128–34.
19. Ford ND, Cox S, Ko JY, Ouyang L, Romero L, Colarusso T, et al. Hypertensive disorders in pregnancy and mortality at delivery hospitalization—United States, 2017–2019. MMWR Morb Mortal Wkly Rep. 2022;71(17):585–91.
20. Harper MA, Espeland MA, Dugan E, Meyer R, Lane K, Williams S. Racial disparity in pregnancy-related mortality following a live birth outcome. Ann Epidemiol. 2004;14(4):274–9.
21. Leonard SA, Formanowski BL, Phibbs CS, Lorch S, Main EK, Kozhimannil KB, et al. Chronic hypertension in pregnancy and racial-ethnic disparities in complications. Obstet Gynecol. 2023;142(4):862–71.
22. Panaitescu AM, Syngelaki A, Prodan N, Akolekar R, Nicolaides KH. Chronic hypertension and adverse pregnancy outcome: a cohort study. Ultrasound Obstet Gynecol Off J Int Soc Ultrasound Obstet Gynecol. 2017;50(2):228–35.
23. Gyamfi-Bannerman C, Pandita A, Miller EC, Boehme AK, Wright JD, Siddiq Z, et al. Preeclampsia outcomes at delivery and race. J Matern-Fetal Neonatal Med Off J Eur Assoc Perinat Med Fed Asia Ocean Perinat Soc Int Soc Perinat Obstet. 2020;33(21):3619–26.
24. Martin JN, Thigpen BD, Moore RC, Rose CH, Cushman J, May W. Stroke and severe preeclampsia and eclampsia: a paradigm shift focusing on systolic blood pressure. Obstet Gynecol. 2005;105(2):246–54.
25. Behrens I, Basit S, Lykke JA, Ranthe MF, Wohlfahrt J, Bundgaard H, et al. Association between hypertensive disorders of pregnancy and later risk of cardiomyopathy. JAMA. 2016;315(10):1026–33.
26. Ross KM, Guardino C, Dunkel Schetter C, Hobel CJ. Interactions between race/ethnicity, poverty status, and pregnancy cardio-metabolic diseases in prediction of postpartum cardio-metabolic health. Ethn Health. 2020;25(8):1145–60.
27. Gad MM, Elgendy IY, Mahmoud AN, Saad AM, Isogai T, Sande Mathias I, et al. Disparities in cardiovascular disease outcomes among pregnant and post-partum women. J Am Heart Assoc. 2021;10(1):e017832.
28. Whitehead SJ, Berg CJ, Chang J. Pregnancy-related mortality due to cardiomyopathy: United States, 1991–1997. Obstet Gynecol. 2003;102(6):1326–31.
29. Sinkey RG, Rajapreyar IN, Szychowski JM, Armour EK, Walker Z, Cribbs MG, et al. Racial disparities in peripartum cardiomyopathy: eighteen years of observations. J Matern-Fetal

Neonatal Med Off J Eur Assoc Perinat Med Fed Asia Ocean Perinat Soc Int Soc Perinat Obstet. 2022;35(10):1891–8.
30. Robbins CL, Hutchings Y, Dietz PM, Kuklina EV, Callaghan WM. History of preterm birth and subsequent cardiovascular disease: a systematic review. Am J Obstet Gynecol. 2014;210(4):285–97.
31. Jackson FM, Rashied-Henry K, Braveman P, Dominguez TP, Ramos D, Maseru N, et al. A prematurity collaborative birth equity consensus statement for mothers and babies. Matern Child Health J. 2020;24(10):1231–7.
32. Martin JA, Hamilton BE, Osterman MJK, Driscoll AK, Mathews TJ. Births: final data for 2015. Natl Vital Stat Rep Cent Dis Control Prev Natl Cent Health Stat Natl Vital Stat Syst. 2017;66(1):1.
33. Schaaf JM, Liem SMS, Mol BWJ, Abu-Hanna A, Ravelli ACJ. Ethnic and racial disparities in the risk of preterm birth: a systematic review and meta-analysis. Am J Perinatol. 2013;30(6):433–50.
34. Osterman MJK, Hamilton BE, Martin JA, Driscoll AK, Valenzuela CP. Births: final data for 2022. Natl Vital Stat Rep. 2024;73(2):33. Available from: https://www.cdc.gov/nchs/data/nvsr/nvsr73/nvsr73-02.pdf [cited 2024 Apr 25]
35. Kistka ZAF, Palomar L, Lee KA, Boslaugh SE, Wangler MF, Cole FS, et al. Racial disparity in the frequency of recurrence of preterm birth. Am J Obstet Gynecol. 2007;196(2):131–6.
36. Shen TT, DeFranco EA, Stamilio DM, Chang JJ, Muglia LJ. A population-based study of race-specific risk for preterm premature rupture of membranes. Am J Obstet Gynecol. 2008;199(4):373.e1–7.
37. Manuck TA, Esplin MS, Biggio J, Bukowski R, Parry S, Zhang H, et al. The phenotype of spontaneous preterm birth: application of a clinical phenotyping tool. Am J Obstet Gynecol. 2015;212(4):487.e1–487.
38. Willis E, McManus P, Magallanes N, Johnson S, Majnik A. Conquering racial disparities in perinatal outcomes. Clin Perinatol. 2014;41(4):847–75.
39. Ncube CN, Enquobahrie DA, Albert SM, Herrick AL, Burke JG. Association of neighborhood context with offspring risk of preterm birth and low birthweight: a systematic review and meta-analysis of population-based studies. Soc Sci Med. 1982;2016(153):156–64.
40. Manuck TA. Racial and ethnic differences in preterm birth: a complex, multifactorial problem. Semin Perinatol. 2017;41(8):511–8.
41. Goldenberg RL, Cliver SP, Mulvihill FX, Hickey CA, Hoffman HJ, Klerman LV, et al. Medical, psychosocial, and behavioral risk factors do not explain the increased risk for low birth weight among black women. Am J Obstet Gynecol. 1996;175(5):1317–24.
42. Rodrigues T, Barros H. Short interpregnancy interval and risk of spontaneous preterm delivery. Eur J Obstet Gynecol Reprod Biol. 2008;136(2):184–8.
43. Lonhart JA, Mayo JA, Padula AM, Wise PH, Stevenson DK, Shaw GM. Short interpregnancy interval as a risk factor for preterm birth in non-Hispanic Black and White women in California. J Perinatol Off J Calif Perinat Assoc. 2019;39(9):1175–81.
44. The 2023 March of dimes report card: the state of maternal and infant health for American families; 2023.
45. Anon. WHO recommendations for the prevention and treatment of postpartum haemorrhage. Geneva: World Health Organization; 2012. [cited 2024 Jun 27]. (WHO Guidelines Approved by the Guidelines Review Committee). Available from: http://www.ncbi.nlm.nih.gov/books/NBK131942/
46. Wormer KC, Jamil RT, Bryant SB. Acute postpartum hemorrhage. In: StatPearls. Treasure Island (FL): StatPearls Publishing; 2024. [cited 2024 Jun 27]. Available from: http://www.ncbi.nlm.nih.gov/books/NBK499988/.
47. Okunlola O, Raza S, Osasan S, Sethia S, Batool T, Bambhroliya Z, et al. Race/ethnicity as a risk factor in the development of postpartum hemorrhage: a thorough systematic review of disparity in the relationship between pregnancy and the rate of postpartum hemorrhage. Cureus. 2022;14(6):e26460.

48. Katz D, Khadge S, Carvalho B. Comparing postpartum estimated and quantified blood loss among racial groups: an observational study. Cureus. 2022;14(5):e25299.
49. Tucker MJ, Berg CJ, Callaghan WM, Hsia J. The Black-White disparity in pregnancy-related mortality from 5 conditions: differences in prevalence and case-fatality rates. Am J Public Health. 2007;97(2):247–51.
50. Meeks M, Voegtline K, Vaught AJ, Lawson SM. Differences in surgery classification and indications for peripartum hysterectomy at a major academic institution. Am J Perinatol. 2024;41(Suppl. 01):e623–9.
51. Vounzoulaki E, Khunti K, Abner SC, Tan BK, Davies MJ, Gillies CL. Progression to type 2 diabetes in women with a known history of gestational diabetes: systematic review and meta-analysis. BMJ. 2020;369:m1361.
52. Janevic T, McCarthy K, Liu SH, Huyhn M, Kennedy J, Tai Chan H, et al. Racial and ethnic inequities in development of type 2 diabetes after gestational diabetes mellitus. Obstet Gynecol. 2023;142(4):901–10.
53. Bower JK, Butler BN, Bose-Brill S, Kue J, Wassel CL. Racial/ethnic differences in diabetes screening and hyperglycemia among US women after gestational diabetes. Prev Chronic Dis. 2019;16:E145.
54. Nguyen BT, Cheng YW, Snowden JM, Esakoff TF, Frias AE, Caughey AB. The effect of race/ethnicity on adverse perinatal outcomes among patients with gestational diabetes mellitus. Am J Obstet Gynecol. 2012;207(4):322–6.
55. Palatnik A, Harrison RK, Walker RJ, Thakkar MY, Egede LE. Maternal racial and ethnic disparities in glycemic threshold for pharmacotherapy initiation for gestational diabetes. J Matern-Fetal Neonatal Med Off J Eur Assoc Perinat Med Fed Asia Ocean Perinat Soc Int Soc Perinat Obstet. 2022;35(1):58–65.
56. Geronimus AT. The weathering hypothesis and the health of African-American women and infants: evidence and speculations. Ethn Dis. 1992;2(3):207–21.
57. Forrester S, Jacobs D, Zmora R, Schreiner P, Roger V, Kiefe CI. Racial differences in weathering and its associations with psychosocial stress: The CARDIA study. SSM Popul Health. 2019;7:100319.
58. VanSickle C, Liese KL, Rutherford JN. Textbook typologies: challenging the myth of the perfect obstetric pelvis. Anat Rec Hoboken NJ 2007. 2022;305(4):952–67.
59. Mathur VA, Morris T, McNamara K. Cultural conceptions of women's labor pain and labor pain management: a mixed-method analysis. Soc Sci Med. 1982;2020(261):113240.
60. Badreldin N, Grobman WA, Yee LM. Racial disparities in postpartum pain management. Obstet Gynecol. 2019;134(6):1147–53.
61. Lee W, Martins MS, George RB, Fernandez A. Racial and ethnic disparities in obstetric anesthesia: a scoping review. Can J Anaesth J Can Anesth. 2023;70(6):1035–46.
62. Thomas CL, Lange EMS, Banayan JM, Zhu Y, Liao C, Peralta FM, et al. Racial and ethnic disparities in receipt of general anesthesia for cesarean delivery. JAMA Netw Open. 2024;7(1):e2350825.
63. Waytz A, Hoffman KM, Trawalter S. A superhumanization bias in whites' perceptions of blacks. Soc Psychol Personal Sci. 2015;6(3):352–9. https://doi.org/10.1177/1948550614553642.
64. Lindahl V, Pearson JL, Colpe L. Prevalence of suicidality during pregnancy and the postpartum. Arch Womens Ment Health. 2005;8(2):77–87.
65. Sidebottom AC, Vacquier M, LaRusso E, Schulte AK, Nickel A. Prenatal and postpartum depression diagnosis in a large health system: prevalence and disparities. Ann Med. 2023;55(2):2281507.
66. Liu S, Ding X, Belouali A, Bai H, Raja K, Kharrazi H. Assessing the racial and socioeconomic disparities in postpartum depression using population-level hospital discharge data: longitudinal retrospective study. JMIR Pediatr Parent. 2022;5(4):e38879.
67. Iturralde E, Hsiao CA, Nkemere L, Kubo A, Sterling SA, Flanagan T, et al. Engagement in perinatal depression treatment: a qualitative study of barriers across and within racial/ethnic groups. BMC Pregn Childbirth. 2021;21(1):512.

68. Ellington S, Strid P, Tong VT, Woodworth K, Galang RR, Zambrano LD, et al. Characteristics of women of reproductive age with laboratory-confirmed SARS-CoV-2 infection by pregnancy status—United States, January 22–June 7, 2020. MMWR Morb Mortal Wkly Rep. 2020;69(25):769–75.
69. Moore JT, Ricaldi JN, Rose CE, Fuld J, Parise M, Kang GJ, et al. Disparities in incidence of COVID-19 among underrepresented racial/ethnic groups in counties identified as hotspots during June 5–18, 2020–22 states, February–June 2020. MMWR Morb Mortal Wkly Rep. 2020;69(33):1122–6.
70. Goldfarb IT, Clapp MA, Soffer MD, Shook LL, Rushfirth K, Edlow AG, et al. Prevalence and severity of coronavirus disease 2019 (COVID-19) illness in symptomatic pregnant and postpartum women stratified by hispanic ethnicity. Obstet Gynecol. 2020;136(2):300–2.
71. Chadha N, Lim B, Kane M, Rowland B. Toward the abolition of biological race in medicine. UC Berkeley: Othering & Belonging Institute; 2020. Available from: https://escholarship.org/uc/item/4gt3n0dd
72. Crear-Perry J, Correa-de-Araujo R, Lewis Johnson T, McLemore MR, Neilson E, Wallace M. Social and structural determinants of health inequities in maternal health. J Women's Health 2002. 2021;30(2):230–5.
73. Balla S, Gomez SE, Rodriguez F. Disparities in cardiovascular care and outcomes for women from racial/ethnic minority backgrounds. Curr Treat Options Cardiovasc Med. 2020;22(12):75.
74. Scharff DP, Mathews KJ, Jackson P, Hoffsuemmer J, Martin E, Edwards D. More than Tuskegee: understanding mistrust about research participation. J Health Care Poor Underserved. 2010;21(3):879–97.
75. Ojanuga D. The medical ethics of the "father of gynaecology", Dr J Marion Sims. J Med Ethics. 1993;19(1):28–31.
76. Baptiste DL, Caviness-Ashe N, Josiah N, Commodore-Mensah Y, Arscott J, Wilson PR, et al. Henrietta lacks and America's dark history of research involving African Americans. Nurs Open. 2022;9(5):2236–8.
77. Grobman WA, Lai Y, Landon MB, Spong CY, Leveno KJ, Rouse DJ, et al. Development of a nomogram for prediction of vaginal birth after cesarean delivery. Obstet Gynecol. 2007;109(4):806–12.
78. Costantine MM, Fox K, Byers BD, Mateus J, Ghulmiyyah LM, Blackwell S, et al. Validation of the prediction model for success of vaginal birth after cesarean delivery. Obstet Gynecol. 2009;114(5):1029–33.
79. Scott KA, Britton L, McLemore MR. The ethics of perinatal care for black women: dismantling the structural racism in "Mother Blame" narratives. J Perinat Neonatal Nurs. 2019;33(2):108–15.
80. Diaz-Tello F. Invisible wounds: obstetric violence in the United States. Reprod Health Matters. 2016;24(47):56–64.
81. Rubashkin N. Epistemic silences and experiential knowledge in decisions after a first cesarean: the case of a vaginal birth after cesarean calculator. Med Anthropol Q. 2023;37(4):341–53.
82. McLemore MR, Altman MR, Cooper N, Williams S, Rand L, Franck L. Health care experiences of pregnant, birthing and postnatal women of color at risk for preterm birth. Soc Sci Med. 1982;2018(201):127–35.
83. Flack JM, Buhnerkempe MG. Race and antihypertensive drug therapy: edging closer to a new paradigm. Hypertens Dallas Tex 1979. 2022;79(2):349–51.
84. Dude AM, Schueler K, Schumm LP, Murugesan M, Stulberg DB. Preconception care and severe maternal morbidity in the United States. Am J Obstet Gynecol MFM. 2022;4(2):100549.
85. Denny CH, Floyd RL, Green PP, Hayes DK. Racial and ethnic disparities in preconception risk factors and preconception care. J Women's Health 2002. 2012;21(7):720–9.
86. Child Health USA 2014. US Department of Health and Human Services, Health Resources and Services Administration; 2015 Mar [cited 2024 Apr 25]. Available from: https://mchb.hrsa.gov/sites/default/files/mchb/data-research/child-health-2014.pdf.

87. Russo M, Krenz EI, Hart SR, Kirsch D. Multidisciplinary approach to the management of placenta accreta. Ochsner J. 2011;11(1):84–8.
88. Wenstrom K, Erickson K, Schulkin J. Are obstetrician-gynecologists satisfied with their maternal-fetal medicine consultants? A survey. Am J Perinatol. 2012;29(8):599–608.
89. Howell EA, Egorova N, Balbierz A, Zeitlin J, Hebert PL. Black-white differences in severe maternal morbidity and site of care. Am J Obstet Gynecol. 2016;214(1):122.e1–7.
90. Lu MC, Chen B. Racial and ethnic disparities in preterm birth: the role of stressful life events. Am J Obstet Gynecol. 2004;191(3):691–9.
91. Howell EA, Egorova NN, Balbierz A, Zeitlin J, Hebert PL. Site of delivery contribution to black-white severe maternal morbidity disparity. Am J Obstet Gynecol. 2016;215(2):143–52.
92. Shaw E, Levitt C, Wong S, Kaczorowski J, McMaster University Postpartum Research Group. Systematic review of the literature on postpartum care: effectiveness of postpartum support to improve maternal parenting, mental health, quality of life, and physical health. Birth Berkeley Calif. 2006;33(3):210–20.
93. Ahmed R, Dunford J, Mehran R, Robson S, Kunadian V. Pre-eclampsia and future cardiovascular risk among women: a review. J Am Coll Cardiol. 2014;63(18):1815–22.
94. Siddiqui R, Bell T, Sangi-Haghpeykar H, Minard C, Levison J. Predictive factors for loss to postpartum follow-up among low-income HIV-infected women in Texas. AIDS Patient Care STDs. 2014;28(5):248–53.
95. Interrante JD, Admon LK, Carroll C, Henning-Smith C, Chastain P, Kozhimannil KB. Association of Health Insurance, Geography, and race and ethnicity with disparities in receipt of recommended postpartum care in the US. JAMA Health Forum. 2022;3(10):e223292.
96. Mi T, Hung P, Li X, McGregor A, He J, Zhou J. Racial and ethnic disparities in postpartum care in the greater Boston area during the COVID-19 pandemic. JAMA Netw Open. 2022;5(6):e2216355.
97. Brislane Á, Larkin F, Jones H, Davenport MH. Access to and quality of healthcare for pregnant and postpartum women during the COVID-19 pandemic. Front Glob Womens Health. 2021;2:628625.
98. DeYoung SE, Mangum M. Pregnancy, birthing, and postpartum experiences during COVID-19 in the United States. Front Sociol. 2021;6:611212.
99. Mazul MC, Salm Ward TC, Ngui EM. Anatomy of good prenatal care: perspectives of low income African-American women on barriers and facilitators to prenatal care. J Racial Ethn Health Disparities. 2017;4(1):79–86.
100. Nawabi F, Krebs F, Vennedey V, Shukri A, Lorenz L, Stock S. Health literacy in pregnant women: a systematic review. Int J Environ Res Public Health. 2021;18(7):3847.
101. Tavakoly Sany SB, Behzhad F, Ferns G, Peyman N. Communication skills training for physicians improves health literacy and medical outcomes among patients with hypertension: a randomized controlled trial. BMC Health Serv Res. 2020;20(1):60.
102. Saftlas AF, Koonin LM, Atrash HK. Racial disparity in pregnancy-related mortality associated with livebirth: can established risk factors explain it? Am J Epidemiol. 2000;152(5):413–9.
103. Grobman WA, Parker CB, Willinger M, Wing DA, Silver RM, Wapner RJ, et al. Racial disparities in adverse pregnancy outcomes and psychosocial stress. Obstet Gynecol. 2018;131(2):328–35.
104. Perry BL, Stevens-Watkins D, Oser CB. The moderating effects of skin color and ethnic identity affirmation on suicide risk among low-SES African American women. Race Soc Probl. 2013;5(1):1–14.
105. Prather C, Fuller TR, Marshall KJ, Jeffries WL. The impact of racism on the sexual and reproductive health of African American Women. J Women's Health 2002. 2016;25(7):664–71.
106. Lin C, Tu P, Terry TC. Moving the needle on racial disparity: COVID-19 vaccine trust and hesitancy. Vaccine. 2022;40(1):5–8.
107. Mehra R, Boyd LM, Magriples U, Kershaw TS, Ickovics JR, Keene DE. Black pregnant women "get the most judgment": a qualitative study of the experiences of black women at

the intersection of race, gender, and pregnancy. Womens Health Issues Off Publ Jacobs Inst Womens Health. 2020;30(6):484–92.
108. van Ryn M, Burgess DJ, Dovidio JF, Phelan SM, Saha S, Malat J, et al. The impact of racism on clinician cognition, behavior, and clinical decision making. Bois Rev Soc Sci Res Race. 2011;8(1):199–218.
109. Arora KS, Shields LE, Grobman WA, D'Alton ME, Lappen JR, Mercer BM. Triggers, bundles, protocols, and checklists—what every maternal care provider needs to know. Am J Obstet Gynecol. 2016;214(4):444–51.
110. Minehart RD, Bryant AS, Jackson J, Daly JL. Racial/ethnic inequities in pregnancy-related morbidity and mortality. Obstet Gynecol Clin N Am. 2021;48(1):31–51.
111. Howell EA, Brown H, Brumley J, Bryant AS, Caughey AB, Cornell AM, et al. Reduction of peripartum racial and ethnic disparities: a conceptual framework and maternal safety consensus bundle. Obstet Gynecol. 2018;131(5):770–82.
112. Kozhimannil KB, Attanasio LB, Jou J, Joarnt LK, Johnson PJ, Gjerdingen DK. Potential benefits of increased access to doula support during childbirth. Am J Manag Care. 2014;20(8):e340–52.
113. Mottl-Santiago J, Dukhovny D, Cabral H, Rodrigues D, Spencer L, Valle EA, et al. Effectiveness of an enhanced community doula intervention in a safety net setting: a randomized controlled trial. Health Equity. 2023;7(1):466–76.
114. Thomas MP, Ammann G, Brazier E, Noyes P, Maybank A. Doula services within a healthy start program: increasing access for an underserved population. Matern Child Health J. 2017;21(Suppl. 1):59–64.
115. Ogunwole SM, Karbeah J, Bozzi DG, Bower KM, Cooper LA, Hardeman R, et al. Health equity considerations in state bills related to doula care (2015–2020). Womens Health Issues Off Publ Jacobs Inst Womens Health. 2022;32(5):440–9.
116. Rising SS. Centering pregnancy. An interdisciplinary model of empowerment. J Nurse Midwifery. 1998;43(1):46–54.
117. Tucker CM, Felder TM, Dail RB, Lyndon A, Allen KC. Group prenatal care and maternal outcomes: a scoping review. MCN Am J Matern Child Nurs. 2021;46(6):314–22.
118. Davis S, O'Brien AM. Let's talk about racism: strategies for building structural competency in nursing. Acad Med J Assoc Am Med Coll. 2020;95(12S):S58–65.
119. Anderson LM, Scrimshaw SC, Fullilove MT, Fielding JE, Normand J, Task Force on Community Preventive Services. Culturally competent healthcare systems. A systematic review. Am J Prev Med. 2003;24(Suppl. 3):68–79.
120. Greenwald AG, Dasgupta N, Dovidio JF, Kang J, Moss-Racusin CA, Teachman BA. Implicit-bias remedies: treating discriminatory bias as a public-health problem. Psychol Sci Public Interest J Am Psychol Soc. 2022;23(1):7–40.
121. Hagiwara N, Elston Lafata J, Mezuk B, Vrana SR, Fetters MD. Detecting implicit racial bias in provider communication behaviors to reduce disparities in healthcare: challenges, solutions, and future directions for provider communication training. Patient Educ Couns. 2019;102(9):1738–43.
122. Greenwood BN, Hardeman RR, Huang L, Sojourner A. Physician-patient racial concordance and disparities in birthing mortality for newborns. Proc Natl Acad Sci U S A. 2020;117(35):21194–200.
123. Acosta DA, Poll-Hunter NI, Eliason J. Trends in racial and ethnic minority applicants and matriculants to US medical schools, 1980–2016. Analysis in Brief. Association of American Medical Colleges; 2017 Nov [cited 2024 Jun 21] p. 1–4. Available from: https://www.aamc.org/media/8816/download?attachment.
124. Sullivan L. Missing persons: minorities in the health professions; 2004 Sep p. 1–19.
125. Okpa A, Buxton M, O'Neill M. Association between provider-patient racial concordance and the maternal health experience during pregnancy. J Patient Exp. 2022;9:23743735221077522.
126. Muse S. Setting the standard for holistic care of and for Black women. Black Mamas Matter Alliance; 2018.

Part III
Cultural Considerations in ART with Diverse Populations

Chapter 10
Orthodox Judaism: Faith and Fertility

Dvora Entin

To be an Orthodox Jew means to be pigeon-holed, to be represented in extremes in movies and on Netflix series, to be assumed to be Chasidic, close minded, old fashioned, cultish, or brainwashed. To be an Orthodox Jew is to be seen as different, insular, and patriarchal. To be an Orthodox Jew means navigating a secular world with a religious identity, constantly adjusting, explaining, and accommodating. To be an Orthodox Jew is to be noticeable, identifiable, and just plain different from others. To be an Orthodox Jew is to have high standards of living, large families and larger tuition bills, expensive kosher food choices, and Jewish holidays that require days off that are often met with frustration and misunderstanding from bosses and colleagues. And to be an Orthodox Jew is to have a firm identity of faith that is deeply woven into religious practice. To be an Orthodox Jew is to have a life filled with ritual and obligation, law and structure, practice and purpose.

To be an Orthodox Jew is to be a part of a community that places significant emphasis on charity and volunteerism, where organizations and charities are created to help outfit new brides, assist couples in navigating financial planning and debt reduction, provide low-cost medical supplies for those in need, and offer support groups for diverse mental health struggles. To be an Orthodox Jew is to support families facing cancer diagnoses and to provide social and emotional support for grieving children who have lost a parent. To be an Orthodox Jew is to be a part of a global family, an interwoven community, to center your life around religious customs and identity, and to understand that you will never be alone when facing life's challenges or difficulties.

When the dream of creating your own family is not unfolding the way you imagined, infertility becomes a part of your language, a foreign and frightening word that puts you and your spouse outside the realm of communal and family norms. The experience of an Orthodox couple when experiencing infertility is incredibly

D. Entin (✉)
Dvora Entin & Associates, Philadelphia, PA, USA

D. A. Kaplan (ed.), *Cultural Responsiveness in Assisted Reproductive Technology*, https://doi.org/10.1007/978-3-031-76204-8_10

vulnerable. The couple, raised with the values of modesty and sexual privacy, is now forced to discuss their sexual life and private, intimate experiences with multiple providers including rabbis, doctors and family [1]. This exposure and vulnerability can be a jarring introduction to the medical landscape of family building, and young couples are usually ill-equipped for these new experiences.

There are unique challenges and opportunities for infertility care providers working within the Orthodox Jewish community. Some distinct factors for Orthodox patients include their religious beliefs and restrictions, potentially limited knowledge about sexual experiences and about their bodies, Orthodox family systems, expectations of the community, and the age of the couple. These are all contributing factors to the experience of infertility, as well as the management of fertility care. The more modern the individual, the more integration one will see between the community and secular spaces. Most communities of today will access standard medical care without hesitation, often seeking the route of those who have faced this challenge before them, and relying on referrals and relationships in seeking out the team that can best address their medical needs. Fertility care for Orthodox patients tends to be clustered in trusted, large group practices where it is easier not to have to explain all the laws or accommodations needed. These practices are likely to have already seen a large number of Orthodox patients, easing the experience for the new patient. The goal of this chapter is to equip reproductive endocrinology & infertility (REIs) and affiliated providers with a more accurate understanding of the tenets of Orthodox Judaism as they relate to fertility and describe the broader social, cultural, and religious context in which Orthodox Jewish patients experience infertility and its care.

Variation in Practice

To meet an Orthodox Jew is to meet ONE Orthodox Jew. The variations in practice that fall under the umbrella of Orthodoxy are vast and often confusing when attempting to capture a community that is diverse in its practices and belief systems. Within any Orthodox community system, you will meet women who cover their hair with scarves, with wigs, or not at all. Men may wear a white button-down shirt or polos or t-shirts, while others wear black hats, baseball caps, or a fur lined *shtreimel*[1]on Shabbat. Some couples will consult with their rabbi for general guidance and support and others only for religious law decisions. All identify as Orthodox. As with any insular system, the myths and theories about the inner workings of the Orthodox community are promulgated through media, pervasive bias, and assumptions. The recent popularity of Orthodox social media influencers has increased broader public awareness and information about common practice and presents a powerful

[1]A *shtreimel* is a fur hat worn by some Orthodox Jewish men, many of whom are Chasidic, on Shabbat, Jewish holidays, and other festive occasions.

opportunity to create a new knowledge base for those outside the community. However, some may highlight the practical or positive aspects of religious practice while others present some of the more non-representative fringe, or even bizarre, faith practices. The mainstream portrayal of Orthodox Judaism and Jews is often flawed and offers little context to the lived experiences of those it seeks to represent.

Terminology is an important starting point for understanding the religious culture and Jewish faith. Judaism is a diverse religion with three main denominations; Orthodox, which makes up about 10% of world Judaism, Conservative, which encompasses about 5%, and Reform, who form the majority, at about 85% [2]. Within each sect, there is a vast continuum of religiosity and heterogeneity.

Orthodoxy is differentiated into various categories, including but not limited to Chasidic, Litvish, and Modern Orthodox. Each of these subcategories has their own meaning, customs, and faith practice. Even within each of these identities, people's countries of origin will further influence the specifics of their religious practice. While each category may hold nuances of practice, identifying as "Orthodox" holds the greatest amount of religious and practical influence on the pursuit of family building.

Orthodox Judaism can be described as a practice of faith that holds tightly to the original script and scripture. The basic tenets of Orthodoxy may be similar to those of other groups within Judaism, but the main difference is in the presence of significantly more structure, and the universality or pervasiveness of religious practice and its influence in daily life.

> Judaism "defines my daily life, who I am, what I do, how I do it, how I approach everything I do… how I run my household, my family and the community is everything." (Miriam) [3]

Religious and cultural rituals impact dress, food choices, language, and family systems. The religious group subcultures with which one identifies are nuanced and will influence almost every aspect of life including where one lives and sends one's children to school. For most Orthodox families, daily life and social experiences are centered around the synagogue and the Jewish Day School communities. A religious lifestyle typically centers around families with children. It often includes numerous child-centered activities in the synagogue and community centers, as well as ceremonies related to childbirth and childrearing, making interactions within the religious community incredibly isolating for couples struggling with infertility [4].

> Ayelet, who had had several miscarriages, said, "I wish they stopped inviting me to the brit[2] parties—every time somebody I know has a boy I shiver and try to think of a pretense for not coming. It is so hard on me watching mothers with babies, and you can't really avoid questions directed at you—all these whys and whens. … Avoiding these gatherings is a kind of self-defense for me [5]".

In Orthodox communities, families will typically send their children to Jewish Day Schools from preschool through high school and often follow this with a year of study and intensive learning in Israel after graduating high school. Schools are

[2] A brit—also referred to as a brit milah or bris—is a communal ceremony in which a baby boy is circumcised, traditionally occurring on the eighth day of life.

often separated by gender from a young age, offering little to no socialization between the sexes until they reach the eligible age for formal dating with intent to marry. Modern Orthodox families sometimes vary from this practice and offer mixed-gender education for children. Men and women marry young, with a significant amount of parental involvement as they begin to live independent lives. Parents frequently participate in connecting their young adults with a potential mate and upon marriage couples usually begin to try to conceive. While there are always exceptions to this plan, and there has been an increased trend of delaying family building to ensure the security of the young couple's relationship, the standard is that couples will attempt to conceive within the first year. For guidance through all these phases and life experiences, couples will typically identify a Rabbi, always male, who will help them make decisions related to religious law.

Young couples will typically have genetic testing done in advance of dating by an organization called "Dor Yeshorim." This remarkable organization was started by parents who were Tay Sachs carriers and worked to create a system where two carriers would not marry each other [6]. This initiative has effectively eliminated Tay Sachs and several other serious inheritable diseases from the Orthodox Jewish community. The Ashkenazi panel they use will screen for fifty-two heritable diseases only. Young men and women will not be told their carrier status—only if they are deemed compatible for a potential marriage match. Many opinions exist about the value of this level of privacy or secrecy, but medical providers should be aware that the screening provided through this service is not comprehensive. While there are other Jewish testing organizations that exist across the world that offer full transparency, most Orthodox families will be using Dor Yeshorim.

Orthodox couples often have limited knowledge and exposure to sexual education in their formative years. School-based sexual education classes are rare, with most education being provided by specialists in religious law and taking place right before marriage. In Modern Orthodox communities, sexual education before marriage is sometimes taught, with a strong emphasis on abstinence-only education, as religious law prohibits sex prior to marriage. The narrow exposure to knowledge means that many have limited information about reproductive biology or how their bodies function; therefore, working with Orthodox couples will likely include psychoeducation around biology, reproduction, and fertility.

Due to the avoidance of talking about sex, some couples may lack knowledge and language for discussing these topics completely while others can feel discomfort and embarrassment while discussing reproduction and sex. In addition to the limited education, the culture has a strong emphasis on modesty and talking about sex or sexual issues like conception can be a source of distress. As counseling continues and a trusting therapeutic alliance builds, there will likely be less discomfort. However, aware providers should notice the language used by the clients, listening for misconceptions and providing psychoeducation to counter gaps in knowledge. Lack of comfort or experience with discussing sex and reproduction can at times lead providers to misunderstand the issues facing Orthodox couples who are having difficulty conceiving. As Haimov-Kochman points out:

With regard to physician-patient communication, modesty could be misinterpreted as a token of discomfort toward the discussion of physical intimacy or as a lack of accurate sexual information. Marriage at young age, avoidance of premarital sexual contacts, as well as ignorance and lack of sexual education may lead to sexual dysfunction sometimes disguised as infertility [7].

The importance of family building in the Jewish community encompasses many facets. The first and arguably the most important commandment from God to Adam is: 'Be fruitful and multiply' (Genesis 1:18). This is considered of paramount importance to an observant Jew. Rabbi Menachem Mendel Schneerson, also known as the Lubavitcher Rebbe, one of the most influential Jewish leaders of the twentieth century, used to say: "Jewish wealth is not houses and money. Jewish wealth, which is eternal, is the observance of Torah and Mitzvot (Jewish commandments) and bringing children and grandchildren into the world who will observe the Torah and its Mitzvot." [8]. When a couple can't fulfill this mitzvah[3] and expectation, it can cause isolation and scrutiny from the community. This imperative to have children can be seen in Israel's approach to infertility care: although geographically small, Israel currently holds the highest number of fertility clinics per capita in the world, and Israel's National Health Insurance Fund provides IVF treatments for up to two live births for childless couples and for women who want to become single mothers [9].

Another factor exclusive to the Jewish community is the traumatic loss of six million Jews in the Holocaust. The decimation of approximately 66% of Europe's Jewish population and the subsequent Jewish community's quest for survival and the replacement of the lost lives is often a driving force in Jewish couples' motivation for having and raising Jewish children [10]. Due to the narrative that procreation is vital for the survival of the Jewish nation, motherhood is what defines an Orthodox woman's identity and grants her place in the community [11].

The Structure of Religious Life and the Laws of Family Purity

A typical initial work-up by a reproductive endocrinologist would likely include assessment of both the female and male patients. In Jewish law, there is a prohibition on ejaculation outside of intercourse. Therefore, semen collection is a significant concern in fertility testing and avoided when possible. Consequently, Orthodox couples may prefer to test only the female partner in the first round of assessments [9]. When necessary, semen analysis is allowed with variations needed to minimize the religious law concerns. Special devices such as non-medicated condoms with a hole in them are accepted by some Rabbis as a permissible method for collecting sperm for testing [12]. Providers can encourage their patients to ask for guidance about a preferred method of collection and consult with the Rabbis if there is

[3] Often incorrectly translated as a good deed, a mitzvah is a biblical commandment from God, the fulfillment of which is a religious duty.

hesitancy about the medically preferred method. As with many aspects of religious law, although there is often a preferred method of proceeding in accordance with religious tenets, variations of interpretation and practice can be employed as needed based on the circumstances. Communication among providers, patients, and trusted religious advisors is the highest priority and value in these situations.

One of the more complex realities for religious couples is the structure of laws related to a woman's menstruation. Family Purity Laws called "Niddah"comprise instructions around physical touch around the menstrual cycle. When a woman is menstruating, the couple is not permitted to touch. The woman must count days after her menstrual flow stops; on the evening of the seventh day, she immerses herself in a ritual bath called the "Mikvah,' 'after which the couple is allowed to be intimate. When a woman is getting a regular monthly period, this creates about 2 weeks during which sexual and casual touch are allowed and about 12 days per month where they are not allowed physical contact. One of the most complex components of the laws of Niddah is unexpected bleeding or spotting between periods and the involvement of a Rabbi in determining if the couple is allowed to resume sexual intimacy or is required to separate for the required time. During fertility treatment, the rabbi and doctors will help the woman determine the origin of the bleeding, such as bleeding from an irregular period or a medical procedure, creating context to whether sexual relations are permitted [13].

As the laws of Niddah are centered around the presence of uterine bleeding, many medical procedures will place a woman "in Niddah," requiring a physical separation from her husband. A patient will likely ask her doctor about the process of each procedure, whether the uterus is opened or accessed, and whether any resultant bleeding would be uterine blood. If blood is not uterine based, it is not generally problematic for the intimate life of the couple, highlighting the importance of accuracy and details in religious life. The nature of medical care will likely not change as a result of the laws of Niddah, but the laws might impact the timing of medical procedures and highlight the importance of proactive communication with patients to determine the issues that might arise [13].

Another aspect of fertility that may be impacted by the laws of Niddah is oocyte retrieval. Oocyte retrieval and transfers must take into account the day the woman is permitted to go to the Mikvah and may be delayed accordingly with hormonal manipulations to ensure the laws are followed [14].

When in Niddah, the couple remains in the same home, eats the same meals, and shares the same relationship but without physical touch. As one can imagine, this may be a source of distress and challenge for couples, or it can be a time for the development of emotional intimacy in the relationship without touch. The inability to "kiss and make-up" after a conflict or when feeling distant forces couples to improve their communication skills and explore ways to feel close without touch. Couples are prepared for this aspect of their married life a few months before the wedding by a teacher who specializes in this area of religious law. Sometimes this education involves basic reproductive biology and function as well as information about sexual and fertility challenges, but there is no standard curriculum and the information discussed is left up to the discretion and comfort level of the teacher.

Consequently, some young couples are ill prepared for possible sexual difficulties as well as the emotional experience of infertility.

One of the most complex components of the laws of Niddah is the involvement of a Rabbi in determining if the couple is allowed to resume sexual intimacy and whether the woman is able to go to the Mikvah. For Orthodox women, this process of religious law can create a significant amount of distress, and even embarrassment, as their private physical functions are under assessment. Too often, women's distress is overlooked and not acknowledged by the teachers who are teaching these laws. Not everyone finds these experiences distressing; for some women, they are an expected part of being a newly married woman. For others, however, this involvement can feel vulnerable and even violating, depending on her history. A young woman who has experienced any kind of child sexual abuse or even one who has had limited interaction with male leadership may struggle with this experience. Strong support and compassion are helpful in managing these new experiences. Additionally, a fairly new trend of having religious women leaders trained in this area of Jewish law has helped to facilitate a way for women to seek guidance from women directly. These women hold the title of "*Yoetzet Halacha*"[4]; several communities across the USA, Canada, and Israel have female leaders who are available for consultation. This is seen as a more modern approach to religious practice and will not be accepted in some communities.

General Medical Approach to Care

The general approach for medical care for Orthodox couples facing infertility is no different than that for the general population. Each relevant medical procedure may involve its own questions or concerns related to religious law; however, there will also be solutions to make interventions work for the couple and their medical needs. Couples and religious authorities will go to all lengths to help couples achieve a healthy pregnancy. Never make the assumption that "the answer will be no" when proposing medical interventions, as you will be surprised at the creativity of the rabbis who are working with these individuals in making care accessible.

Young Married Couples Will Likely Seek Infertility Care Early in Their Relationship

Young couples who are attempting to conceive may show up in infertility clinics more quickly and at much younger ages than the general population. Couples who failed to conceive within 6 months of marriage may seek the advice of infertility

[4] Literally, "one who answers questions." In this context, the title refers to a woman who is certified in answering questions related to the law of Niddah.

specialists. The conception gap regarding the basic definition of infertility and the speed with which some couples seek treatment may lead to communication dissonance between the couple and their caregiver [9].

> People who get married are expected to get pregnant in their first year… people start looking at your stomach, thinking that you have something in there. (Rina) [3]

Physicians may question why such a young couple is seeking intervention and even question the wisdom of testing or treatment. Couples have heard the clinical team make comments such as, "just go home and enjoy your newly married life and come back in a few years," disrespecting the desire and autonomy of these couples to pursue care. When cultural norms include marrying young and having large families, the medical team's support of these choices is vital for a respectful experience. Unless there is a known concern about reproductive capacity, couples will likely be told to wait a year before seeking medical treatment when they have not conceived.

Parents of the Couple May Be Involved in Decision Making

It may surprise or even annoy the medical team when a young couple has parents involved in decision making related to the course of treatment. It is not unusual for patients to defer to parents' suggestions or to consult with them before making decisions. Part of the culture of young marriages is the ongoing emotional and often financial support that parents will provide. It is not unusual for parents to help the couple with regular financial needs as well as more significant involvement in decisions that feel particularly "grown up."

Rabbis are Likely to be an Active Party in the Decisions and Processes Related to Treatment Plans

Rabbis are also the "guardians" of the kinship ties between ART users and their resulting children to ensure that the processes of ART align with Jewish law at the highest standard, as Jewish identity is primarily claimed by birthright [15]. In the structure of Orthodox religious practice, the rabbi will contribute in varying degrees to family building decisions of couples. A rabbi can hold different functions within different families but is typically focused on guidance around religious law in terms of what is permitted and what is not. The rabbi may also play the role of consultant and provide advice or opinions on decisions that are not necessarily related to law. The rabbi may have a long-term relationship with the couple or may be chosen for his specific expertise in the laws of fertility treatment. It is common that rabbis will be asked to collaborate with the medical team to determine the best way to proceed within the construct of religious law.

> We became closer to our Rabbi because it is a much more emotional conversation… we spoke to our Rabbi about how to handle moods… and to advise us on how to protect dignity. (Rebecca) [3]

Of greatest importance is the recognition that one rabbi's opinion may not be the same as that of another rabbi. Physicians may hear conflicting opinions or even disagreements about how to proceed, which can create confusion for the medical team. Ultimately, trusting the couple is of the utmost value in this triadic relationship. They will have to be comfortable with the decision of *their* rabbi. Introducing alternatives to the religious opinions offered by the couple's trusted rabbi would be inappropriate and out of the bounds of the culturally sensitive medical team.

The Number of Desired Children Will Be Determined by the Specific Community in Which the Patient Lives

One of the challenges of working with a culture that is not your own is the need to understand the desire to have a large family. Even the definition of the word "large" takes on a new meaning when working with religious families. The family size in which you were raised is often the guiding feature of what you hope to create in your own family with your spouse. If you were raised in an Orthodox household, you imagine that family from a young age, the children with matching outfits, sitting around a Shabbat table, and the general chaos and busyness of life as your family and responsibilities grow. For many couples, it is the silence of the home that is the most profound when the family size is not what they hoped for. For others it is the constant reminder about what's missing when visiting their family of origin or going to synagogue. Asking about and noticing the spaces in their lives that are triggering is an important part of understanding how Orthodox patients see the world with a small family size.

Providers working with Orthodox patients may feel conflicted about the motivating factors behind their desired family size and may question if a woman has choice or agency in determining family size. The gap in cultural expectations between patients and their providers may impact the way clients' desires are understood and acted on. As with any strong religious community, the norms for family size are determined by the nuances within the subculture. Chasidic families are more likely to have significantly larger families, often 10–12 children on average, and the presence of a small family size often indicates "a problem" versus a choice [16–19].

One can deduce that when a couple has a smaller family, when there *have* been challenges in conceiving, it can further highlight the distress that couples experience. While the provider may not be able to fully understand the desire to have large families, ascribing it to pressure rather than choice, it is imperative for clinicians to notice the biases and opinions that may interfere with meeting the client in their own reality. It is deeply important to trust the couple in how they experience the desire to have a large family. Listening to their truth, even if it's subjective, is a critical point of alignment that is often missed when the therapist and client have different values or perspectives. Even a religious therapist can find it challenging to see the world through the eyes of a couple who have differing views or perspectives on family size. Often an individual or couple seeking support from a therapist or medical care from a physician will be met with annoyance at their desire to continue with treatments once they have a child or two, especially when the pregnancies were hard won. They are commonly told to reconsider, or to just "enjoy the ones you have" without respect for the communal norms or the couple's desire for a family that matches their hopes and dreams.

> There is an assumption I think that if people chose to have a family in the Jewish community it is very likely that it will not just be one child… I felt there was an expectation that we should have more than one child, I felt other people were expecting it of us. (Sandra) [3]

> I had a hard time … I was told at least you have one child, but they don't understand that having one makes you just stick out so much in a religious community even if you are modern and it doesn't matter how modern you are, without children you stick out. (Andrea) [3]

Birth Control Is Allowed But in Some Communities, It Will Be Discouraged Unless for Very Specific or Extreme Situations

The growth of a religiously oriented family is a significant part of a family identity. For some, decisions about family size are not typically discussed prior to marriage, with the assumption that family size will be determined naturally as the marriage continues rather than through determining a specific number of desired children in advance. The cultural norms around birth control are probably among the most misunderstood practices within the Jewish community. The myth is that birth control is forbidden and not allowed to be used by religious couples [20]. The truth is far from this. The culture of religious communities is to build families and to have children. This comes from traditional religious law and the religious obligation of men (note, not women!) to have a male and female child. This outcome is obviously not always in the control of the couple but expected norms for family building begin with this obligation and with the desire to create homes similar to the ones in their cultural community.

The limitations on birth control center around type and frequency of use. Most couples will begin married life without birth control. After the first child is born, or in case of medical necessity, a couple will seek guidance from their chosen Rabbi about the choice to use contraception and for how long. A rabbi might suggest the use of contraception for between 6 months and 2 years to prevent pregnancy with the potential to revisit the conversation as needed. The rabbi will likely guide the couple on the preferred choices that are available as well. Under usual circumstances, the intrauterine device (IUD), the vaginal ring, and oral contraceptive pills will be the choices endorsed with the least amount of hesitation [21]. All options will focus on decreasing risks of staining or spotting as the complications within religious law are many and stressful. Some couples will be encouraged to use spermicide without a barrier method, which decreases its efficacy. The diaphragm is not a common choice; condoms are the least approved option and would only be used in extreme circumstances [21].

The greater challenge with birth control usage is the related stigma or internal conflict that many women experience. The cultural pressures around family building and limited education about birth control norms and prevalence of use can lead women who use contraception to experience a sense of failure or the perception of not living up to personal or community expectations of welcoming "whatever GOD gives me" instead of listening to their own voice and needs. Only once women become willing to forego privacy to discuss the use of contraception within their own communities and begin to hear how common this practice is can they change their internal narrative of pressure, failure, and distress. Each smaller subsect within Judaism will have its own norms of use and rabbis within each sect will be more limited or expansive in their flexibility around whether and what kind of contraception is allowed.

Beyond stigma and community expectations is the reality that many women and spouses don't even ask questions about birth control and don't consult with the Rabbi about the possibility of its use. Many couples do not feel that they should be asking for a "break" by considering the option of using contraception, believing that their life circumstances have to be atypically stressful for birth control to be under consideration. This can lead to significant difficulty in persuading women to accept the help needed when struggling postpartum, as the request to use contraception may feel completely out of the bounds of their religious life experiences. Be mindful of the context of birth control use when recommending or encouraging a couple to prevent pregnancy, especially in the aftermath of a pregnancy loss. Be concrete about the physical and emotional need that you see as a medical provider and why emotional wellness is a crucial part of wellness to consider when planning for another attempt at pregnancy.

In the context of infertility treatment, the use of birth control for the purpose of regulating or preparing for a treatment cycle would not be problematic, assuming that the kind recommended is aligned with religious law.

Termination of Pregnancy and Complications

Jewish law places extreme value on human life above almost any religious obligation. This deeply held value and religious core belief impacts decisions related to organ donation, removing a person from life support, and many other complex end of life decisions. Abortion is typically not supported or endorsed, aligning with the deep foundational belief in life above all else. However, abortion has always been a complex space in religious law with differences of opinion about what is allowed. The life of the mother always holds primacy over the life of the fetus with no disagreement in rabbinic discourse [22]. If the life of the mother is at risk, the decision will be made to end the pregnancy to keep her safe. Mental health is also a significant consideration and when it is determined that a woman's emotional health is at risk if she continues the pregnancy, termination will be permitted. For women undergoing abortion care, this decision will likely bring significant distress as it feels so outside of the traditional values upholding life above all else. The need to terminate a pregnancy may bring about confusion and emotional difficulty. The recent growth in support services around abortion specifically for the Orthodox couple is creating a forum for this conversation as well as a space in which to acknowledge grief and receive the education around abortion that is so deeply needed.

When a pregnancy has a confirmed fetal anomaly, there are vast disagreements about what is permitted and what is forbidden. Some rabbis will allow termination of pregnancy when a fetus has a life-limiting diagnosis, with no specific gestational age limitations. Other rabbis do not allow for terminations under these circumstances and the pregnancy will continue [22].

Providers need to be aware that for many religious couples the idea of termination for medical reasons will feel deeply antithetical to their belief system as this is not an area of regular discussion. When facing options counseling, suggestions about termination may be met with a response of "you don't understand my faith". The decision to terminate for medical reasons will always require consultation with the patient's rabbinic authority. Of note, providers who are accustomed to options counseling may use the term "compassionate choice" when discussing the ending of a pregnancy with fetal anomalies. This idea holds no weight in the religious world as the decision is made based on religious law—what is allowed and what is not allowed rather than on emotion or feelings. Ending a pregnancy with fetal anomalies would be done in collaboration with a rabbi and typically left up to the discretion and choice of the pregnant couple.

Options for Family Development—Donor, Surrogacy

Orthodox couples who have been unsuccessful with the standard fertility treatments using their own gametes may have limited options for use of donor gametes. This is another area in religious law that comprises many different opinions. As with the non-Jewish world, the option to use donor eggs has opened up doors for religious families when there is rabbinic support. Most of the rabbis who support or allow the use of donor eggs prefer that the donor herself be Jewish according to traditional laws of matrilineal descent [5, 9, 23]. There are several Jewish donor egg banks in the United States, with limited oversight or restrictions. Many of the donors associated with these egg banks come from other countries, primarily Israel, to donate multiple times. Often couples who are using donor eggs choose not to disclose to their children with the knowledge that the current cultural norms within their communities could call into question the validity of the child's Jewish identity. Even given current ASRM recommendations and best practices related to disclosure [24, 25], this population may have concerns about the consequences of disclosure that counterbalance and even outweigh current best practice guidelines. While medicine and science allow for these options, and some rabbis permit it as well, the larger community may not be as receptive to these choices.

Sperm donation is less commonly allowed due to complex laws related to a married woman being "impregnated" by someone other than her husband [2]. Gestational surrogacy will similarly be allowed by some Orthodox subgroups and not by others. Some of the religious-based organizations that assist in fertility care funding will not financially support third party reproduction. Of utmost importance is asking the patient what would be allowed for them in their infertility journey, as they may have never considered having a conversation with their rabbi about his position on the use of donors and gestational surrogacy. Knowing what means for family building would be acceptable can be helpful for couples who are not having success with traditional fertility options. While you as a provider may be uncomfortable with the restrictions related to religious law, respecting choice and the reality of these couples needing to and wanting to live within these laws is an important part of meeting their needs.

Fertility Preservation

Considerations for fertility preservation for unpartnered women are expanding and even being supported with funding from religious organizations. There is more openness around the realities of reproductive aging, changing the conversation for many women. This may be seen as an empowered position, but it also may be filled with sadness for women who have not yet met their marriage partner in a world that prizes this relationship [26]. For men facing fertility preservation, likely due to illness, the process will be more complicated for an unmarried man, primarily because of restrictions around ejaculation outside of intercourse. Each individual will explore how best to approach these procedures through conversations with their rabbi.

Procedures in Medical Care That Have Special Consideration

Most medical procedures that involve sperm or eggs outside of the body will require a partnership with an organization that provides oversight of these procedures. Specially trained religious women will oversee the process of intrauterine insemination (IUI) and sperm treatments, egg retrievals and fertilization, and the thawing of embryos and transfers. The term for this process is "*hashgacha,*" and these individuals are there to add a layer of protection against mistakes that could have catastrophic outcomes for couples. There are no religious blessings and no traditions associated with hashgacha, only oversight to ensure that the correct eggs, sperm, and embryos are being created and transferred. "In IVF clinics dealing with orthodox Jewish patients, Orthodox women called "*mashgichot*",[5] are present in the clinics. They observe the laboratory technicians to make sure that the correct sperm and correct egg are being united – so as not to produce a *mamzer*, or an illegitimate child" [27, 28]. Any lab working with a religious couple will need to allow these trained individuals laboratory access, and at times access to the procedure room during retrievals and transfers, for the purpose of patient care.

Themes in Therapy

While each person's experience of infertility will be unique, many religious individuals will likely express similar themes in therapy. Strong, religiously focused communities tend to create a fishbowl effect, especially when differences are obvious to others. If the norm is to have children quickly after marriage, then not having children exposes a couple to the scrutiny and opinions of others. The emotional experience of standing out in a crowd is particularly highlighted in this communal space. Religious life requires engagement in synagogue services and activities. As the fertility struggle persists, it becomes increasingly difficult to continue to participate in spaces that have children everywhere and experience the sermons and activities that are family focused [29].

> In the Jewish community, specifically where we are, there is such a pressure to have kids that people want to have many more kids… some people would feel pressured to have more kids… as much as you try not to focus on it all the time and when you are going through it, everywhere you look there is someone with a buggy or someone pregnant or some other event. (Ana) [3]

Couples may also feel the pressure and responsibility of ensuring Jewish continuity and the continuation of legacy and heritage, especially in the aftermath of the Holocaust and the decimation of so many families. The imperative to rebuild what was lost is a common experience for the younger generations. This imperative may not be presented as an overt message, but it remains a strong and powerful subtle one.

For any individual experiencing infertility, isolation and disconnection from peers and family deeply impact their social experience. When living in a religious community, this aspect of the lived experience is particularly difficult to navigate as the focus of those around you is mostly about family life. As the peer group quickly builds families, the absence of people at the same stage of life but without children becomes more apparent and more lonely, leaving couples in the in-between space of being married but with limited friends who share current life experiences.

> Although I know it's not my fault, I can't help feeling inferior to other women. It's only a few close friends whom I told about this, and my parents of course. ...I did not tell it to people I work with since I don't want to hear their words of sympathy and tons of free

[5] This word, used here in the feminine version of the plural, means "supervisors" or "overseers."

advice—where to seek treatment, what other women did in this situation, etc. I am sure they will feel superior since they are all mothers and I am not." Miri [3]

Childlessness means that during holidays, when families gather multiple times a year, the emotional pressures and exhaustion are highlighted. Orthodox Jewish traditional holidays mean multiple days and meals with extended families. Couples will express the anxiety of going home to their parents and worrying about how much they can tolerate sitting around the table with their pregnant siblings or their nieces and nephews for several days. The absence is made louder when their younger siblings have children first, being the first to claim the treasured grandparent's name or making their parents grandparents for the first time. Holidays are often deeply focused on the transmission of spiritual legacy and education to the next generation, creating a greater sense of absence, of missed purpose, and helplessness for the childless couple [29].

My husband has four siblings that have gotten married since we got married and three of them have kids and the one that got married last year has also had a baby since then and this is quite pressuring and they all live here as well. So, when we get together every Shabbat at my in-laws, for Hannukah or this or that party, it's always about the kids and you feel a bit left out.—Maya [3]

For religious couples, the experience of infertility opens up conversations around aspects of their lives that would typically be considered immodest to discuss with others. Infertility means opening up about sexual issues, sexual practices, and schedules for mikvah, all of which would typically be treated as private matters. Especially for more sheltered couples, these conversations are particularly complex and often intermingle with shame and discomfort. "I shouldn't be talking about these things" is a common refrain in the therapy space, as patients may hold a general feeling of being inappropriate when discussing these issues. Even if the therapist has a high comfort level, the clients may need to take more time developing a comfort level that allows for conversation and expression. For example, the mikvah experience is prized as a spiritual refresh and beautiful experience for a woman. Fertility challenges mean that often this experience becomes associated with anger, disappointment, hopelessness, and frustration about having to go month after month when pregnancy does not occur. It may feel inappropriate for a woman to express her true feelings about mikvah, and patients may need prompting to explore the distress that is often experienced but feels wrong to share.

Resources for the Religious Community

The religious Jewish community is incredibly well resourced when facing life's challenges. There are organizations like A TIME and Yesh Tikva to support couples impacted by infertility, with support groups that are specific to the parents of the couple, male factor, female factor, genetic issues, failed cycles, and other topics.

Knafayim is an organization focusing exclusively on pregnancy and reproductive losses.

With the cultural and religious expectations to grow families, several organizations exist within the Jewish world that help fund fertility treatment, most notably Bonei Olam. These organizations will have criteria that couples will be required to meet prior to qualifying for funding and most funding is exclusively for primary infertility. While there is some overlap, the community has created multiple means of support and creative networks to raise awareness, sensitivity, and support. These programs are nuanced and culturally specific to the Orthodox individual, increasing comfort levels and access points. Collaboration with these organizations is an important community partnership that any reproductive endocrinology practice serving the religious community should develop. Affiliated providers should also be aware of these resources and have them available to share with patients who may benefit from their support.

Conclusion

To be an Orthodox Jew is to be a part of a huge community of family. To be Orthodox is to be networked across states and languages with the unifying identity of beliefs and faith practice. To be Orthodox is to know that someone actually cares about the difficult life experience you are facing; there may even be a nonprofit that's already functioning to offer you connection and support. To be an Orthodox, Jew means that family holds a very high priority and having children is deeply rooted in this priority and identity. To be Orthodox without children leaves a couple feeling disconnected from the future and continuity of the family. To be without children is a lonely and difficult space to sit as an Orthodox Jew.

While this chapter discusses the therapeutic themes of the Orthodox Jewish couple facing infertility, one can easily and appropriately expand the content to working with other religious populations. The specifics of cultural and spiritual practice will be different, but the broader experience of living in a cultural space that emphasizes family growth, where there is strong interdependence between young couples and their parents, and where there is a cultural narrative that is full of expectation both inside the family as well as in the community, transcends the specific practices of Judaism and is equally relevant to individuals and couples in other communities where childbearing is both prized and viewed as a cultural expectation. Guiding principles of increased curiosity, attentive communication and clarification, and minimizing assumptions based on media influences will help support both therapists and medical providers in navigating infertility care with these individuals.

References

1. Ribner DS, Rosenbaum TY. Evaluation and treatment of unconsummated marriages among orthodox Jewish couples. J Sex Marital Ther. 2005;31:341–53.
2. Silber S. Infertility, IVF and Judaism. In: Rizk B, Garcia-Velasco J, Sallam H, Makrigiannakis A, editors. Infertility and assisted reproduction. Cambridge University Press; 2008. p. 728–31.
3. Mouyal, Alegria. Hidden voices: orthodox Jewish women and infertility; 2021.
4. Weizmann G. (2009) "Give me children or else I dead": Orthodox Jewish perspectives on fertility. In: Blyth E, Landau R, editors. Faith and fertility: attitudes towards reproductive practices in different religions from ancient to modern times. London: Jessica Kingsley Publishers; 2009. p. 205–24.
5. Remennick L. Childless in the land of imperative motherhood: Stigma and coping among infertile Israeli women. Sex Roles J Res. 2000;43(11–12):821–41. https://doi.org/10.1023/A:1011084821700.
6. Our Mission. Dor Yeshorim. Available from: https://doryeshorim.org/our-mission/.
7. Haimov-Kochman R, Rosenak D, Orvieto R, Hurwitz A. Infertility counseling for Orthodox Jewish couples. Fertil Steril. 2010;93(6):1816–9. https://doi.org/10.1016/j.fertnstert.2008.03.025.
8. Hayom Yom Nissan 9. Menachem Mendel Schneerson. Available from: https://www.chabad.org/therebbe/article_cdo/aid/6151/jewish/Hayom-Yom-Nissan-9.htm.
9. Schenker JG. Assisted reproductive practice: religious perspectives. RBM Online. 2005;3:310.
10. Gold M. And Hannah wept. Philadelphia: The Jewish Publication Society; 1988.
11. Berkowitch N. Motherhood as a national mission: the construction of womanhood in the legal discourse in Israel. Women's Studies Int Forum. 1997;20(5–6):605–19.
12. Sallam HN, Sallam NH. Religious aspects of assisted reproduction. Facts Views Vis Obgyn. 2016;8(1):33–48.
13. Shenker JS. Religious aspects of reproduction. In: Seibel MM, editor. Infertility: a comprehensive text. Stanford, CT: Appleton & Lange; 1997.
14. Reichman DE, Brauer AA, Goldschlag D, Schattman G, Rosenwaks Z. In vitro fertilization for Orthodox Jewish couples: antagonist cycle modifications allowing for mikveh attendance before oocyte retrieval. Fertil Steril. 2013;99:1408–12.
15. Ivry T. Kosher Medicine and Medicalized Halacha: an exploration of triadic relations among Israeli Rabbis, doctors and infertility Patients. Am Ethnol. 2010;37(4):662–80.
16. Kasstan B. Making bodies Kosher. The politics of reproduction among Haredi Jews in England. Fertility, reproduction and sexuality. Berghahn Books, New York and Oxford Publishing; 2019.
17. Taragin-Zeller L. "Conceiving god's children": toward a flexible model of reproductive decision-making. Med Anthropol. 2019;38(4):370–83.
18. Birenbaum-Carmeli D. Your faith or mine—family planning intervention in an ultra-orthodox Jewish community in Israel. Reprod Health Matters. 2018;16(32):185–91.
19. Teman E, Ivry T, Bernhardt BA. Pregnancy as a proclamation of faith: Ultra-Orthodox Jewish women navigating the uncertainty of pregnancy and prenatal diagnosis. Am J Med Genet. 2011;155:69–80.
20. Mayer YJ. I'm an Orthodox med student. My community needs real sex education. The Forward; 2021 [cited 2024 Aug 8]. Available from: https://forward.com/opinion/480106/im-an-orthodox-med-student-my-community-needs-real-sex-education/#:~:text=Currently%2C%20we%20entrust%20the%20sex,in%20traditional%20pre%2Dmarriage%20classes.
21. Meyers MR, Tenfelde SM. Providing culturally sensitive evidence-based care for Orthodox Jewish women. December 2022. npwomenshealthcare.com.
22. Stadlan N. Abortion from the perspective of orthodox Judaism. In: Abortion: global positions and practices, religious and legal perspectives; 2021. p. 23–35.
23. Silber S. Infertility, IVF and Judaism. In: Rizk B, Garcia-Velasco J, Sallam H, Makrigiannakis A, editors. Infertility and assisted reproduction. Cambridge University Press; 2008. p. 728–73.

24. Practice Committee of the American Society for Reproductive Medicine, Practice Committee for the Society for Assisted Reproductive Technology. Guidance regarding gamete and embryo donation. Fertil Steril. 2021;115(6):1395–410.
25. ESHRE Working Group on Reproductive Donation, Kirkman-Brown J, Calhaz-Jorge C, Dancet EA, Lundin K, Martins M, Tilleman K, Thorn P, Vermeulen N, Frith L. Good practice recommendations for information provision for those involved in reproductive donation. Hum Reprod Open. 2022;2022(1):hoac001.
26. Birenbaum-Carmeli D, Inhorn MC, Vale MD, Patrizio P. Cryopreserving Jewish motherhood: egg freezing in Israel and the United States. Medical Anthropol Quart. 2021;35(3):346–63.
27. Kahn SM. Reproducing Jews: a cultural account of assisted conception in Israel; 2000.
28. Wahrzman MZ. Jewish medical ethics: assisted reproduction and Judaism. Jewish Virtual Library; 1997.
29. Kohane I. Empty cribs: infertility challenges for orthodox jewish couples. (Doctoral dissertation, Antioch University); 2020.

Chapter 11
Catholic Patients and Reproductive Healthcare

Danielle A. Kaplan

Alice and Jeremy are a married couple who have been trying to conceive for 18 months. Alice is a practicing Catholic and Jeremy was raised in the Catholic church but currently does not consider himself religious. Alice attended a conservative Catholic high school, where she grew up hearing that IVF was against the teachings of the Church and that having a baby was a gift from God rather than a right. Nevertheless, she attends an initial consultation with an REI and is surprised to learn that her antral follicle count is high and her bloodwork is similarly encouraging. The REI informs her that she and Jeremy are good candidates for success with IVF and tells the couple that "you might not need to do too many retrievals to get a good number of embryos." The REI is surprised to see that although Jeremy looks encouraged, Alice seems increasingly troubled as the consultation progresses. Alice and Jeremy do not make a follow-up appointment and ultimately do not pursue treatment at the clinic.

What cultural factors might have influenced Alice and Jeremy's decision making? What alternatives could the REI have offered the couple to increase their comfort with treatment? What options are open to Alice and Jeremy if they decide not to pursue IVF?

Introduction

An estimated 1.375 billion people worldwide identify as Catholic. Of these, approximately 7% live in the United States, where they represent about 24% of the US population. Internationally, the largest numbers of self-identified Catholics live in

D. A. Kaplan (✉)
Department of Psychiatry, NYU Langone Medical Center, New York, NY, USA

D. A. Kaplan (ed.), *Cultural Responsiveness in Assisted Reproductive Technology*, https://doi.org/10.1007/978-3-031-76204-8_11

Latin America and the Caribbean, with the most rapidly growing Catholic populations located in sub-Saharan Africa[1] [1, 2]. Catholicism comprises adherents of all races, ethnicities, genders, and sexual orientations.

Unlike other major world religions, Catholicism has a hierarchical structure, with the Pope serving as the titular, spiritual, and doctrinal head of the Church and nonclerical adherents to the faith at the bottom of the hierarchy. Regardless of their geographic location and their position in the hierarchy, adherents to the Catholic religion are bound by canon law, a body of law drawn from scripture, decisions made by ecclesiastical councils, and papal decrees [3]. Thus, all Catholics are exposed to some degree to the same Church doctrines on reproductive health and fertility care. As will be discussed below, there is often a striking disjunction between Church teachings and the actual reproductive health practices of Catholics, regardless of their level of self-professed religious adherence. For some practicing Catholics facing reproductive health choices, Church doctrine may limit their options and increase their sense of isolation. For others, Catholicism can serve as both a source of comfort and a framework for decision-making. This chapter aims to discuss the complexities of reproductive health and infertility for Catholic patients in the hopes that providers can better support these patients in any of their reproductive health choices.

Contraception and Abortion

The Catholic Church views heterosexual marriage—the only relationship within which sexual intercourse is permissible—as a relationship with both unitive and procreative ends. In other words, the Church "teaches that it is necessary that each and every marriage act remain ordered per se to the procreation of human life" [4]. All contraceptive and sterilization practices except for Natural Family Planning, which involves charting of cervical mucus and basal body temperature to identify windows of peak fertility [5] are therefore considered inconsistent with Church teachings.

There is a consistent and striking contrast between the Church's views on birth control and abortion and the actual practices of Catholics in these areas. A recent Guttmacher Institute survey suggests that 99% percent of self-identified Catholics in the USA practice some form of birth control other than the rhythm method, with 25% using permanent contraceptive methods, 15% using long-acting reversible contraception such as intrauterine devices (IUDs), and 25% using hormonal contraception [6]. Notably, the disparity between religious self-identification and contraceptive choices dates back at least to the mid-1960s, when methods of oral contraception became widely available. An early study on nonconformity to

[1] For completists and trivia fans, it must be noted that the country with the highest percentage of Catholic citizens is Vatican City, a nation of 800 inhabitants of whom 100% are Catholic.

Catholic teachings on birth control documented a 49% rate of contraceptive use among practicing Catholic women in 1965, a percentage that jumped to 65% in 1970. This led the authors to conclude that Catholic women of all ages and levels of education and church attendance were "increasingly just ignoring Church teaching on birth control" [7 , p. 42].

Similarly, the Catholic Church has had a longstanding philosophical prohibition on abortion. The question of abortion was first addressed by the Church as early as the first century; however, definitions of abortion and its consequences varied greatly over time, with the termination of pregnancy variously considered to represent the end of life, the deprivation of property of a husband by his wife, and a crime to be judged by God but not by the courts [8]. The current Church's position of absolute prohibition of abortion as a violation of the sanctity of life was ultimately codified into canon law in 1917 [9].

In spite of the absolute Church prohibition on abortion, the relationship between religiosity and support for abortion among practicing Catholics is complex [10]. In a 2022 study conducted by the Pew Research Center, there was an inverse relationship between the frequency with which participants attended Mass and their support for legal abortion, with only 30% of those who attended Mass once a week or more supporting abortion in all or some cases. Overall, however, over three-quarters of US Catholics surveyed supported some form of legal abortion, endorsing the procedure when a pregnancy threatens the pregnant person's life or health or is the result of rape, or if the abortion is performed in the early stages of pregnancy. In the same survey, 13% of practicing Catholics supported legal abortion without exception [11]. Similarly, the majority of US Catholic voters in the 2020 election opposed efforts to overturn *Roe v Wade*, citing the personal nature of the decision to continue or terminate a pregnancy [12].

The discrepancy between Church teaching on abortion and the attitudes of practicing Catholics is also evident in self-reported behavior. In a 2020 survey, 24% of the people presenting for abortion care self-identified as Roman Catholic [6]. Related data suggest that Catholic women are as likely to have abortions as women from any other religious group [13]. The majority of US Catholics of all racial and ethnic groups also indicate that they are likely to support a friend or family member who chooses abortion care [14, 15].

The studies cited here pertain primarily to self-identified Catholics in the United States. Uptake of reproductive health options including contraception and abortion vary widely on an international basis, with variations in the legality and availability of reproductive health services in predominantly Catholic countries worldwide. However, recent studies conducted in Mexico, Poland, and the Philippines suggest similarly increasing rates of uptake of contraceptive technology among Catholics, the majority of whom appear to support contraceptive use and the termination of pregnancy under certain circumstances either for themselves or for their reproductive-aged children [16–18].

Access to Care

In the United States, an estimated one in six hospital beds are located in Catholic hospitals [19]. Close to 40% of all reproductive-age women in the US live in counties with a high Catholic hospital market share [20]. The religious affiliation of the setting in which patients receive reproductive healthcare may influence both the nature and quality of the care they receive.

In a survey of OB-GYN residency directors at Catholic hospitals, all directors surveyed reported that their programs provided adequate training in contraceptive care [19]. However, medical students who completed rotations in obstetrics and gynecology at Catholic hospitals scored lower on structured clinical exams assessing their competency in contraceptive counseling, suggesting that their academic knowledge was not complemented by sufficient clinical encounters to achieve competency [21]. Similarly, training programs at Catholic hospitals were more likely to report poor abortion training by ACGME standards, with one-third of programs offering this training as an elective rather than a requirement and the majority arranging for clinical experience in providing abortions by partnering with off-site facilities [22]. Up to one-fifth of directors of programs affiliated with Catholic hospitals reported that their program had received citations for failing to provide residents with the required amount of abortion training [19].

The limitations to contraceptive training and care provided in Catholic healthcare settings have direct implications for the patients who seek treatment there. Women surveyed about their reproductive healthcare experiences at faith-based hospitals reported that they were often unaware of the limitations to the care that they would be provided. Further, they reported that a lack of explicit information on hospital websites and marketing materials made it difficult to research restrictions on care in advance of their treatment [23]. Restrictions on reproductive care are inconsistent across Catholic-affiliated institutions and the specific nature of the care that is sought. Thus, patients of reproductive age who are treated in healthcare settings with a Catholic affiliation may be exposed to different information about and options for reproductive healthcare, including postpartum contraception and abortion care, without being aware of the wide disparities in treatment options that exist [24, 25].

Notably, however, limited access to reproductive healthcare for patients in Catholic healthcare settings may not extend to infertility treatment. In a survey of OB-GYN clinics affiliated with Catholic and non-Catholic hospitals, the religious affiliation of the clinic did not have a significant impact on the range of infertility services offered, with only two of the practices surveyed citing religious affiliation as the reason for denial of infertility services. Among those practices offering infertility evaluations and ovulation induction, the methods of infertility treatment that are deemed acceptable by the Church, Catholic hospital affiliation did not prevent clinics from offering services to same-sex couples [25]. These findings led the researchers to conclude that practitioners in Catholic healthcare settings may view some infertility treatment as consistent with the "pro-life" doctrine of the Church and that these clinics are more likely to follow a policy of antidiscrimination than they are to adhere to doctrinal teachings about same-sex family building.

IVF and Associated Treatments

The Catholic Church places an emphasis on procreation, with conception and childrearing seen as integral to the lifecycle of a family and as the ultimate reflection of God's love. The Church professes a particular compassion for couples experiencing infertility, with as many as 21 different saints being viewed as providing intercession for infertile individuals and couples [26, 27]. However, the Catholic doctrine on infertility is best summarized as "Yes to Life, No to IVF" [28]. Although Church doctrine supports medical intervention with the goal of enhancing fertility, its support is limited to those interventions that take place solely within the body of the patient. For example, doctrinal support can be found for general medical evaluation for infertility, medications that treat ovulatory dysfunction, and surgical intervention to alleviate tubal blockage, sometimes referred to as NaPro technology [28]. Even within the guidelines laid out by the Church for allowable technologies and interventions, there are specific modifications suggested to adhere to the principles laid out in these doctrinal instructions. For example, urologists obtaining a semen specimen for a male-factor infertility workup might instruct Catholic patients to ejaculate into a condom during vaginal intercourse rather than masturbating [29].

The official opposition of the Catholic Church to fertility treatment extends to the use of intrauterine insemination (IUI), IVF, gestational surrogacy, and donor gametes. The objections of the Church were articulated in 1987 in the Domus Vitae (Respect for Human Life in its Origin and on the Dignity of Procreation) and reaffirmed in the Dignitas Personae (The Dignity of a Person) in 2008 [30]. These objections follow three primary lines of reasoning. The first is the perceived inextricability of procreative activity (i.e., fertilization) from unitive activity (i.e., heterosexual intercourse). Thus, any conception that is divorced from the sexual act itself is viewed as a severing of two functions that are meant to be inseparable. Church teachings also consider human life to begin at fertilization; thus, the creation of embryos that may not be selected for transfer or are subject to medical intervention through preimplantation genetic testing is seen as violating the sanctity of life even as it aims to create it. Finally, Church doctrine objects to what it classifies as the commodification of reproduction through ART, the use of donor gametes, and gestational surrogacy, which it contrasts with the right of the child "to be the fruit of the specific act of the conjugal love of his parents" [28, p. 452].

By extension, it should be noted that the Church's position on reproductive technology definitionally excludes all but cisgender, heterosexual couples from reproduction. This prohibition continues despite recent instructions from Pope Francis allowing baptism for transgender men and women and priestly blessings for same-sex couples [31]. Despite its resounding objections to the use of most reproductive technology, however, it is the position of the Catholic Church that Catholics who avail themselves of these treatments and the children born from them are welcomed wholeheartedly into the community of the church and can participate fully in church sacraments.

GIFT

Although Catholic doctrine does not support the use of IVF, some interpretations of Church teachings support the use of GIFT, or Gamete Intrafallopian Transfer. In this procedure, eggs are retrieved, mixed with sperm, and placed in the fallopian tubes in the hopes of achieving fertilization [32]. In the empirical literature, data on the prevalence and outcomes of GIFT are often intermingled with those from other procedures involving oocyte retrieval, including zygote intrafallopian transfer (ZIFT) and IVF [33–35]. Clear information about the frequency with which this procedure is currently used is therefore difficult to obtain, though advances in IVF technology mean that this is an increasingly rare method of treatment that is not currently offered in the majority of IVF clinics. However, some Catholic patients who have sought out information on reproductive technology that is consistent with the teachings of the Church might be aware of this method of medically aided conception, and a discussion of the reasons that it is rarely offered in practice might be indicated [36].

Disposition of Supernumerary Embryos

Infertility patients who have completed their desired family building through IVF are often faced with the choice of what to do with supernumerary embryos. Options for embryo disposition include thawing and discarding, maintaining them in perpetual cryostorage, donating them for research, or donating them to another individual or couple for transfer [37]. Some patients may also seek religious burial for their embryos through a private organization or by contacting a local Catholic cemetery.

From a Catholic perspective, the donation of supernumerary embryos for use by other infertile individuals or couples represents a clash of ethical principles. Viewed from one angle, donating embryos might appear to be a preferable alternative to discarding them or donating them to research, both of which run counter to the Catholic teaching that embryos are a form of unborn life [28]. At the same time, however, the official Church position on the donation of embryos is that this practice encourages the creation of embryos through IVF. Thus, official Catholic teaching frowns on embryo donation as representing a tacit endorsement of technology that the Church considers unacceptable.

Limited data exist on the decisions that Catholic infertility patients actually make regarding embryo disposition. One recent study of factors influencing patients' ultimate decision-making about donating embryos to recipient parents (as opposed to their intentions at the time of embryo creation) suggests that religiosity is one of many factors influencing patients' decisions regarding embryo donation, and that it interacts in a complex way with other factors such as concerns about children conceived via embryo donation being raised in other families, concerns about anonymity, and beliefs about the similarities between embryo donation and adoption [38]. Other data [39] suggest that patients who identified as Catholic were significantly more likely to discard their supernumerary embryos than they were to donate them for research, a finding that is perhaps consistent with the official Church caution against the comingling of reproduction and technology.

Compassionate Transfer

Compassionate transfer refers to the transfer of potentially viable embryos when pregnancy is not the desired outcome. It involves the transfer of the embryos at a time or to a location in the patient's body (for example, the cervix, endometrium, or vagina) that is unlikely to result in pregnancy [40]. Some Catholic patients who have completed their family building may consider this a more ethical alternative than the discarding of cryopreserved embryos. Further, there remains some minority of IVF clinics in which the thawing and discarding of embryos is not offered as an option due to the clinic's own religious affiliation or interpretation of ethical practices in embryo disposition [41].

Although compassionate transfer has long been acknowledged as a theoretical alternative to discarding supernumerary embryos or maintaining them in perpetual cryopreservation, access to this option in practice is far from universal. In a 2018 survey, 45% of REIs reported having offered this option for embryo disposition to a patient. Significantly more, however, cited a lack of perceived demand for this option and indicated that they would be willing to offer compassionate transfer if they perceived it as consistent with patient desires and ASRM guidance [42].

It should also be noted that despite the intention to transfer embryos with suboptimal timing or placement for pregnancy, clinical pregnancies and subsequent live births have been known to occur as a result of compassionate transfer [41]. REIs are advised to counsel individuals and couples who have completed their desired family building that compassionate transfer may be available as an alternative to embryo disposal. Patients should also be informed that this option may require the transfer of embryos to a clinic where the procedure is available. Finally, however, all patients should also be informed of the possibility of a resultant pregnancy and the need to make decisions related to this outcome.

For all patients, but particularly for those whose faith impacts the ways that they view the status of the embryo, a discussion of the possibility of supernumerary embryos should occur prior to the initiation of treatment. Providers should also consider introducing the possibility of cycles in which some of the oocytes retrieved are used in embryo creation and some cryopreserved for possible future use, thereby decreasing the likelihood that patients will be faced with choices for embryo disposition that are inconsistent with their religious beliefs.

Catholic patients—and, indeed, all patients—who do find themselves with supernumerary embryos will require decisional support in clarifying their desires for disposition. Interactive decisional aids such as the one developed by VARTA [43] can help patients articulate their beliefs about the status and meaning of their embryos and arrive at clearer preferences for their ultimate disposition. It should be noted that patients' conceptualization of their embryos can change throughout the process of fertility treatment and subsequent parenting of a living child, suggesting that counseling at the time of embryo creation alone is likely to be insufficient to support patients at the time when decisions about disposition are ultimately made [44].

Psychosocial Considerations in Working with Catholic Infertility Patients

Across most major world religions, religiosity is associated with an increased desire to bear children and an increase in desired and actual family size [45–47]. In this context, infertility is seen as both a painful event at the individual level and one that can isolate the couple from the larger community. For Catholic patients, the primary importance placed on procreation and the Church prohibition on many fertility treatments can create a "double bind [in which devout Catholics] face pressures from society and their religious community to have children, but… feel judged by their Church community and isolated from secular society for refusing ARTs" [48, p. 726]. Many devout Catholic women describe feeling alienated from their church communities by religious leaders' silence around infertility from the pulpit and fear that their childlessness will be viewed by other members of the congregation as a sign that they are using contraception.

Catholic patients who do choose to pursue IVF may differ from members of other religious groups in their beliefs and concerns about fertility treatment. In a survey of patients receiving treatment at a Midwestern fertility clinic, Catholic patients were significantly more likely than their nonreligious counterparts to worry that fertility treatment would result in miscarriage, ectopic pregnancy, or birth defects. They were also more likely to report that pursuing infertility treatment violated their religious beliefs and that infertility would compromise their relationship with their partner [49]. The differences in Catholic patients' beliefs and concerns about ART suggest that even those who make the decision to pursue IVF could benefit from psychoeducation about the risks and probabilities of adverse outcomes. Practitioners should offer their patients a chance to freely express all doubts and concerns and be mindful of times when patients would benefit from referral to a qualified mental health professional or an appropriate cultural broker to discuss their feelings related to beginning treatment.

The culturally aware practitioner should also take note of the fact that presentation for treatment at a fertility clinic does not indicate that all Catholic patients have entirely resolved their moral and relational qualms about pursuing treatment. Catholic patients who do pursue IVF may find that their ability to disclose their treatment to their family and community is limited by the anticipation of stigma and judgment [48]. One patient poignantly described being visited at home by a cousin during her pregnancy and purging all evidence of treatment from her apartment, hiding sharps containers and medication vials and taking down the picture of the embryo given to her at transfer, which she had hopefully displayed on the refrigerator.

For religious Catholic patients who experience a pregnancy loss after conceiving via ART, there may be an additional layer of complexity to their grief. Having already struggled to reconcile their decision to undergo ART treatment with the doctrines of their faith, patients may struggle with the question of whether their loss was a punishment for having engaged in treatment that was not supported by their religion. They may also differ in the degree to which they find comfort in pursuing traditional Catholic sacraments, such as baptism and religious burial, to commemorate the loss of the pregnancy [50].

Different Patients, Different Choices: Choosing Not to Pursue IVF

The information available on Catholic patients and IVF is, of course, limited to the self-identified Catholics who have decided that pursuing ART is consistent with their religious beliefs, or that their desire to have a family overrides their desire to act in a manner consistent with Church teaching. As one researcher points out, "those who are most conflicted about ARTs never make it to the clinic, or leave" [48], p. 46]. However, there is a subset of Catholic men and women experiencing infertility who eschew IVF as inconsistent with their moral and religious beliefs. Their experiences serve as a useful reminder that for some infertility patients across religions, coping with and integrating infertility is not achieved solely through the use of ART. A comprehensive discussion of Catholics and infertility should therefore include both patients who pursue ART and recognition of those patients experiencing infertility who choose to cope with the diagnosis through other means.

The positive impact of religiosity on perceived social support and well-being has been extensively documented. Individuals who are higher in religiosity generally report improved coping with stressful life events as diverse as cancer, being diagnosed with HIV, and natural disasters [51–54]. Even absent a period of acute crisis, religiosity is associated with improved mental and physical health outcomes across multiple domains [55, 56]. Studies have demonstrated a correlation between religiosity and improved cardiovascular functioning, decreased rates of hospitalization, and lower levels of self-reported pain [57–59]. Although findings on the mental health benefits of religiosity are mixed, there is some support for the idea that participation in public religious events such as church services and communal celebrations is associated with an increase in self-reported psychological well-being [60]. Higher levels of religiosity have also been associated with lower levels of substance abuse, depression, and suicidality, and can serve as a buffer against post-traumatic stress [61, 62].

The connection between spirituality and religiosity and improved health outcomes is the product of many possible pathways. Some authors have proposed a relationship between religiosity and virtues like altruism, gratitude, and forgiveness. Others point to the behavioral correlates of religiosity, including prohibitions on substance use, adherence to health-promoting behaviors, and participation in communal gatherings, all of which have direct implications for mental health and functioning. Finally, spirituality and religiosity provide adherents to a faith with a framework within which to make meaning from adverse events [63]. The literature on spirituality and coping provides a useful starting point in understanding the experiences of Catholics experiencing infertility who do not choose ART.

For many religious women, infertility can evoke a crisis of faith and the sense of having been betrayed or abandoned by God. For others, however, spirituality can provide a useful source of support. Engaging with spiritual beliefs and practices can help with the process of grieving and integrating an infertility diagnosis—as well as with strengthening marital connections [64]. In one study [65], spiritual coping was associated with improved well-being among women with a POI diagnosis, with most of the benefit deriving from the ability to use spiritual beliefs to make meaning from the diagnosis.

For Catholic women who choose not to pursue IVF, the belief that infertility is part of God's plan for them informs their treatment choices and reaffirms their commitment to Church teachings. Seen in this light, the decision not to pursue IVF or other medicalized technologies is viewed as a moral choice to resist the commodification and technologization of pregnancy through infertility treatment. Belief in Catholic doctrine can also help infertile individuals and couples find meaning in their suffering. In contrast to those espousing the medical model, in which "suffering is not something to be understood, but something to be conquered" [66, p. 173], devout Catholic women who chose not to pursue IVF "not only [find] their suffering meaningful but also [critique] the notion that all suffering should be avoided" [67. p. 39]. Devout Catholics experiencing infertility may also use their faith to reconceptualize motherhood, a process that Czarnecki [67] refers to as the construction of "moral femininity." In interviews with devout Catholic women who decided against pursuing IVF, Czarnecki identified the decision not to use ART as a way in which Catholic women strengthened their sense of self-worth in the face of infertility. By focusing on their marriages, extended families, and alternatives to biological kinship like adoption, these women were able to construct a narrative in which infertility served to reaffirm rather than challenge their identity as devout Catholics.

Summary and Conclusions

Catholicism provides its adherents with a clear set of guidelines on reproductive healthcare, including contraception, abortion, and technology to aid in procreation. Practicing Catholics, however, vary widely in the degree to which they follow these guidelines. The culturally aware practitioner should be cognizant of the areas in which the services they offer may be inconsistent with the limitations imposed by Church teachings and of the concerns that may impact Catholic patients' uptake of available services. Attention should also be paid to supporting Catholic IVF patients in their decision-making regarding embryo creation and the disposition of supernumerary embryos, both of which may be influenced by religiously derived beliefs about the nature of the embryo.

Additional awareness of and research into the experiences of devout Catholics whose reproductive health choices are heavily informed by Church doctrine is also needed. For these patients, addressing infertility may require practitioners to adopt a stance that is focused on support and the provision of alternative options rather than achieving pregnancy through ART. Care providers should also be aware of the complex role of faith in relation to infertility, contributing as it does in some cases to stigma and isolation and in others providing patients with solace and meaning. It is hoped that an increased awareness of the issues faced by Catholics making reproductive healthcare decisions will help practitioners approach all their patients, regardless of their ultimate treatment choices, with increased understanding and compassion.

References

1. N.A. Highest Catholic Population 2024 [Internet]. World Population Review. https://worldpopulationreview.com/country-rankings/highest-catholic-population. Accessed 23 Mar 2024.
2. Agencia Fides. Vatican, Catholic Church Statistics 2023 [Internet]. Agencia Fides. https://www.fides.org/en/news/74319VATICAN_CATHOLIC_CHURCH_STATISTICS_2023. Accessed 23 Mar 2024.
3. Cornell Law School Legal Information Institute. Canon Law [Internet]. Cornell.edu. https://www.law.cornell.edu/wex/canon_law#:~:text=Canon%20law%20originated%20as%20a,well%20as%20secular%20Roman%20law. Accessed 14 Feb 2024.
4. US Catholic Church. Catechism of the Catholic Church. Image; 2003.
5. Obelenienė B, Narbekovas A, Juškevičius J. Anthropological and methodical differences of natural family planning and fertility awareness–based methods. Linacre Q. 2021;88(1):14–23.
6. Jones RK. People of all religions use birth control and have abortions. Guttmacher Institute; 2020.
7. Westoff CF, Bumpass L. The revolution in birth control practices of US Roman Catholics. Science. 1973;179(4068):41–4.
8. Ciobanu P. INCURRUNT IN EXCOMMUNICATIONEM: brief history of canonic punishment of abortion. Dialog Teologic. 2020;23(46):18.
9. Přibyl S. Human person in the Code of Canon Law of John Paul II. Philosophy Canon Law. 2021;2(7):1–9.

10. Murawski CM. Diverse religious perspectives on abortion politics in the US. Feminist Pedagogy. 2023;3(2):8.
11. Smith GA. Like Americans overall, Catholics vary in their abortion views, with regular Mass attenders most opposed [Internet]. Pew Research Center. https://www.pewresearch.org/short-reads/2022/05/23/like-americans-overall-catholics-vary-in-their-abortion-views-with-regular-mass-attenders-most-opposed/. Accessed 1 Mar 2024.
12. Agne K. How Catholics voted. Conscience. 2020;1(2):1.
13. Catholics for Choice. Abortion. https://www.catholicsforchoice.org/issues/abortion/. Accessed 14 Feb 2024.
14. Holman M, Podrazik E, Mohamed HS. Choosing choice: how gender and religiosity shape abortion attitudes among Latinos. J Race Ethnicity Politics. 2020;5(2):384–411.
15. Eilerman N. Pro-understanding: understanding the pro-choice Catholic. 2022. Honors Thesis: University of Dayton. Accessed from: ecommons.udayton.edu.
16. Küng SA, Saavedra-Avendano B, Vélez EA, Piñeros MC, Metcalfe GM, Darney BG. Factors associated with support for adolescent access to contraception among Mexican Catholic parents. J Relig Health. 2021;60:1600–12.
17. Kościańska A, Ignaciuk A, Chełstowska A. Catholic intimacies: negotiating contraception in late Communist Poland. J Relig Hist. 2022;46(3):483–502.
18. Casas KD. Between doctrine and democracy: examining church-state relations and reproductive health policies in The Philippines, 1990-–2017. Br J Multidiscip Adv Stud. 2023;4(3):52–75.
19. Guiahi M, Teal S, Kenton K, DeCesare J, Steinauer J. Family planning training at Catholic and other religious hospitals: a national survey. Am J Obstet Gynecol. 2020;222(3):273–e1.
20. Drake C, Jarlenski M, Zhang Y, Polsky D. Market share of US Catholic hospitals and associated geographic network access to reproductive health services. JAMA Netw Open. 2020;3(1):e1920053.
21. Bringley J, Zu V, Javlekar A, Yilmaz FD, Flink-Bochacki R. Effects of rotating at a Catholic hospital on medical student contraceptive objective structured clinical exam scores. Contraception. 2022;106:64–7.
22. Go VA, Steinauer J, Guiahi M. Work-arounds at faith-based obstetrics and gynecology residency programs to accomplish family planning training. Contraception. 2022;115:59–61.
23. Wascher JM, Stulberg DB, Freedman LR. Restrictions on reproductive care at Catholic hospitals: a qualitative study of patient experiences and perspectives. AJOB Empirical Bioethics. 2020;11(4):257–67.
24. Wong ZJ, Thompson L, Boulware A, Chen J, Freedman L, Stulberg D, Hasselbacher L. What you don't know can hurt you: patient and provider perspectives on postpartum contraceptive care in Illinois Catholic hospitals. Contraception. 2022;107:62–7.
25. Stein LE, Goldman KN, Takimoto S, Neshek B, Guiahi M. Provision of fertility services to women in same-sex relationships at Catholic and non-Catholic clinics in the United States. Perspect Sex Reprod Health. 2022;54(3):109–15.
26. Olmos Alvarez AL, Johnson MC. Biomedical treatment and divine assistance: complementary reproductive itineraries among catholic women users of assisted reproduction technology in Argentina. Anthropol Med. 2022;29(4):383–98.
27. Jones LG. Holiness, saints, and sanctity in Christianity. In: Saints and sanctity in Judaism, Christianity, and Islam. Routledge; 2020. p. 42–64.
28. McTavish J. Why the church says "yes" to life and "no" to IVF. Linacre Q. 2022;89(4):450–4.
29. Donnenfeld SR, Mehta A. The urologist's guide to religion and male factor fertility treatment. Urology. 2022;167:128–31.
30. Bindeman J. Sex, religion, and infertility: the complications of Gd in the bedroom. In: Psychological and medical perspectives on fertility care and sexual health. Elsevier; 2022. p. 237–61.
31. Horowitz J. Francis urges ban on surrogacy, calling it "despicable." https://www.nytimes.com/2024/01/08/world/europe/pope-francis-surrogacy-ban.html.

32. Oyelowo T. Mosby's guide to women's health: a handbook for health professionals. Elsevier Health Sciences; 2007.
33. Dever J. Infertility and assisted reproductive technology. Female Biol. 2023;361:361–72.
34. De Jongh SF. GIFT and ZIFT: is there a place for these procedures in a new era of assisted reproduction? (Doctoral dissertation). University of the Witwatersrand, Faculty of Health Sciences; 2021.
35. Dongarwar D, Mercado-Evans V, Adu-Gyamfi S, Laracuente ML, Salihu HM. Racial/ethnic disparities in infertility treatment utilization in the US, 2011–2019. Syst Biol Reprod Med. 2022;68(3):180–9.
36. Dierks KE. Begotten not made: the Catholic church's stance on the morality of IVF and reproductive technology. Et in ArcAdiA Ego 26.
37. Rinehart LA. Storage, transport, and disposition of gametes and embryos: legal issues and practical considerations. Fertil Steril. 2021;115(2):274–81.
38. Barishansky SJ, Devine K, O'Brien JE, Rothwell E, Lawson AK. One size does not fit all: the personal nature of completed embryo donation. J Assist Reprod Genet. 2024;4:1–4.
39. Alexander VM, Riley JK, Jungheim ES. Recent trends in embryo disposition choices made by patients following in vitro fertilization. J Assist Reprod Genet. 2020;37:2797–804.
40. Hairston JC, Kohlmeier A, Feinberg EC. Compassionate embryo transfer: physician practices and perspectives. Fertil Steril. 2020;114(3):552–7.
41. Ethics Committee of the American Society for Reproductive Medicine. Compassionate transfer: patient requests for embryo transfer for nonreproductive purposes. Fertil Steril. 2020;113(1):62–5.
42. Hairston JC, Feinberg EC. Compassionate transfer: provider practices and perspectives. Fertil Steril. 2018;110(4):e374.
43. What to do with your unused embryos? VARTA [Internet]. 2021. Varta.org.au. Available from: https://www.varta.org.au/resources/information-sheets/what-do-your-unused-embryos
44. Hayford SR, Morgan SP. Religiosity and fertility in the United States: the role of fertility intentions. Soc Forces. 2008;86(3):1163–88.
45. Frejka T, Westoff CF. Religion, religiousness and fertility in the US and in Europe: religion, religiosité et fécondité aux Etats-Unis et en Europe. Eur J Population. 2008;24:5–31.
46. Westoff CF, Frejka T. Religiousness and fertility among European Muslims. Popul Dev Rev. 2007;33(4):785–809.
47. Czarnecki D. Moral women, immoral technologies: how devout women negotiate gender, religion, and assisted reproductive technologies. Gend Soc. 2015;29(5):716–42.
48. Galic I, Swanson A, Warren C, Negris O, Bozen A, Brown D, Lawson A, Jain T. Infertility in the Midwest: perceptions and attitudes of current treatment. Am J Obstet Gynecol. 2021;225(1):61–e1.
49. Reimann JG. Re-riting ritual for reproductive loss: an inclusive support resource for catholics experiencing reproductive loss (Doctoral dissertation). 2022.
50. Kelly EP, Paredes AZ, Tsilimigras DI, Hyer JM, Pawlik TM. The role of religion and spirituality in cancer care: an umbrella review of the literature. Surg Oncol. 2022;42:101389.
51. Czarnecki D. Modern crosses: how Christian women navigate gender, religion, and assisted reproductive technologies (Doctoral dissertation). 2017.
52. Bukhori B, Hidayanti E, Situmorang DD. Religious coping strategies for people with HIV/AIDS (PLWHA) Muslims in Indonesia: a qualitative study with a telling-the-stories. Heliyon. 2022;8(12):e12208.
53. Wood ZB, Wang DC, Lee C, Barnes H, Abouezzeddine T, Aten J. Social support, religious coping, and traumatic stress among Hurricane Katrina survivors of southern Mississippi: a sequential mediational model. Traumatology. 2021;27(4):336.
54. Van Nieuw Amerongen-Meeuse JC, Schaap-Jonker H, Anbeek C, Braam AW. Religious/spiritual care needs and treatment alliance among clinical mental health patients. J Psychiatr Ment Health Nurs. 2021;28(3):370–83.

55. Louws-Hendriksen M, Amerongen-Meeuse JC, Hommes M, Kuntze J, Schaap-Jonker H. Positive and negative religiousness and search for meaning: impact on treatment of substance abuse after 6 months. Drug Alcohol Depend. 2022;230:109182.
56. Abu HO, Ulbricht C, Ding E, Allison JJ, Salmoirago-Blotcher E, Goldberg RJ, Kiefe CI. Association of religiosity and spirituality with quality of life in patients with cardiovascular disease: a systematic review. Qual Life Res. 2018;27:2777–97.
57. Elhag M, Awaisu A, Koenig HG, Mohamed Ibrahim MI. The association between religiosity, spirituality, and medication adherence among patients with cardiovascular diseases: a systematic review of the literature. J Relig Health. 2022;61(5):3988–4027.
58. Illueca M, Doolittle BR. The use of prayer in the management of pain: a systematic review. J Relig Health. 2020;59(2):681–99.
59. Garssen B, Visser A, Pool G. Does spirituality or religion positively affect mental health? Meta-analysis of longitudinal studies. Int J Psychol Relig. 2021;31(1):4–20.
60. Carroll TD, McCormick WH, Smith PN, Isaak SL, Currier JM. PTSD, religious coping, and interpersonal antecedents of suicidal desire among military veterans: an initial examination of moderation models. Psychol Relig Spiritual. 2020;12(3):304.
61. Walker HE, Wamser-Nanney R, Howell KH. Relationships between childhood interpersonal trauma, religious coping, post-traumatic stress symptoms, and resilience. J Interpers Violence. 2022;37(13–14):NP11296–314.
62. Lucchetti G, Koenig HG, Lucchetti AL. Spirituality, religiousness, and mental health: a review of the current scientific evidence. World J Clin Cases. 2021;9(26):7620.
63. Chamberlain AM. The spiritual identity of women coping with infertility in a religion stressing fertility (Doctoral dissertation). Fielding Graduate University; 2022.
64. Greil AL. Not yet pregnant: infertile couples in contemporary America. Rutgers University Press; 1991.
65. Ventura JL, Fitzgerald OR, Koziol DE, Covington SN, Vanderhoof VH, Calis KA, Nelson LM. Functional well-being is positively correlated with spiritual well-being in women who have spontaneous premature ovarian failure. Fertil Steril. 2007;87(3):584–90.
66. Varzoni TC. Religiosity and spirituality as a mediator of perceived social support in couples with fertility issues 2023. Doctoral dissertation, Fielding Graduate University.
67. McDonald IR, Welt CK, Dwyer AA. Health-related quality of life in women with primary ovarian insufficiency: a scoping review of the literature and implications for targeted interventions. Hum Reprod. 2022;37(12):2817–30.

Chapter 12
Islam, Assisted Reproduction, and the Bioethical Aftermath

Marcia C. Inhorn and Soraya Tremayne

Introduction

Since the 1980s, in vitro fertilization (IVF) and other forms of assisted reproductive technology (ART) have rapidly globalized, spreading into many parts of the Muslim world. This is due in large part to the enthusiastic reception of these technologies by Islamic religious authorities over the past 45 years. In this article, we intend to show how IVF and related ARTs emerged in the Muslim Middle East, leading to multiple social and cultural transformations in the reproductive lives of Muslims. Through this account of Islam and assisted reproduction, we hope to debunk the widespread Western myth of Islam as biomedically backward or anti-scientific. Far from it, Islam is a religion that can be said to encourage science and technology, including medical developments to overcome human suffering. Islam, as we will argue, is scientifically agentive, encouraging the pursuit of high-tech medicine and science.

Editor's note: This chapter is a reprint of a 2016 article by the authors, who have graciously allowed for its republication in this volume. This work represents a seminal contribution to our understanding of ARTs in the Islamic world, and I am grateful to Drs. Inhorn and Tremayne and to Springer Nature, for consenting to give it new life as a chapter in this book. The original article can be found at:
Inhorn MC, Tremayne S. Islam, assisted reproduction, and the bioethical aftermath. Journal of religion and health. 2016 Apr;55:422–30, Springer Nature.

M. C. Inhorn (✉)
Anthropology and International Affairs, Yale University, New Haven, CT, USA
e-mail: marcia.inhorn@yale.edu

S. Tremayne
Institute for Social and Cultural Anthropology, Oxford University, Oxford, UK
e-mail: soraya.tremayne@anthro.ox.ac.uk

D. A. Kaplan (ed.), *Cultural Responsiveness in Assisted Reproductive Technology*, https://doi.org/10.1007/978-3-031-76204-8_12

Indeed, the continual emergence of new ARTs has led to the concomitant emergence of interesting Islamic bioethical discourses on how these technologies should be appropriated and used by Muslim physicians and their patients.

Overall, the theme of this chapter is *emergence*: the emergence of the ARTs themselves; the emergence of Islamic bioethical discourses surrounding ARTs; the emergence of an ART industry in the Muslim Middle East; the emergence of third-party reproductive assistance in the Shia-dominant countries of Iran and Lebanon; and finally, the emergence of what we will call the "bioethical aftermath," or a number of unanticipated and troubling consequences, which are presenting social and ethical challenges in the contemporary Muslim world.

Because we are both anthropologists, we base our chapter on long-term field research undertaken in IVF clinics in four Middle Eastern countries, including Egypt [1], Lebanon [2], the United Arab Emirates [3], and Iran [4, 5]. Together, we have traced the significant differences between the Sunni and Shia Muslim religious discourses surrounding the ARTs, particularly in the realm of third-party reproductive assistance [6].

The Emergence of ARTs

In his seminal essay, "Dominant, Residual, and Emergent," social theorist Raymond Williams [7] defined "emergence" as "new meanings and values, new practices, new relationships and kinds of relationship, which are continually being created" (p. 123). The term emergence has great relevance in the world of ARTs. Since the birth in 1978 of England's Louise Brown, the world's first "test-tube baby," there has been a veritable explosion of ARTs related to IVF. These include (1) intracytoplasmic sperm injection (ICSI) to overcome male infertility; (2) third-party reproductive assistance (with donor eggs, sperm, and embryos) to overcome problems of poor gamete quality; (3) gestational surrogacy to help women who are unable to carry a pregnancy in their own uterus; (4) cryopreservation (freezing) and storage of unused sperm, embryos, eggs, and now ovaries; (5) mitochondrial transfer from a healthy human egg to the diseased egg of another woman; (6) preimplantation genetic diagnosis (PGD) to determine whether embryos have genetic defects, to select embryos of a specific sex, or to select embryos that can grow into "savior siblings" through the donation of their umbilical cord blood; (7) human embryonic stem cell (hESC) research on unused embryos for the purpose of therapeutic intervention; and (8) the future possibility of human reproductive cloning or asexual, autonomous reproduction, which has already occurred in other mammals (e.g., Dolly the sheep) [8]. With virtually all of these technologies, sperm and eggs are retrieved from bodies, embryos are returned to bodies, and sometimes they are donated to other bodies or used for the purposes of stem cells and other forms of medical research.

The Emergence of Sunni Islamic Bioethical Discourses

IVF globalized quickly, moving to the Middle East within 8 years of Louise Brown's birth. Today, the Middle East is host to a booming and high-tech ART industry [9]. Egypt alone boasts more than 50 IVF clinics, Iran has nearly 70 clinics, and Turkey has the largest number, with more than 100 clinics. Even a small country such as the United Arab Emirates boasts more than a dozen IVF centers, including two supported by the Emirati state [3].

The development of a Middle Eastern IVF industry is not surprising: Islam encourages the use of science and medicine as solutions to human suffering and is a religion that can be described as "pronatalist," encouraging the growth of an Islamic "multitude." Yet, relatively little is known about Islam and technoscience, if technoscience is defined broadly as the interconnectedness between science and technology. As noted by Mayzar Lotfalian [10, p. 6], in his monograph on *Islam, Technoscientific Identities, and the Culture of Curiosity*, there is a glaring lacuna in the literature on science and technology in cross-cultural perspective, particularly from the Islamic world, where there are "really only two strains of relevant work"—one on the Islamic medieval sciences and one on philosophical arguments for a so-called clash of civilizations between science and technology in the Islamic and Western worlds. This dearth of relevant scholarship on Islamic techno-science applies to the cross-cultural study of ARTs. For example, in the seminal volume on *Third Party Assisted Conception Across Cultures: Social, Legal, and Ethical Perspectives* [11], not a single Muslim society is represented among the 13 country case studies.

IVF was first practiced in 1986 in the Sunni Muslim-majority countries of Egypt, Saudi Arabia, and Jordan. Egypt's early entry into assisted reproduction was especially important from an Islamic standpoint [1, 12]. The Grand Shaykh of Egypt's renowned religious university, Al-Azhar, issued the first widely authoritative *fatwa* on assisted reproduction on March 23, 1980—only 2 years after the birth of the first IVF baby in England but a full 6 years before the opening of Egypt's first IVF center.[1] Nearly 45 years later, this original Al-Azhar *fatwa* has proved to be quite authoritative and enduring. It has been reissued many times in Egypt and subsequently reaffirmed by *fatwa*-granting authorities in other parts of the Sunni Muslim world, from Morocco to Saudi Arabia to Indonesia.

In general terms, the Sunni Islamic religious authorities have been very permissive in granting the use of ARTs to Muslim IVF physicians and their patients. The Sunni *fatwas* on ARTs have allowed:

1. Artificial insemination with a husband's sperm
2. In vitro fertilization of an egg from a wife with the sperm of her husband

[1] Although a *fatwa* is non-legally binding, it is generally regarded as an authoritative Islamic religious decree, offered by an Islamic cleric who is considered to be an expert in Islamic jurisprudence.

3. Intracytoplasmic sperm injection (ICSI), in which the sperm of a husband is injected into the egg of his wife
4. Cryopreservation, or freezing, of any excess embryos, as well as sperm and eggs to be used later by a married couple
5. Postmenopausal pregnancy using a wife's own cryopreserved embryos or oocytes, in combination with the sperm of her husband
6. Preimplantation genetic diagnosis for couples at high risk of genetic disorders in their offspring
7. Multifetal pregnancy reduction, a form of selective abortion, which eliminates one or more fetuses in a high-risk IVF pregnancy with triplets, quadruplets, or beyond. In general, Islam is permissive when it comes to therapeutic abortion since it does not consider life to begin at the moment of conception.
8. Embryo research on excess embryos that are donated by couples for the advancement of scientific knowledge and the benefit of humanity; and
9. Uterine transplantation, a newly emergent technique in which a healthy uterus is transplanted from a willing donor to another woman who lacks a competent uterus.

This clearly represents a substantial list of permissions, thereby fueling the development of a robust IVF industry across much of the Sunni Muslim world [6]. However, the Sunni religious authorities have not condoned every possible ART practice. The list of ART restrictions is equally long.

1. Most importantly, third-party donors are not allowed, whether they are providing donor sperm, eggs, embryos, or uteruses, as in surrogacy. The use of a third party is tantamount to *zina*, or adultery.
2. Therefore, all forms of surrogacy are forbidden.
3. A donor or surrogate child conceived through any of these illegitimate forms of assisted reproduction cannot be made legitimate through adoption. The child who results from a forbidden method belongs to the mother and is considered to be a *walad il-zina*, or an illegitimate child.
4. Assisted reproduction cannot be performed on an ex-wife or widow using sperm from a divorced or dead husband.
5. Sperm banks for the purposes of sperm donation are forbidden. Sperm may only be cryopreserved before cancer treatment and used later in life by that same individual.
6. PGD or sperm sorting techniques for the purposes of sex selection are forbidden.
7. Human reproductive cloning for the creation of a cloned child- who would theoretically be the genetic twin of the cloning parent- is forbidden.
8. Genetic alteration of embryos is forbidden. However, in the future, gene therapy may be approved to remediate inherited genetic diseases and pathological conditions.

This is a long list, but it clearly summarizes which technologies are *haram*, or forbidden in Sunni Islam. Most importantly from a clinical perspective, all forms of third-party donation are *haram,* including sperm donation, egg donation, embryo donation, and surrogacy. As noted by Ebrahim Moosa [13],

> In terms of ethics, Muslim authorities consider the transmission of reproductive material between persons who are not legally married to be a major violation of Islamic law. This sensitivity stems from the fact that Islamic law has a strict taboo on sexual relations outside wedlock (*zina*). The taboo is designed to protect paternity (i.e., family), which is designated as one of the five goals of Islamic law, the others being the protection of religion, life, property, and reason (p. 23).

With regard to the first issue, Islam is a religion that can be said to privilege- even mandate- heterosexual marital relations. As is made clear in the original Al-Azhar *fatwa*, reproduction outside of marriage is considered *zina*, or adultery, which is strictly forbidden in Islam. Although third-party donation does not involve the sexual body contact ("touch or gaze") of adulterous relations, nor presumably the desire to engage in an extramarital affair, it is nonetheless considered by most Islamic religious scholars to be a form of adultery, by virtue of introducing a third party into the sacred dyad of husband and wife. It is the very fact that another man's sperm or another woman's eggs enter a place where they do not belong that makes a donation of any kind inherently wrong and threatens the marital bond.

The second aspect of third-party donation that troubles marriage is the potential for incest among the offspring of anonymous donors. If an anonymous sperm donor, for example, "fathers" hundreds of children, the children could grow up, unwittingly meet each other, fall in love, and marry. The same could be true for the children of anonymous egg donors. Thus, moral concerns have been raised about the potential for incest to occur among donor children who are biological half-siblings.

The final moral concern is that third-party donation confuses issues of kinship, descent, and inheritance. As with marriage, Islam is a religion that can be said to privilege- even mandate- biological inheritance. Preserving the *nasab*, or genealogical "origins" of each child, meaning his or her relationships to a known biological mother and father, is considered not only an ideal in Islam but a moral imperative. The problem with third-party donation, therefore, is that it destroys a child's *nasab* and violates the child's legal rights to known parentage, which is considered immoral, cruel, and unjust.

Muslim IVF patients use the term "mixture of relations" to describe this untoward outcome. Such a mixture of relations, or the literal confusion of lines of descent introduced by third-party donation, is described as being very "dangerous," "forbidden," "against nature," "against God"—in a word, *haram*, or morally unacceptable. It is argued that donation, by allowing "a stranger to enter the family," confuses lines of descent. For men in particular, ensuring paternity and the "purity" of lineage through "known fathers" is of paramount concern. This is because virtually all Muslim societies are organized patrilineally—that is, descent and inheritance are traced through fathers and the "fathers of fathers" through many generations. Thus, knowing paternity is of critical concern [14].

Accordingly, at the ninth Islamic law and medicine conference, held under the auspices of the Kuwait-based Islamic Organization for Medical Sciences (IOMS) in

Casablanca, Morocco, a landmark five-point declaration included recommendations to prohibit all situations in which a third party invades a marital relationship through donation of reproductive material [13]. Such a ban on third-party reproductive assistance is effectively in place in the Sunni-dominant countries. Not a single Sunni Muslim-majority country allows gamete donation and surrogacy,[2] and couples who need these technologies are told firmly that third-party donation is "against the religion."

The Emergence of Shia Islamic Third-Party Reproductive Assistance

However, the situation is changing for Shia Muslims, whose leading clerics have taken a step in a different direction. Shia Islam is the minority branch, constituting less than 10% of the world's Muslim population. Iran is the current epicenter of the Shia world, where it constitutes the majority religion. Shia majorities are also found in Lebanon, Iraq, and Bahrain, and significant Shia minority groups are found in eastern Saudi Arabia, Syria, Turkey, as well as Afghanistan, Pakistan, and India.

Many Shia religious authorities support the majority Sunni Islamic view: namely, they agree with Sunni *fatwas* that prohibit altogether third-party reproductive assistance. However, in the 1990s, some Shia clerics began supporting third-party reproductive assistance, particularly egg donation, but also sperm donation. By the end of that decade, the Supreme Leader of the Islamic Republic of Iran, Ayatollah Ali al-Husseini al-Khamene'i, the handpicked successor to Iran's Ayatollah Khomeini, had issued an authoritative *fatwa* effectively permitting both egg and sperm donation to be used [6]. Ayatollah Khamene'i's *fatwa* justified these donor technologies as a "marriage savior," preventing the "marital and psychological disputes" that would otherwise arise from remaining childless indefinitely.

With regard to egg donation specifically, Ayatollah Khamene'i argued that egg donation "is not in and of itself legally forbidden." However, he stated that *both* the egg donor and the infertile mother must abide by the religious codes regarding parenting. Thus, the child of the egg donor has the right to inherit from her, as the infertile woman who received the eggs is considered to be like an adoptive mother. With regard to sperm donation, Ayatollah Khamene'i stated in his *fatwa* that the baby born of sperm donation belongs to the biological father (i.e., the sperm donor) and thus can only inherit from him. But the infertile father is considered to be like an adoptive father, and thus the child takes his name from him.

Indeed, these Shia *fatwas*—culminating in the 1999 *fatwa* of Ayatollah Khamene'i—have led to an "Iranian ART revolution" [16]. Since the new millennium, all forms of sperm donation, egg donation, embryo donation, and gestational

[2] The possible exception is Mali, where at least one IVF clinic is performing third-party reproductive assistance [15].

surrogacy have been taking place in Iran. Iran is also leading the way in the Middle Eastern stem cell industry [17].

This "millennial moment" in Iran has also had a major impact on Shia-dominant Lebanon [2]. By 2003, one of the major Shia-serving IVF clinics in Beirut had developed a full-fledged egg donation program and had begun to cater to so-called reproductive tourists coming from other parts of the Middle East. Soon, other IVF clinics in Lebanon began providing egg donation services, as market demand increased among both Shia and Sunni Muslims, as well as Middle Eastern Christian couples.

Indeed, it is fair to state that this development of third-party reproductive assistance programs in both Iran and Lebanon has weakened the regional Sunni Muslim ban on donor technologies. In particular, husbands sympathetic to their wives' infertility problems are active participants in obtaining egg donation, sometimes engaging in *mut'a*, or temporary marriages, in order to undertake egg donation within the remit of a temporary polygamous marriage [2].

The Emergence of an ART Bioethical Aftermath

This use of temporary marriage as a way to make egg donation morally permissible is a creative solution to the moral challenges posed by third-party reproductive assistance within an Islamic framework. Yet, in the aftermath of the widespread Shia "opening" to third-party reproductive assistance, other bioethically troubling issues have continued to emerge.

The aftermath of sperm donation is a case in point. Outside of Iran, not a single Muslim cleric, either Sunni or Shia, approves of this particular donor technology. As a result, sperm donation has provoked a particularly strong bioethical reaction from many conservative quarters in both the Shia and Sunni Muslim worlds. In Iran, sperm donation is largely shrouded in secrecy, practiced primarily in private clinics beyond the scrutiny of the state. This is because sperm donation is seen as defying deeply rooted patriarchal values in Iran, including patrilineal kinship reckoning, in which the father assumes priority and rights of ownership over the child. According to Twelver Shia Islam, the child takes his lineage from both parents (mother and father) but the father remains the sole "owner" of the child, with the mother's role viewed primarily as that of caretaker [18]. Thus, from a Shia bioethical perspective, using a sperm donor is tantamount to conceiving another man's child. Indeed, most Shia Muslim men, as well as Sunni Muslim men who oppose sperm donation, often argue that a sperm-donor child "won't be my son." For them, it would be the equivalent of raising another man's child [2, 19].

Egg donation, on the other hand, has been more easily accommodated in Shia bioethical discourses, with the majority of Shia jurists now allowing the practice. For infertile women who receive a donated egg, the fact that they can gestate, give birth to, and breastfeed the egg-donor child creates the bonds of *rida'*, or milk kinship [20, 21]. These elements of perceived biogenetic relatedness between mother and child are not available to infertile men who seek to become fathers using donor sperm. As a result, infertile men's reactions to their sperm-donor children are not straightforward. In fact, in Iran, men's reaction to sperm donation has ranged from reluctant acceptance of their donor child, to major depression, to acts of physical violence against both mother and child [4, 5].

To prevent these untoward outcomes, many infertile Shia Muslim couples prefer to use their close relatives, especially same-sex siblings, for gamete donation. Thus, brothers donate sperm to their brothers' wives, while sisters donate their eggs or uteruses (via surrogacy) to their infertile sisters and sisters-in-law. Indeed, if a sister donates her eggs to her brother's infertile wife the child so produced would be the biological offspring of the actual brother and sister—a form of biological incest not only in Islamic societies but in most if not all societies around the world. Furthermore, under Islamic law, this kind of intra-familial donation may lead to peculiar forms of relatedness and the possibility of committing incest or adultery according to the Islamic laws governing association between the sexes.

Namely, the extent of social and sexual interaction between men and women is regulated through the concept of *mahramiat* (closeness/privacy), which determines the boundaries of the interaction between men and women in society. Accordingly, men and women are divided into two groups- the *mahram* and *na-mahram*. The *maharem* (plural for *mahram*) are relatives, who are not potential marriage partners and with whom one may undertake free but not sexual interaction. Any sexual relationship between the *maharem* therefore constitutes incest. The *mahram* group includes one's siblings, parents, grandparents, aunts and uncles, children, and grandchildren. *Na-mahram*, on the other hand, are nonfamily members, who are potential marriage partners and with whom neither sexual nor social contact is permitted. Social contact with *na-mahram* individuals is supposed to remain limited and guarded. This latter category includes all nonfamily members, as well as those members of the kin group who are not part of the *mahram* category. There also exists a third category, namely those who are *mahram* at some point, but who become *na-mahram* due to changes in the individuals' marital status (see also [22]).

In the case of gamete donation within the kin group, egg and sperm donation between brothers and sisters and their spouses may violate the rules of *mahramiat*, while also leading to both incest and adultery. Yet, infertile couples who recruit their own relatives as gamete donors typically do not see their actions in this light. Because there is no sexual contact occurring during the donation process—in which gametes retrieved from individuals' bodies are placed in petri dishes and made into embryos there—ARTs allow family members to bypass the rules of *mahramiat,* as well as feelings of incest or adultery. Instead, by using a relative's gamete, the "purity" of the lineage can be maintained, and the donation can be kept "all in the family," strengthening those social bonds. Furthermore, the financial aspect of familial donation is also advantageous, as it typically does not entail payment to the donor.

Finally, the use of ARTs in Iran, Lebanon, and other Sunni-dominant countries of the Middle East has led to other bioethical conundrums. For example, even though son preference and daughter discrimination are anathema in Islam—with the Prophet Muhammad explicitly forbidding the pre-Islamic practice of female infanticide—the emergence of ARTs, particularly PGD, is leading to new forms of female "embryocide" in the Muslim world. Namely, in some Middle Eastern IVF clinics, couples who want sons, especially after the birth of only daughters, are using PGD to perform sex selection, culling female embryos in an attempt to produce male-only progeny [3, 12]. Furthermore, new forms of "fetal reduction" are occurring in many clinics, through selective abortion of fetuses in higher-order multiple pregnancies (i.e., triplets and beyond) [3, 12].

Like the ART-abetted forms of biological incest occurring in Iran, these "selective" practices of embryo and fetal "culling," especially of female offspring, are deeply troubling. However, these are part of the "bioethical aftermath" of ARTs in the Muslim world, a world where the widespread acceptance and use of ARTs have not been entirely unambiguous. Indeed, the emergence of ARTs has led to a bioethical "slippery slope," where technologies intended for one use may morph into another, as shown in the case of PGD and the "new" sex selection.

Conclusion

Having said this, it is fair to state that the Muslim world has nonetheless embraced ARTs with considerable enthusiasm while, at the same time, attempting to regulate them in accordance with local religious moralities. In Sunni Muslim countries such as Egypt, the prohibition on third-party reproductive donation has clearly led to an entrenchment of deeply held religious beliefs about the importance of marriage, biological kinship, and family life, which no third party should tear asunder. For this reason, donor gametes continue to be morally shunned and clinically banned in the Sunni Muslim world, with donation itself equated to *zina*, or adultery.

Yet, having said this, the globalization of these technologies to other parts of the Shia Muslim world has fundamentally altered our understanding of the ways in which families *can* be made and how marriages *can* be saved through the use of ARTs. The permission of donor technologies in Shia-dominant Iran and Lebanon has led to a brave new world of reproductive possibilities never imagined when these technologies were first introduced to the Middle East nearly 40 years ago. This emergence of donor technologies has led to, among other things, significant reproductive tourism from the Sunni to Shia regions of the Middle East, the mixing of gametes across familial, ethnic, national, and religious lines, and the birth of thousands of donor children to devout infertile Muslim couples. Many infertile Muslim couples have also begun to reconsider traditional notions of biological kinning, even if the "social parenthood" of a donor child is still not widely embraced.

Moreover, the availability of donor technologies has weakened the Sunni Muslim ban on third-party reproductive assistance across the region, with at least some infertile Sunni Muslim couples reconsidering their anti-donation moral stances. As a result, Shia Muslim donor gametes are making their way into Sunni Muslim bodies—an exchange of gametes that defies stereotypes about the rifts within Islam and the inter-sectarian tensions that are currently causing great pain to the Muslim body politic as a whole.

References

1. Inhorn MC. Local babies, global science: gender, religion and in vitro fertilization in Egypt. Routledge; 2012.
2. Inhorn MC. The new Arab man: Emergent masculinities, technologies, and Islam in the Middle East. Princeton University Press; 2003.
3. Inhorn MC. Cosmopolitan conceptions: IVF sojourns in global Dubai. Duke University Press; 2015.
4. Tremayne S. Law, ethics, and donor technologies in Shia Iran. In: Assisting reproduction, testing genes: Global encounters with new biotechnologies, vol. 18. Berghahn Books; 2009. p. 144–63.
5. Tremayne S. The "down side" of gamete donation: challenging "happy family" rhetoric in Iran. In: Islam and assisted reproductive technologies: Sunni and Shia perspectives, vol. 20. Berghahn Books; 2012. p. 130–56.
6. Inhorn MC, Tremayne S, editors. Islam and assisted reproductive technologies: Sunni and Shia perspectives. Berghahn Books; 2012.
7. Williams R. Marxism and literature. Oxford University Press; 1977.
8. Franklin S. Dolly mixtures: the remaking of genealogy. Durham: Duke University Press; 2007.
9. Inhorn MC, Patrizio P. Infertility around the globe: new thinking on gender, reproductive technologies and global movements in the 21st century. Hum Reprod Update. 2015;21(4):411–26.
10. Loftalian M. Islam, technoscientific identities, and the culture of curiosity. Washington, DC: University Press of America; 2004.
11. Blyth E, Landau R. Third party assisted conception across cultures: social, legal and ethical perspectives. Jessica Kingsley Publishers; 2004.
12. Serour GI. Islamic perspectives in human reproduction. Reprod Biomed Online. 2008;17:34–8.
13. Moosa E. Human cloning in Muslim ethics. Voices Across Boundaries. 2003;2(2):23–6.
14. Clarke M. Islam and new kinship: reproductive technology and the Shariah in Lebanon. Berghahn Books; 2009.
15. Hörbst V. 'You cannot do IVF in Africa as in Europe': the making of IVF in Mali and Uganda. Reprod Biomed Soc. 2016;2:108–15.
16. Abbasi-Shavazi MJ, Inhorn MC, Razeghi-Nasrabad HB, Toloo G. The "Iranian ART Revolution": infertility, assisted reproductive technology, and third-party donation in the Islamic Republic of Iran. J Middle East Women's Stud. 2008;4(2):1–28.
17. Saniei M. Human embryonic stem cell research in Iran: the significance of the Islamic context. In: Islam and assisted reproductive technologies: Sunni and Shia perspectives, vol. 20. Berghahn Books; 2012. p. 194–217.
18. Mir-Hosseini Z. Marriage on trial: a study of Islamic family law. Bloomsbury Publishing; 2000.
19. Inhorn MC. He won't be my son: Middle Eastern Muslim men's discourses of adoption and gamete donation. Med Anthropol Q. 2006;20(1):94–120.
20. Khatib-Chahidi J. Milk kinship in Shi'ite Islamic Iran. In: The anthropology of breast-feeding: natural law or social construct. Routledge; 1992. p. 109–32.
21. Altorki S. Milk-kinship in Arab society: an unexplored problem in the ethnography of marriage. Ethnology. 1980;19(2):233–44.
22. Behman J. The social structures of family in Iran. Tehran: Tehran University Press; 1973.

Chapter 13
Black Patients and the Historical Context of Racism in Medical Care

Karima Ann Forbes

"Her blood pressure is too low; she could die if we cut her open." I lay there in the hospital bed feeling nauseous, dizzy, out of control of my own body, and reflecting on how I even got here, as I waited for my first bundle of joy to arrive. Like most, I had planned for a vaginal birth, and had romanticized what it could look like—hoping to go to term, hoping to have a natural birth, and hoping to hold my little one and take one of those first pictures that I always see that people have posted from the delivery room; you know, the one with the baby covered in a combination of things like vernix, blood, and amniotic fluid. As I lay there, I thought about the regular blood pressure monitoring that I had undergone throughout pregnancy and the latest blood pressure reading that landed me in labor and delivery 6 weeks early: 150/96. I was admitted and started on magnesium sulfate. While the details are blurry, after 2 days of inpatient admission and difficulty regulating my blood pressure, I was informed by my OB that labor would be induced. There was a flood of emotions as I worried about the health of our little one. Once in the delivery room, as we waited for the progression of my dilation, there was so much beeping. *Our sweet girl was in distress; I was in distress.*

The medical team came in to discuss options as they needed to get our little one out right away. The Black doctor I had hand-selected, intentionally—one who looked like me—had rotated off shift. I scanned the room…no one looked like me. My anxiety increased though I didn't have the energy for it to manifest visually. As a Black woman, I know the experience of racism and discrimination in many contexts intimately and as a psychologist, I understood the history and impact of it in

K. A. Forbes (✉)
WorkHaven, LLC, New York, NY, USA

Bloom Psychological & Wellness Consulting, LLC, Montclair, NJ, USA

New York, NY, USA

D. A. Kaplan (ed.), *Cultural Responsiveness in Assisted Reproductive Technology*, https://doi.org/10.1007/978-3-031-76204-8_13

the medical context. Stats were flying through my mind as I wondered if I would be one of the Black women referenced in discussions where they mention that the maternal mortality rate for Black women is three times higher than that of White women [1]. We were told that I would likely have a C-section. An attending physician came in and revisited this suggestion with the team present, warning, "*Her blood pressure is too low; she could die if we cut her open.*" At that moment, I was terrified, and I could see the fear in my partner's eyes as these words were stated. Things moved fast after that. I was eventually able to deliver our child vaginally, though her distress continued, resulting in a Neonatal Intensive Care Unit (NICU) stay. I didn't see her in person or hold her for 2 days and only saw her in pictures as I continued to be treated for preeclampsia. She is now a thriving healthy girl, but sometimes I look at her and can't help but think about the traumas related to her arrival.

In my later reflections, I realized my fear for my pregnancy-related health started as soon as I found out I was pregnant. I sought out a Black provider because I thought my health would be valued differently given the biases that exist within systems, including the healthcare system. If I had not, would my blood pressure have been checked regularly during appointments due to the potential risk? How would all this have been different if I didn't have health insurance and access to choice? I think a lot about my labor and delivery experience and whether bias impacted the suggestion of a C-section and the related risk of mortality. What if the attending had not spoken up? Would this suggestion have been made if I looked different? I lived when so many women who look like me have not. I carried that fear through my first pregnancy, and it was further exacerbated in my second pregnancy by my lived experience. I can't help but also wonder, *if I weren't Black, would I even be plagued by these questions? Would I still wonder?* There is a privilege in not having to wonder.

Setting the Frame

Why do I bring up this experience in a chapter discussing the history of racism in medicine? I recognize that my behaviors and choices, including my choice of a Black obstetrician, demonstrated a distrust of the medical system. This is a shared reaction by many individuals who share my racial identity. Black individuals have been subjected to systemic injustices for centuries, injustices that have continued over the 150 years since slavery was abolished [2–4]. These injustices serve to disenfranchise Black people [5, 6] and have been demonstrated and perpetuated in systems including, but not limited to, education [7, 8], housing [9–11], criminal justice [5, 6], employment [8, 9], and healthcare [12–14].

Beginning in early childhood, disparities exist in the educational opportunities available to Black children. Per The Education Trust [15] funding discrepancies can be seen between schools in predominantly Black communities and those in predominantly White communities. Additionally, statistics indicate that Black students are more likely to face disciplinary actions, such as suspensions and expulsions, compared to their White counterparts for similar behaviors [16, 17]. Persistent disparities also exist in the context of housing; research indicates that Black people continue to be impacted by redlining, which was a discriminatory practice in the 1930s that facilitated the denial or limitation of financial services, such as loans and mortgages, to people living in predominantly Black neighborhoods or areas with high minority populations [18, 19]. Due to this practice, we continue to see economic disparities and poverty perpetuated in certain communities, continued racial segregation, and inequitable access to housing financing [18].

Perhaps the most glaring inequities exist in the area of criminal justice. As indicated in *The New Jim Crow: Mass Incarceration in the Age of Colorblindness* [5], Black individuals are disproportionately arrested, incarcerated, and sentenced compared to White individuals charged with similar offenses. Additionally, according to The Sentencing Project [20], Black people are incarcerated at nearly five times the rate of White Americans. The most recent report of The Sentencing Project [20] suggests that while laws and policies appear "race-neutral," in actuality, they have a disproportionate impact on communities of color, and particularly on Black Americans, resulting in higher rates of arrests, convictions, and longer sentences compared to their White counterparts.

Unsurprisingly, given the disparities in education and treatment by the criminal justice system, statistics indicate that Black people often face higher rates of unemployment and underemployment compared to White individuals with similar qualifications [21–23]. Studies have also shown that in the context of employment, there is a persistent racial wage gap, where Black workers earn less than White workers for similar work [24, 25]. The wage gap tends to be worse for Black women than for Black men. According to the Economic Policy Institute (EPI), Black women earn significantly less than their White, non-Hispanic male counterparts [26]. Specifically, Black women earn only 62 cents for every dollar earned by White, non-Hispanic men, whereas Black men earn 72 cents for every dollar earned by White, non-Hispanic men [26]. This disparity is compounded by the intersection of both racial and gender discrimination. The National Partnership for Women & Families highlights that Black women face a more severe wage gap due to both systemic racial biases and gender discrimination. These factors contribute to higher poverty rates among Black women compared to Black men [27].

The focus of the current chapter is racism in the context of medical care. However, to understand the context in which these systemic injustices exist, it is important to appreciate that these injustices are not unique to the healthcare system. Systems of inequity frequently reinforce each other; for example, housing disparities can inform and perpetuate disparities that exist within education or access to healthcare by limiting Black individuals' access to well-funded schools and high-quality medical care close to where they live [28].

Healthcare Disparities Experienced By Black Patients

Numerous well-documented disparities are faced by Black patients within the United States healthcare system [29]. These disparities include limited access to healthcare services, the presence of implicit biases among healthcare providers affecting treatment decisions and diagnoses [30], and an increased prevalence of chronic health conditions like diabetes, hypertension, obesity, and asthma among the Black population [31]. Studies have highlighted the poorer management of these chronic conditions within Black communities, leading to higher rates of mortality and morbidity compared to other racial or ethnic groups [29]. Furthermore, significant disparities persist in access to mental health care for Black individuals, contributing to unmet mental health needs within this demographic [31].

COVID Pandemic. Healthcare disparities faced by Black communities were thrown into stark relief by the COVID-19 pandemic. Black communities have been disproportionately affected by COVID-19, experiencing higher infection rates, hospitalizations, and mortality rates compared to other racial groups [32]. Yancy cited factors including socioeconomic status, access to healthcare, and underlying health conditions as contributors to this disparity [32]. Inequities faced by Black communities were further manifested in the context of the COVID-19 vaccination rollout. At various points during the rollout, Black individuals were vaccinated at lower rates than other racial and ethnic groups in the United States [32]. Reasons documented by Artiga et al. related to the disparity included access barriers and vaccine hesitancy. While there were general concerns among the US population about the safety and efficacy of the vaccines fueled by misinformation or misconceptions about the COVID-19 vaccines, for Black patients the hesitancy was also related to historical distrust of the healthcare system [33, 34]. As Dr. Uché Blackstock noted in her book "Legacy," the pandemic brutally exposed the deep racial fault lines in our society [34].

Pain Management. Another example of a disparity issue experienced by Black patients in healthcare is the way in which Black patients' pain is understood and managed. The phenomenon of Black Americans being undertreated for pain compared to their White counterparts has been documented in various studies and has garnered significant attention in recent years [35–37]. A landmark study published in 2016 highlighted that half of White medical students and residents held false beliefs about biological differences between Black and White patients [38]. These beliefs included misconceptions about pain tolerance, with some incorrectly believing that Black people have less sensitive nerve endings or higher pain thresholds than White individuals. This study suggested that these false beliefs might lead to the undertreatment of pain in Black patients. Relatedly, a review written by Hoffman and colleagues [39] indicated that Black patients with chronic pain were less likely to be prescribed opioid medications despite reporting similar pain levels to White patients. This disparity in opioid prescribing patterns persisted even when controlling for factors such as income, insurance status, and pain severity [39].

In another study conducted by Goyal and colleagues, results indicated that Black patients with abdominal pain were less likely than White patients to receive analgesics in emergency departments, even when presenting with similar symptoms [40]. These disparities in pain management can be attributed to various factors, including implicit biases held by healthcare providers, stereotypes about racial differences in pain perception, historical mistrust of healthcare systems among Black communities, and inadequate cultural competence in medical care [39–42]. Undertreatment of pain can have detrimental effects on patient outcomes, leading to prolonged suffering, decreased quality of life, and delayed recovery from illnesses or injuries [43].

Implicit Bias and Diagnostic Disparities. Implicit bias among healthcare providers has been identified as a significant factor contributing to diagnostic disparities experienced by Black patients in physical health care. Multiple studies reveal that these disparities are pervasive and detrimental. For example, one study found that Black patients presenting with similar symptoms to White patients were less likely to receive appropriate diagnostic imaging for conditions such as back pain or chest pain [44]. A second study reported that Black patients were significantly less likely to receive referrals for this potentially life-saving procedure compared to their White counterparts, increasing their risk of significant cardiac complications [45]. Yet a third study reported that Black patients with heart disease symptoms were less likely to be referred for cardiac catheterization, even after adjusting for clinical factors [46].

Trauma care is not immune to these biases. Haider and colleagues [47] found that Black trauma patients were less likely to be transferred to specialized trauma centers than White patients, adversely affecting their chances of survival and recovery. Additional studies emphasize that implicit racial biases can lead to underdiagnosis or delayed diagnosis of critical conditions across various medical fields [48, 49]. These biases stem from unconscious stereotypes and prejudices, causing clinicians to misinterpret symptoms or apply different diagnostic criteria based on a patient's race. The cumulative effect of these biases is profound, resulting in prolonged suffering, decreased quality of life, and increased mortality for Black patients. Addressing these implicit biases is crucial to ensuring equitable healthcare for all individuals, regardless of race.

Healthcare Access and Structural Barriers. Racial minorities continue to face barriers to quality healthcare services, including economic disparities, limited insurance coverage, and geographic obstacles to accessing healthcare facilities. Structural barriers, such as the lack of healthcare facilities in minority neighborhoods, contribute to reduced access to essential treatments and preventive care, perpetuating health disparities [50].

Assistive Reproductive Technologies. Disparities within the realm of assistive reproductive technologies (ART) have been observed and documented in the realms of access, quality of care, and treatment outcomes. For instance, access to ART services is significantly skewed, with minority populations in the United States, particularly Black and Hispanic women, facing greater barriers. This is attributable to factors including socioeconomic disparities and insurance coverage issues [51]. The quality of care in ART also varies by race. Studies indicate that minority women often receive different and inferior ART care when compared to their White counterparts, which can stem from biases in treatment recommendations or a lack of culturally sensitive care [52]. Specifically, minority women are less likely to receive advanced ART treatments like preimplantation genetic diagnosis (PGD) and are more often counseled towards less effective treatments or natural conception, highlighting disparities in the types of services provided [52]. This disparity extends to treatment outcomes as well. Research shows that Black women, for instance, have lower pregnancy and live birth rates from in vitro fertilization (IVF) treatments compared to White women, a disparity that might be linked to both healthcare quality and underlying health issues [53].

Bias also permeates the research used to develop and evaluate ART procedures. Historically, the focus has been predominantly on White populations, leading to a potential oversight of specific issues or treatment responses in other racial groups. The downstream effect of this bias is exemplified in a study of the Society for Assisted Reproductive Technology (SART) database in which their findings revealed that out of the 80,390 ART cycles, approximately 4.6% were performed on African American women, 85.4% on Caucasian women, and 11.9% on women from other racial backgrounds [54]. This lack of diversity in the populations able to access ART care and therefore available for research on treatment outcomes can result in less effective treatment protocols for non-White patients. These medical practices are not just clinical but intersect with broader ethical and societal issues. They raise questions about who has access to these advanced technologies and how societal biases and structural inequalities manifest in reproductive healthcare [55, 56].

Maternal Mortality Disparities. Maternal mortality disparities among African American women in the United States represent a stark example of medical racism and healthcare inequalities. Multiple studies have consistently demonstrated that African American women face significantly higher maternal mortality rates compared to their White counterparts. For instance, a study published in the journal *Health Affairs* found that African American women were three to four times more likely to die from pregnancy-related causes than White women [57, 58]. Related research reports the rate as being two to three times more likely [59].

Furthermore, high-profile cases like that of tennis legend Serena Williams have drawn attention to the dismissive attitudes and systemic biases that African American women often encounter in healthcare settings. Williams shared her experience of having her concerns downplayed during childbirth, leading to a delay in diagnosis and treatment for a life-threatening condition. Such dismissive attitudes can contribute to delayed or inadequate care, potentially exacerbating maternal mortality disparities [57]. These persistent disparities highlight the urgent need for addressing systemic racism in healthcare, improving access to quality prenatal and obstetric care, and promoting cultural competence among healthcare providers to ensure equitable reproductive and maternal health outcomes for all.

How Did We Get Here? Understanding the History

While finding solutions to these disparities is an important part of the conversation, there is a need to understand the broader context that informs how providers navigate treatment with Black patients in the context of the disparities that persist. The deep-seated influence of historical racism on present healthcare disparities forms a crucial backdrop for understanding the intricate history of racial biases within medical care. Centuries of systemic racism have perpetuated inequalities in healthcare access, especially affecting marginalized groups like Black and other minority communities. This historical context sheds light on the origins of distrust and inequity within healthcare systems, stemming from past injustices such as segregation, discriminatory policies, and notorious incidents like the Tuskegee Syphilis Study. These injustices have profoundly shaped Black patients' healthcare-seeking behaviors and outcomes, emphasizing the urgency of exploring the nuanced history of racism in medical care comprehensively.

The Transatlantic Slave Trade, spanning roughly four centuries from the sixteenth to the nineteenth centuries, involved the forcible transportation of millions of Africans to the Americas for labor exploitation. Historically, it remains one of the largest and most brutal forced migrations in human history [60, 61]. European powers, including Portugal, Spain, Britain, France, and the Netherlands, actively participated in this trade, profoundly affecting the demographics, economies, and societies of Africa and the Americas. Estimates suggest that between 10 and 12 million Africans were captured and transported across the Atlantic, enduring unimaginable horrors during the Middle Passage, where mortality rates were devastatingly high due to disease, malnutrition, and harsh conditions on the slave ships [62]. The Transatlantic Slave Trade not only stripped millions of Africans of their freedom but also laid the groundwork for deeply entrenched systems of racial oppression, leaving a lasting legacy of trauma and systemic inequality that continues to reverberate in present-day social, economic, and political structures.

Slavery and Medical Racism

The transatlantic slave trade inflicted unspeakable medical atrocities upon enslaved individuals, from their abduction in Africa to their arrival in the Americas. This traumatic journey, documented in academic research [60], subjected captives to harrowing conditions aboard slave ships characterized by abysmal overcrowding, filthy environments, and a dire scarcity of provisions. Shackled and packed in confined spaces, enslaved people endured this passage under horrific circumstances, fostering the rampant transmission of diseases such as dysentery, smallpox, and various other communicable illnesses. The appalling lack of adequate medical care and unsanitary living conditions precipitated extensive suffering and a substantial loss of life during the voyage. Upon reaching the Americas, many enslaved individuals, already debilitated from the arduous journey, faced further exploitation and mistreatment. This marked the inception of their enslavement in a milieu that persistently disregarded their health and well-being, perpetuating a legacy of systemic neglect and maltreatment that reverberated throughout their lives and those of subsequent generations [60–62].

Enslaved individuals faced grueling labor on plantations, experiencing frequent injuries, fatigue, and an array of health challenges while receiving minimal healthcare support [63, 64]. Basic medical interventions, such as rudimentary wound care or traditional herbal remedies, were often the full extent of medical aid available. For more severe injuries or illnesses, access to adequate healthcare was scarce and often delayed, and was primarily geared towards maintaining the labor force rather than addressing individual health needs. Fear of repercussions and mistreatment deterred many enslaved individuals from disclosing injuries or illnesses, creating a climate of silence and concealment regarding their health status [64, 65]. Seeking medical aid risked severe consequences such as punishment, increased work demands, or familial separation, amplifying the pervasive fear of retribution [65].

Enslaved individuals confronted systemic dismissal and allegations of malingering when reporting authentic illnesses or injuries within the oppressive structures of slavery. The concept of malingering involves the fabrication or exaggeration of symptoms, and it became a recurrent accusation wielded by overseers and plantation owners to undermine legitimate health grievances arising from the demanding working conditions endured by enslaved individuals [65–67]. This accusation of feigned illness or injury served as a tool to discredit their genuine health concerns, systematically obstructing their access to adequate medical care within the plantation system. Moreover, brutal physical punishment, particularly whipping, was commonly employed as a punitive measure against those accused of malingering [65]. This practice of "treating" individuals reporting ailments with physical abuse further perpetuated an environment of fear and intimidation. The widespread use of physical punishment aimed at curbing health-related complaints contributed significantly to the systemic devaluation of enslaved people's health and well-being, reinforcing the cycle of mistreatment and neglect pervasive within the oppressive system of slavery. It also laid the groundwork for a system of thought by medical providers within which Black patients' ailments could be dismissed as exaggerated or wholly fabricated.

The adverse living conditions endured by enslaved individuals also impacted their health and well-being, contributing significantly to widespread sickness and adverse health outcomes [67, 68]. Enslaved individuals typically resided in overcrowded and unsanitary living quarters, lacking adequate shelter, clean water, and proper sanitation facilities. The nutritionally deficient diets provided to them resulted in chronic malnutrition, weakened immune systems, and heightened susceptibility to various illnesses and diseases [69]. The compounded stress and trauma related to harsh working conditions, constant exposure to extreme weather conditions, frequent physical, mental, and emotional abuse, malnutrition, and poor living conditions, compromised the health of the enslaved and exacerbated their vulnerability to illnesses, significantly impacting their overall health and life expectancy.

Reproductive Exploitation. Pregnant enslaved women faced dire circumstances, receiving inadequate prenatal care and frequently being coerced to continue labor-intensive work until close to childbirth. This physical strain not only jeopardized the health of these women but also posed substantial risks to the well-being of their unborn children, contributing to elevated maternal and infant mortality rates within enslaved communities [55]. Enslaved women were systematically exploited for their reproductive capabilities, serving to augment the enslaved population and fulfill the economic interests of slaveowners [70]. Slave owners impregnated enslaved women forcibly or through coercion to bolster the population of enslaved individuals [55]. These women had no control over their reproductive decisions and often suffered sexual exploitation and assault by enslavers and overseers. The offspring of enslaved women, including those conceived through assault by their enslavers, were deemed the property of enslavers, perpetuating the cycle of enslavement across generations and ensuring a steady labor supply [55, 70].

Experimentation. During the era of slavery in the United States, the enslaved were often subjected to medical experiments without their consent or any regard for their dignity. Enslaved individuals were seen as expendable and were used as subjects for various medical procedures, surgeries, and experiments conducted by physicians and scientists seeking to advance medical knowledge [65, 71].

J. Marion Sims, a nineteenth-century American physician, is often acclaimed as a trailblazer in gynecology. Yet his pioneering work stemmed from deeply unethical experimentation on enslaved Black women. Sims conducted his controversial experiments in the 1840s and 1850s in Montgomery, Alabama, and later in New York City. His focus was on developing a surgical approach to addressing vesicovaginal fistulas, a condition resulting in an abnormal tract between the bladder and the vagina, that usually occurred as a result of childbirth trauma [55, 65, 70, 72]. Sims conducted infamous surgical experiments on enslaved Black women, notably Anarcha, Betsey, and Lucy. Records indicate that Lucy was the first subject; she nearly died from blood poisoning after the initial procedure and took months to heal. Despite this, Sims' experimentation on Lucy continued. After 4 years, Sims ultimately succeeded in repairing her fistula [72].

Upon relocating to New York City in 1853, Sims advanced his medical career and gained acclaim in the field of gynecology. Although there is no documented evidence of him directly perpetuating similar experimental practices or surgeries on enslaved individuals in New York City, Sims' legacy remains controversial. Many accounts note that Sims continued his experimentation on seven or eight other enslaved women, in front of audiences of up to 12 people. The women held each other down due to the difficulty of remaining still in the context of extreme pain, and opium was provided to control their movement, rather than to treat their pain [55, 65]. The ethical controversies arising from Sims' experiments continue to provoke discussions in medical ethics, particularly concerning consent and the historical mistreatment of marginalized communities. While there is no debate about the exploitation of slaves in the context of Sims' work, some, like Dr. Irwin Kaiser in 1978, argue that his behavior was justified. Kaiser published statements such as, "Be skeptical of judging 1850 decisions by 1975 norms" and referred to Sims as a "product of his era" [72]. In 1894, a statue of Dr. Sims was erected in New York City's Bryant Park and relocated to Central Park in 1934. The contentious legacy of Sims led to the removal of his statue from Central Park in April 2018 [73].

Medical experimentation on enslaved people extended beyond the infamous Dr. Sims. Thomas Hamilton, a physician based in South Carolina, sought to find a cure for sunstroke [74]. Documents indicate that he was known for buying and raising slaves solely for experimentation [65]. Among them was an enslaved man named John Brown. Hamilton created various medical concoctions that he believed would treat sunstroke. To test these medications, after a full day of labor on the plantation, John Brown was administered the medication and forced to sit naked in a pit on a stool placed on a plank of wood above a fire [65]. Hamilton observed Brown, noting blisters, fainting, and flayed skin. Brown's accounts reveal that Hamilton's ongoing experimentation aimed to examine the depth of his black skin, resulting in repeated bleeding and blistering [74].

Medical Training. During the era of slavery in the United States, medical schools and institutions frequently acquired the bodies of deceased enslaved individuals through grave robbing, theft, and other unethical means, for anatomical dissection and educational purposes. These bodies were used not only to train medical students but also to conduct scientific research and study supposed anatomical differences between racial groups, often based on erroneous and racist theories [65]. This exploitative practice highlights the deep-seated racial prejudices and dehumanization prevalent in the medical profession's history.

The concept of "night doctors" emerged from the genuine fears prevalent among Black communities during and after slavery [75]. This phrase referred to the very real threat posed by White medical practitioners or individuals associated with medical institutions who would abduct or harm Black individuals, particularly at night, for medical experimentation, dissection, or forced treatment without consent [75]. These fears were well-founded, rooted in the horrific practices of the time. The legacy of "night doctors" has contributed to the mistrust of the medical profession within Black communities, a mistrust that continues to resonate through generations.

Jim Crow Era

The Jim Crow era, extending from the late nineteenth to the mid-twentieth century, was characterized by a multitude of state and local statutes that enforced racial segregation and institutionalized systemic discrimination against Black Americans and other minority groups [76]. These laws mandated segregation in public facilities, including schools, transportation, restaurants, and other public accommodations, establishing separate facilities for White and Black individuals on the grounds that segregated institutions could provide services of equal quality to the groups they were designated to serve. Many described these laws as a ruse, noting that no public accommodations provided "equal" facilities [77, 78]. Black schools, hospitals, and public amenities received inferior resources, funding, and support compared to those designated for White communities. Laws passed during this era also imposed restrictions on voting rights through literacy tests, poll taxes, and other discriminatory measures, effectively disenfranchising Black voters and limiting their political participation [79]. Examples of Jim Crow Laws include the following [80]:

> *Lunch Counters*: No persons, firms, or corporations, who or which furnish meals to passengers at station restaurants or station eating houses, in times limited by common carriers of said passengers, shall furnish said meals to White and colored passengers in the same room, or at the same table, or the same counter. *South Carolina*
>
> *Education*: [The County Board of Education] shall provide schools of two kinds; those for White children and those for colored children. *Texas*
>
> *Mental Hospitals*. The Board of Control shall see that proper and distinct apartments are arranged for said patients, so that in no case shall Negroes and White persons be together. *Georgia*
>
> *Militia*. The White and colored militia shall be separately enrolled and shall never be compelled to serve in the same organization. No organization of colored troops shall be permitted where White troops are available and where Whites are permitted to be organized, colored troops shall be under the command of White officers. *North Carolina*
>
> *Nurses*. No person or corporation shall require any White female nurse to nurse in wards or rooms in hospitals, either public or private, in which negro men are placed. *Alabama*.

The Jim Crow era was also characterized by racial violence, including lynchings, mob attacks, and acts of intimidation directed against Black individuals by White supremacist groups [81]. These violent acts aimed to maintain racial dominance and instill fear within Black communities, contributing to an atmosphere of terror and oppression [79, 82]. While Black people made efforts to challenge these laws, an example of their denied efforts can be reflected in the 1896 Supreme Court ruling in *Plessy v. Ferguson,* which ruled that "separate but equal" facilities—including public transport and schools—were constitutional [83, 84]. In 1892, Plessy, who was classified as Black due to Louisiana's "one-drop rule," intentionally boarded a Whites-only railway car and was subsequently arrested. His arrest and subsequent legal challenge were part of a planned challenge to Louisiana's Separate Car Act, which required separate railway cars for Blacks and Whites [83, 84]. This ruling set the stage for the institutionalization of Jim Crow laws throughout the United States, perpetuating racial segregation and inequality for several decades until the laws were eventually overturned by the Supreme Court in the case of *Brown v. Board of Education* in 1954 [83].

Like Jim Crow Laws, the Black Codes were laws that emerged during Reconstruction, after the Civil War [85, 86]. Black Codes were laws passed by Southern states that were designed to control and restrict the freedom of newly freed Blacks and to maintain White supremacy. Black Codes varied by state but generally aimed to limit the rights of Black citizens, including their ability to own property, work in certain occupations, and move freely [85]. While Black Codes had their primary influence in the post-Civil War period, they and the subsequent Jim Crow laws continued and expanded upon the principles of segregation and discrimination, shaping the social and legal landscape of the Southern states for decades until the

Civil Rights Movement challenged and eventually led to the dismantling of these laws in the mid-twentieth century [87, 88].

Jim Crow Era and Medicine. During the Jim Crow era, Black individuals encountered substantial medical disparities and discriminatory practices. Segregation laws birthed separate and unequal medical facilities, where Black patients received inferior care compared to their White counterparts. Founded in 1862 under initiatives of the Freedmen's Bureau, Freedmen's Hospital, operating in Washington, D.C., faced chronic underfunding, resulting in limited resources, outdated equipment, and insufficient staffing to care for its Black patient population. Despite these challenges, Freedmen's Hospital, in collaboration with Howard University, played a critical role in training Black physicians and nurses, providing opportunities for individuals excluded from medical education elsewhere due to racial segregation [89]. Redlining further marginalized Black neighborhoods, curtailing access to quality housing and well-funded healthcare facilities. This lack of investment in Black communities led to fewer hospitals, clinics, and medical services available to these populations.

Eugenics

The term "Eugenics," introduced by Sir Francis Galton in the late nineteenth century, espoused a theory advocating for selective breeding to amplify desirable traits while eliminating those deemed "undesirable." The eugenics movement promoted the idea of racial hierarchy and advocated for the manipulation of human genetics through selective mating [90, 91]. During the Jim Crow era, the eugenics movement's influence intersected with prevailing racist policies, perpetuating systemic racism and further marginalizing Black people and other minority groups. The eugenics movement continued the harm perpetuated by laws and behaviors designed to curtail enslaved women's reproductive choices, employing measures like forced sterilization to manipulate the gene pool and control reproduction thereby violating Black individuals' reproductive autonomy and rights [55, 65].

Forced Sterilization. During the early twentieth century, several states implemented eugenics-based programs and laws that disproportionately targeted marginalized communities [55, 65, 91]. The notorious *Buck v. Bell* case in 1927, in which the Supreme Court upheld Virginia's sterilization law, significantly legitimized these practices. Carrie Buck, institutionalized at the Virginia State Colony for Epileptics and Feeble-Minded, became the focal point of the case due to her perceived intellectual disabilities and her mother's similar classification. The court's 8-1 decision, notably Justice Oliver Wendell Holmes Jr.'s opinion stating, "Three generations of imbeciles are enough," set a precedent for allowing sterilization without consent [90, 91].

These procedures, often lacking medical or ethical considerations, were implemented by healthcare providers, social workers, and government agencies. Black women were disproportionately affected, as evidenced by the dramatic rise in sterilization rates among these women during the 1970s. Victims of involuntary sterilization were often subjected to coercive tactics or misinformation [65]. The term "Mississippi Appendectomies," popularized by Fannie Lou Hamer, refers to the involuntary sterilization of African American women in Mississippi during the Jim Crow era, highlighting discriminatory practices within the healthcare system. Hamer, a prominent civil rights leader, shared her personal experience of involuntary sterilization during a 1961 surgery meant to remove a uterine tumor. Hamer underwent a hysterectomy without her knowledge or consent, exposing systemic exploitation and reproductive rights violations faced by numerous African American women [55, 92].

Laws in 31 states and the District of Columbia allow permanent forced sterilizations for people with disabilities, subject to judicial determination. In other contexts, sterilization has been offered as an incentive for reduced prison sentences [93]. In May 2017, inmates in White County, Tennessee were offered a reduction in their jail sentences in exchange for undergoing procedures providing long-term birth control, including vasectomies for males or Nexplanon implants for females. Judge Sam Benningfield signed an order allowing inmates to receive jail credit, with the potential for a 30-day reduction in their sentence if they underwent these procedures. The order was implemented to address concerns about children born addicted to drugs or neglected due to their parent's drug use. The order faced criticism from civil rights attorneys, health officials, and the public for potentially infringing on reproductive autonomy and bodily integrity, with concerns about the permanence of the procedures and the ethical implications of linking sentence reductions to specific health services. Despite the judge's claim of collaboration with the Tennessee Department of Health, the Department denied involvement in developing such a policy. The initiative stirred controversy surrounding inmates' autonomy and the ethical implications of incentivizing medical procedures in exchange for sentence reductions [93]. These instances, albeit arguably voluntary, pose concerns due to the disproportionate impact on people of color within the criminal justice system [5, 94, 95].

Margaret Sanger & Planned Parenthood. Margaret Sanger, an advocate for birth control and the founder of Planned Parenthood, played a significant role in the eugenics movement. While her primary focus was on promoting women's reproductive rights and access to birth control, she also aligned herself with eugenicists, believing that birth control could lead to what she saw as "better births" and healthier children by allowing families to plan and limit the size of their families [55, 96]. Sanger's birth control clinics, including those in predominantly Black neighborhoods, aimed to provide reproductive health information and services to underserved communities. While some Black leaders supported her efforts to provide birth control education and access, others criticized her views on eugenics and expressed concerns about the potential for birth control programs to be coercive or to target specific racial groups for population control [55, 97].

Additional Noteworthy Medical Research

The Tuskegee Syphilis Study, a pivotal case illustrating medical racism, was conducted by the United States Public Health Service (USPHS) from 1932 to 1972 in Tuskegee, Alabama [55, 65, 98, 99]. Approximately 600 African American men, predominantly poor sharecroppers, were recruited for the study. Investigations extensively document this research aimed at observing the untreated progression of syphilis. The participants were initially told they were receiving treatment for "bad blood," a term used locally for various ailments including syphilis, but also anemia and fatigue. However, the men were deceived about the actual nature of the study and were not informed that they had syphilis. Despite the discovery in the 1940s of penicillin's efficacy as a treatment for syphilis, researchers intentionally withheld treatment from the participants for four decades. This breach of ethical standards included the denial of informed consent, leading to immense suffering, severe health complications, and fatalities among the participants. Public revelation of the Tuskegee Study's unethical nature, brought to light in 1972 by investigative journalist Peter Buxtun, triggered widespread public outcry, congressional hearings, and a significant reevaluation of ethical guidelines in medical research. The exposure led to the establishment of stringent regulations and ethical protocols for research involving human subjects, including the formation of Institutional Review Boards (IRBs) to safeguard participants' rights and ensure informed consent [99–101].

The case of Henrietta Lacks, explored in further detail elsewhere in this volume, stands as yet another stark example of medical exploitation. The use of Lacks' cells to form a self-regenerating cell line known as HeLa contributed significantly to scientific advancements. However, these cells were obtained by the researchers who studied them without Lacks' knowledge or consent or that of her family. This raised profound ethical concerns, highlighting systemic issues regarding medical ethics, patient autonomy, and equitable compensation [65, 102].

Another case of medical exploitation involved Dr. Albert Kligman, who conducted unethical experiments on predominantly Black incarcerated individuals [103, 104]. Dr. Kligman conducted dermatological experiments at Holmesburg Prison in Philadelphia from the 1950s to the 1970s, using prisoners as subjects for testing various substances, including skin care products and chemicals, without their informed consent. These experiments led to the development of products like Retin-A, which became commercial successes in the skincare and pharmaceutical industries. However, the foundation of these advancements was built on the backs of incarcerated men, a majority of whom were Black. Participants in these experiments, many lured by the promise of financial gain or better living conditions within the prison, were often uninformed about the nature and potential risks of the tests they underwent. They were subjected to various trials, including the infamous "milkshake tests" in which participants lived in an isolated cellblock and received their only nutrients in the form of milkshakes with unknown ingredients for 6 months. Participation in these experiments resulted in physical and psychological trauma that haunted inmates long after their release [103, 104]. The ethical implications of conducting medical experiments in prison settings have sparked debates regarding the coercion involved, the lack of true informed consent, and the profound disregard for the well-being of incarcerated individuals. While regulations have been introduced to govern prison-based research, questions persist about the true agency of incarcerated persons in consenting to trials and the ethical boundaries of such experimentation.

The cases mentioned above significantly contribute to the pervasive mistrust of the healthcare system among African Americans, affecting perceptions of medical research, healthcare access, and patient–provider relationships within African American communities for decades. Of note, these are the cases accessible; the power of the system is that it silences the voices of the oppressed. How many voices have been silenced? These are the atrocities that we know of; imagine the depth of those we do not know and how they have also impacted the disparities that we see impacting Black patients.

Understanding the Impact of Medical Racism

Medical racism casts a long and dark shadow across our healthcare system, inflicting disproportionate harm on Black patients. Its roots lie in a troubling history marked by unethical medical experiments and pervasive racial biases ingrained in healthcare delivery. These injustices have eroded the trust between Black communities and the medical establishment, forming a barrier to effectively addressing healthcare disparities. Despite strides in medicine and efforts at increasing equity, medical racism's persistence is evident through the enduring struggles faced by marginalized communities. Instances of medical racism continue to be stark reflections of systemic biases and disparities within the healthcare system, which directly impact the health outcomes of minority populations. In the twenty-first century, medical racism persists in various forms, including disparities in maternal mortality, the harsh impact of the COVID-19 pandemic on minority communities, implicit biases that sway diagnostic and treatment decisions, structural obstacles obstructing equitable healthcare access, and the ongoing challenge of achieving diversity in medical research. Delving into the multifaceted impact of medical racism on Black individuals demands more than surface-level recognition.

The impact of medical racism on Black patients' mental health is especially pronounced. Research has shown the connection between experiences of racial discrimination and adverse mental health outcomes among African Americans [105]. Persistent encounters with biased healthcare practices, such as misdiagnoses or undertreatment, can engender mistrust of the medical system and heightened anxiety when seeking care. This, in turn, results in delays in seeking medical attention that hamper effective treatment. Additionally, the stress associated with navigating a healthcare system that frequently invalidates marginalized patients' concerns contributes to chronic stress and depression. Chronic stress, especially when worsened by ongoing experiences of discrimination, can significantly harm physical health, including reproductive health. Research has shown that chronic stress can affect fertility in both women and men by disrupting hormonal balance. When the body is under constant stress, it releases higher levels of cortisol, a stress hormone. This hormone can interfere with the normal function of the hypothalamic-pituitary-ovarian (HPO) axis in women, leading to menstrual irregularities and ovulation issues [106, 107]. For men, chronic stress affects the production and quality of sperm by disrupting testosterone levels, which are crucial for sperm health [108].

Race Based Traumatic Stress

According to a report by the American Psychological Association, the cumulative effects of racism and discrimination can lead to higher rates of PTSD and other mental health disorders among Black individuals [105]. Research on race-based traumatic stress further elucidates how these experiences of discrimination and racism can lead to significant psychological distress, manifesting in symptoms akin to PTSD [109].

Race-based traumatic stress refers to the psychological and emotional distress experienced by individuals due to racial discrimination, racism, and other forms of racial oppression. Unlike general traumatic stress, which can result from various types of distressing events to which individuals from most groups are equally vulnerable, race-based traumatic stress is specifically tied to experiences of racism. This can include direct experiences such as racial slurs, physical violence, and microaggressions, as well as systemic issues like discriminatory policies and institutional racism [109].

The effects of race-based traumatic stress can be profound and pervasive, impacting mental health, physical health, and overall well-being. Individuals may experience symptoms similar to those of post-traumatic stress disorder (PTSD), including anxiety, depression, hypervigilance, intrusive thoughts, and avoidance behaviors [110]. Additionally, chronic exposure to racism can lead to increased stress levels, which can, in turn, contribute to various health problems such as hypertension, cardiovascular disease, and weakened immune function [111].

Research indicates that race-based traumatic stress is not only a response to individual acts of racism but also to the cumulative impact of living in a society where racial discrimination is prevalent. This cumulative stress can affect one's sense of identity, self-worth, and belonging. For instance, being repeatedly exposed to negative stereotypes and biases can lead to internalized racism, where individuals begin to accept and believe harmful stereotypes about their racial group [112]. Understanding race-based traumatic stress is essential in the fertility context, given the well-documented impact of chronic stress on reproductive health. Historical and ongoing experiences of racism contribute to significant stress for marginalized communities, potentially impacting fertility outcomes.

Intergenerational Trauma

Intergenerational trauma refers to the transmission of historical trauma and its associated stressors across multiple generations within a family or community. This phenomenon particularly impacts communities that have experienced profound and sustained injustices, such as slavery, colonization, and systemic discrimination [113, 114]. The impact of centuries of medical racism can manifest in intergenerational trauma, where the cumulative effects of historical injustices reverberate across generations, profoundly affecting Black individuals on a psychological, emotional, and physiological level [115].

Intergenerational trauma can manifest in a complex web of stressors and disparities, including heightened susceptibility to mental health issues such as depression, anxiety, and post-traumatic stress disorder (PTSD) [116, 117]. Additionally, it can influence behavioral patterns, coping mechanisms, and overall health outcomes within affected communities. The trauma experienced by previous generations can influence the way subsequent generations perceive the world, react to stress, and interact with others.

Examples of the impact of intergenerational trauma include:

- Family Dynamics and Parenting: A parent who has experienced trauma may have difficulty forming secure attachments with their children, potentially leading to attachment issues and emotional difficulties in the next generation [118]. For instance, a parent who endured racial violence or systemic discrimination might be overprotective or excessively fearful for their child's safety, affecting the child's sense of autonomy and security.
- Health Disparities: The legacy of intergenerational trauma can contribute to health disparities seen in Black communities. For example, higher rates of hypertension and diabetes among Black individuals can be linked to chronic stress responses inherited from generations that lived under oppressive conditions, combined with ongoing discrimination and limited access to quality healthcare [31, 119].
- Cultural Transmission: Cultural narratives and collective memory play a crucial role in intergenerational trauma. Stories of suffering and resilience passed down through generations can shape a community's identity and worldview. This transmission can maintain a collective sense of vigilance and mistrust towards societal structures perceived as oppressive, impacting how individuals engage with institutions such as education and healthcare [120, 121].

Dr. Joy DeGruy has extensively explored the concept of Post Traumatic Slave Syndrome (PTSS), proposing that the psychological and emotional toll of slavery persists in contemporary society. PTSS suggests that the legacy of slavery has contributed to ongoing mental health challenges faced by Black communities [115]. This syndrome underscores how historical trauma can shape contemporary experiences and health outcomes.

Summary and Conclusions

The convergence of systemic racism, intergenerational trauma, and ongoing racial disparities in healthcare creates a multifaceted burden on the mental health of Black patients. This underscores the pressing need for culturally sensitive and equitable healthcare services. Healthcare providers embracing cultural humility can help address these unique challenges by acknowledging the historical context of trauma, fostering trust, and providing tailored interventions that consider the lived experiences of Black individuals [122, 123].

Confronting these challenges necessitates resolute efforts to combat systemic biases, enhance cultural competency among healthcare providers, ensure equitable access to healthcare resources, and prioritize inclusivity in medical research for the development of a more equitable healthcare system [123]. It is necessary for healthcare professionals to recognize the historical context and ongoing ramifications of medical racism so they can work toward mitigating its impact. Through continuous education, self-reflection, and systematic efforts to dismantle biases, healthcare providers can contribute to cultivating an environment marked by trust, respect, and inclusivity in healthcare interactions [31]. Such an approach is not only vital for individual patient care but also for advancing equitable and inclusive healthcare practices that prioritize the physical and mental health and well-being of Black communities.

References

1. Abbasi J. US maternal mortality is unacceptably high, unequal, and getting worse—what can be done about it? JAMA. 2023;330(4):302–5.
2. Broussard PA. Black women's post-slavery silence syndrome: a twenty-first century remnant of slavery, Jim Crow, and systemic racism-who will tell her stories. J Gen Race Just. 2013;16:373.
3. Feagin J. Systemic racism: a theory of oppression. Routledge; 2013.
4. McCluney CL, King DD, Bryant CM, Ali AA. From "Calling in Black" to "Calling for Antiracism Resources": the need for systemic resources to address systemic racism. Equal Divers Inclusion Int J. 2021;40(1):49–59.
5. Alexander M. The new Jim Crow: mass incarceration in the age of colorblindness. Revised ed. New York: New Press; 2012.
6. Marable M. Introduction: racializing justice, disenfranchising lives. In: Racializing justice, disenfranchising lives: the racism, criminal justice, and law reader. New York: Palgrave Macmillan US; 2007. p. 1–14.
7. Brown AF, Bloome D, Morris JE, Power-Carter S, Willis AI. Classroom conversations in the study of race and the disruption of social and educational inequalities: a review of research. Rev Res Educ. 2017;41(1):453–76.
8. Cooper Brathwaite A, Versailles D, Juüdi-Hope D, Coppin M, Jefferies K, Bradley R, Campbell R, Garraway C, Obewu O, LaRonde-Ogilvie C, Sinclair D. Tackling discrimination and systemic racism in academic and workplace settings. Nurs Inq. 2022;29(4):e12485.
9. Banaji MR, Fiske ST, Massey DS. Systemic racism: individuals and interactions, institutions and society. Cogn Res Princ Implic. 2021;6(1):82.

10. Feagin JR. Excluding blacks and others from housing: the foundation of white racism. City. 1999;1:79–91.
11. Lloyd CM, Shaw S, Alvira-Hammond M, DeMand A. Racism and discrimination contribute to housing instability for Black families during the pandemic. Child Trends; 2021.
12. Berger JT, Miller DR. Health disparities, systemic racism, and failures of cultural competence. Am J Bioeth. 2021;21(9):4–10.
13. Maness SB, Merrell L, Thompson EL, Griner SB, Kline N, Wheldon C. Social determinants of health and health disparities: COVID-19 exposures and mortality among African American people in the United States. Public Health Rep. 2021;136(1):18–22.
14. Ombongi S. Racial disparities in healthcare: a problem due to systemic racism. 2021.
15. Morgan I. Equal is not good enough: an analysis of school funding equity across the US and within each state. Education Trust; 2022.
16. Chadwick NJ. Teacher perceptions of Black male students and the effect on student classroom behavior (Doctoral dissertation). Texas Wesleyan University. 2023.
17. Del Toro J, Wang MT. Longitudinal inter-relations between school cultural socialization and school engagement: the mediating role of school climate. Learn Instr. 2021;75:101482.
18. Lynch EE, Malcoe LH, Laurent SE, Richardson J, Mitchell BC, Meier HC. The legacy of structural racism: associations between historic redlining, current mortgage lending, and health. SSM Populat Health. 2021;14:100793.
19. Swope CB, Hernández D, Cushing LJ. The relationship of historical redlining with present-day neighborhood environmental and health outcomes: a scoping review and conceptual model. J Urban Health. 2022;99(6):959–83.
20. Nellis A. The color of justice: racial and ethnic disparity in state prisons [Internet]. The Sentencing Project. 2021. https://www.sentencingproject.org/reports/the-color-of-justice-racial-and-ethnic-disparity-in-state-prisons-the-sentencing-project/.
21. Ajilore O. The persistent Black-White unemployment gap is built into the labor market [Internet]. Center for American Progress. 2020. https://www.americanprogress.org/article/persistent-black-white-unemployment-gap-built-labor-market/.
22. Moore KK. Unemployment rates remained low through the third quarter of 2023 though labor market disparities persist [Internet]. Economic Policy Institute. Nov 2023. https://www.epi.org/indicators/state-unemployment-race-ethnicity/.
23. US Bureau of Labor Statistics. Labor force characteristics by race and ethnicity, 2021 [Internet]. US Bureau of Labor Statistics. Jan 2023. https://www.bls.gov/opub/reports/race-and-ethnicity/2021/home.htm.
24. Miller S. Black workers still earn less than their White counterparts: employers can examine their pay policies to root out inequities [Internet]. SHRM. 11 June 2020. https://www.shrm.org/topics-tools/news/benefits-compensation/black-workers-still-earn-less-white-counterparts.
25. Wilson V, Darity W. Understanding Black-White disparities in labor market outcomes requires models that account for persistent discrimination and unequal bargaining power [Internet]. Economic Policy Institute. 25 Mar 2022. https://www.epi.org/unequalpower/publications/understanding-black-white-disparities-in-labor-market-outcomes/.
26. Economic Policy Institute. Black-White wage gaps expand with rising wage inequality. Retrieved from EPI. 2021.
27. National Women's Law Center. The wage gap: the who, how, why, and what to do. National Women's Law Center; 2020.
28. Swope CB, Hernández D. Housing as a determinant of health equity: a conceptual model. Soc Sci Med. 2019;243:112571.
29. Williams DR, Mohammed SA. Racism and health I: pathways and scientific evidence. Am Behav Sci. 2013;57(8):1152–73.
30. Gee GC, Ford CL. Structural racism and health inequities: old issues, new directions1. Du Bois Rev. 2011;8(1):115–32.
31. Bailey ZD, Krieger N, Agénor M, Graves J, Linos N, Bassett MT. Structural racism and health inequities in the USA: evidence and interventions. Lancet. 2017;389(10077):1453–63.

32. Artiga S, Orgera K, Pham O, Corallo B. Racial disparities in COVID-19 impacts and vaccinations among older adults. Kaiser Family Foundation; 2020.
33. Khan MS, Ali SA, Adelaine A, Karan A. Rethinking vaccine hesitancy among minority groups. Lancet. 2021;397(10288):1863–5.
34. Blackstock U. Legacy: a Black physician reckons with racism in medicine. Viking; 2022.
35. Burgess DJ, Nelson DB, Gravely AA, Bair MJ, Kerns RD, Higgins DM, Van Ryn M, Farmer M, Partin MR. Racial differences in prescription of opioid analgesics for chronic noncancer pain in a national sample of veterans. J Pain. 2014;15(4):447–55.
36. Goyal MK, Kuppermann N, Cleary SD, Teach SJ, Chamberlain JM. Racial disparities in pain management of children with appendicitis in emergency departments. JAMA Pediatr. 2015;169(11):996–1002.
37. Waytz A, Hoffman KM, Trawalter S. A superhumanization bias in Whites' perceptions of Blacks. Soc Psychol Personal Sci. 2015;6(3):352–9.
38. Hollingshead NA, Meints SM, Miller MM, Robinson ME, Hirsh AT. A comparison of race-related pain stereotypes held by White and Black individuals. J Appl Soc Psychol. 2016;46(12):718–23.
39. Hoffman KM, Trawalter S, Axt JR, Oliver MN. Racial bias in pain assessment and treatment recommendations, and false beliefs about biological differences between blacks and whites. Proc Natl Acad Sci. 2016;113(16):4296–301.
40. Goyal MK, Johnson TJ, Chamberlain JM, Cook L, Webb M, Drendel AL, Alessandrini E, Bajaj L, Lorch S, Grundmeier RW, Alpern ER. Racial and ethnic differences in emergency department pain management of children with fractures. Pediatrics. 2020;145(5):e20193370.
41. Burgess DJ, Gravely AA, Nelson DB, Van Ryn M, Bair MJ, Kerns RD, Higgins DM, Partin MR. A national study of racial differences in pain screening rates in the VA health care system. Clin J Pain. 2013;29(2):118–23.
42. Odonkor CA, Esparza R, Flores LE, Verduzco-Gutierrez M, Escalon MX, Solinsky R, Silver JK. Disparities in health care for black patients in physical medicine and rehabilitation in the United States: a narrative review. PM R. 2021;13(2):180–203.
43. Brennan F, Lohman D, Gwyther L. Access to pain management as a human right. Am J Public Health. 2019;109(1):61–5.
44. Todd KH, Deaton C, D'adamo AP, Goe L. Ethnicity and analgesic practice. Ann Emerg Med. 2000;35(1):11–6.
45. Schulman KA, Berlin JA, Harless W, Kerner JF, Sistrunk S, Gersh BJ, Dube R, Taleghani CK, Burke JE, Williams S, Eisenberg JM. The effect of race and sex on physicians' recommendations for cardiac catheterization. N Engl J Med. 1999;340(8):618–26.
46. Green AR, Carney DR, Pallin DJ, Ngo LH, Raymond KL, Iezzoni LI, Banaji MR. Implicit bias among physicians and its prediction of thrombolysis decisions for black and white patients. J Gen Intern Med. 2007;22:1231–8.
47. Haider AH, Chang DC, Efron DT, Haut ER, Crandall M, Cornwell EE. Race and insurance status as risk factors for trauma mortality. Arch Surg. 2008;143(10):945–9.
48. Sabin JA, Nosek BA, Greenwald AG, Rivara FP. Physicians' implicit and explicit attitudes about race by MD race, ethnicity, and gender. J Health Care Poor Underserved. 2009;20(3):896–913.
49. Cooper LA, Roter DL, Carson KA, Beach MC, Sabin JA, Greenwald AG, Inui TS. The associations of clinicians' implicit attitudes about race with medical visit communication and patient ratings of interpersonal care. Am J Public Health. 2012;102(5):979–87.
50. Arcaya MC, Schnake-Mahla A. Health in segregated cities [Internet]. NYU Furman Center. https://furmancenter.org/research/iri/essay/health-in-the-segregated-city%20#:~:text=Access%20to%20quality%20health%20care%20in%20the%20segregated%20city&text=Predominantly%20Black%2C%20racially%20isolated%20neighborhoods,supply%20of%20surgeons%20(9).

51. Dieke AC, Zhang Y, Kissin DM, Barfield WD, Boulet SL. Disparities in assisted reproductive technology utilization by race and ethnicity, United States, 2014: a commentary. J Womens Health. 2017;26(6):605–8.
52. Wellons MF, Fujimoto VY, Baker VL, Barrington DS, Broomfield D, Catherino WH, Richard-Davis G, Ryan M, Thornton K, Armstrong AY. Race matters: a systematic review of racial/ethnic disparity in Society for Assisted Reproductive Technology reported outcomes. Fertil Steril. 2012;98(2):406–9.
53. McCarthy-Keith DM, Schisterman EF, Robinson RD, O'Leary K, Lucidi RS, Armstrong AY. Will decreasing assisted reproduction technology costs improve utilization and outcomes among minority women? Fertil Steril. 2010;94(7):2587–9.
54. Armstrong A, Plowden TC. Ethnicity and assisted reproductive technologies. Clin Pract. 2012;9(6):651.
55. Roberts DE. Killing the black body: race, reproduction, and the meaning of liberty. New York: Vintage Books; 1999.
56. Thompson TA, Young YY, Bass TM, Baker S, Njoku O, Norwood J, Simpson M. Racism runs through it: examining the sexual and reproductive health experience of Black women in the South: study examines the sexual and reproductive health experiences of Black women in the South. Health Aff. 2022;41(2):195–202.
57. Howell EA. Reducing disparities in severe maternal morbidity and mortality. Clin Obstet Gynecol. 2018;61(2):387–99.
58. Hoyert DL. Maternal mortality rates in the United States, 2022. NCHS Health E-Stats. 2024;230:440.E1–E13. https://doi.org/10.15620/cdc/152992.
59. MacDorman MF, Thoma M, Declcerq E, Howell EA. Racial and ethnic disparities in maternal mortality in the United States using enhanced vital records, 2016–2017. Am J Public Health. 2021;111(9):1673–81.
60. Eltis D. A brief overview of the Trans-Atlantic Slave Trade. In: Voyages: The trans-Atlantic slave trade database. Slave Voyages; 2007. p. 1700–810.
61. Eltis D, Richardson D, editors. Routes to slavery: direction, ethnicity and mortality in the transatlantic slave trade. Routledge; 2013.
62. Eltis D. The US transatlantic slave trade, 1644–1867: an assessment. Civil War History. 2008;54(4):347–78.
63. Savitt TL. Medicine and slavery: the diseases and health care of blacks in antebellum Virginia. University of Illinois Press; 2002.
64. Bankole K. Slavery and medicine: enslavement and medical practices in Antebellum Louisiana. Routledge; 2019.
65. Washington HA. Medical apartheid: the dark history of medical experimentation on Black Americans from colonial times to the present. Doubleday Books; 2006.
66. Alozai UU, McPherson PK. Malingering. In: StatPearls. StatPearls Publishing; 2023.
67. Blassingame JW. The slave community: plantation life in the antebellum South. New York: Oxford University Press; 1972.
68. Otto JS, Burns AM. Black folks and poor Buckras: archeological evidence of slave and overseer living conditions on an antebellum plantation. J Black Stud. 1983;14(2):185–200.
69. Margo RA, Steckel RH. The heights of American slaves: new evidence on slave nutrition and health. Soc Sci Hist. 1982;6(4):516–38.
70. Owens DC. Medical bondage: race, gender, and the origins of American gynecology. University of Georgia Press; 2017.
71. Wailoo K. Historical aspects of race and medicine: the case of J. Marion Sims. JAMA. 2018;320(15):1529–30.
72. Ojanuga D. The medical ethics of the 'father of gynaecology', Dr J Marion Sims. J Med Ethics. 1993;19(1):28–31.
73. Wall LL. The controversial Dr. J. Marion Sims (1813–1883). Int Urogynecol J. 2020;31(7):1299–303.

74. Savitt TL. The use of blacks for medical experimentation and demonstration in the Old South. J South Hist. 1982;48(3):331–48.
75. Halperin EC. The poor, the black, and the marginalized as the source of cadavers in United States anatomical education. Clin Anat. 2007;20(5):489–95.
76. Packard JM. American nightmare: the history of Jim Crow. Macmillan; 2003.
77. Pilgrim D. What was Jim Crow. Ferris State University; 2007.
78. Pilgrim D. Understanding Jim Crow: using racist memorabilia to teach tolerance and promote social justice. PM Press; 2015.
79. Epperly B, Witko C, Strickler R, White P. Rule by violence, rule by law: lynching, Jim Crow, and the continuing evolution of voter suppression in the US. Perspect Polit. 2020;18(3):756–69.
80. Jim Crow Museum. Examples of Jim Crow Laws—Oct. 1960—Civil Rights [Internet]. Jim Crow Museum. 2020. https://jimcrowmuseum.ferris.edu/links/misclink/examples.htm.
81. Tolnay SE, Beck EM. Racial violence and black migration in the American South, 1910 to 1930. Am Sociol Rev. 1992;57:103–16.
82. Thompson-Miller R, Feagin JR, Picca LH. Jim Crow's legacy: the lasting impact of segregation. Rowman & Littlefield; 2014.
83. Bartz DE, Kritsonis WA. Racism, the white power structure, and the tragic history of the education of African American children in the United States. Schooling. 2019;10(1):1–9.
84. Levine RS. Reconstructions: Frederick Douglass, Albion Tourgée, and Plessy v. Ferguson. New North Star J Life Times Frederick Douglass. 2022;4(1):83–8.
85. Wallenfeldt J. Black Code | United States History [Internet]. Encyclopedia Britannica. 4 June 2015. https://www.britannica.com.
86. Zeki E. History of Black codes and Jim Crow laws. Soc Mental Res Thinkers J. 2022;5(26):2026–41.
87. Blackmon DA. Slavery by another name: the re-enslavement of Black Americans from the Civil War to World War II. Anchor; 2009.
88. Hansan JE. Jim Crow laws and racial segregation [Internet]. Social Welfare History Project. 2011. https://socialwelfare.library.vcu.edu/eras/civil-war-reconstruction/jim-crow-laws-andracial-segregation/.
89. Cobb WM. A short history of Freedmen's hospital. J Natl Med Assoc. 1962;54(3):271.
90. Lombardo PA. Medicine, eugenics, and the Supreme Court: from coercive sterilization to reproductive freedom. J Contemp Health L Pol'y. 1996;13:1.
91. Lombardo PA, editor. A century of eugenics in America: from the Indiana experiment to the human genome era. Indiana University Press; 2011.
92. Dixon Omere ZO, King J. America's history of health disparities: how does this affect the future of healthcare in Mississippi? University of Mississippi; 2022.
93. Adams EB. Voluntary sterilization of inmates for reduced prison sentences. Duke J Gender L Pol'y. 2018;26:23.
94. Sawyer W. Visualizing the racial disparities in mass incarceration. Prison Policy Initiative. 2020;27:27.
95. Weidner RR, Schultz J. Examining the relationship between US incarceration rates and population health at the county level. SSM Populat Health. 2019;9:100466.
96. Roberts D. Margaret sanger and the racial origins of the birth control movement. In: Racially writing the republic: Racists, race rebels, and transformations of American identity. Duke University Press; 2009. p. 196–213.
97. Green TL. The negro project: Margaret Sanger's eugenic plan for Black Americans. Life Education and Resource Network: Fayetteville, NC; 2004.
98. Alsan M, Wanamaker M. Tuskegee and the health of black men. Q J Econ. 2018;133(1):407–55.
99. Reverby SM. Examining Tuskegee: the infamous syphilis study and its legacy. University of North Carolina Press; 2009.
100. Jones JH. Bad blood. Simon and Schuster; 1993.

101. Gamble VN. A legacy of distrust: African Americans and medical research. Am J Prev Med. 1993;9(6 Suppl):35–8.
102. Skloot R. The immortal life of Henrietta lacks. Crown Publishers; 2010.
103. Adamson AS, Lipoff JB. Reconsidering named honorifics in medicine—the troubling legacy of dermatologist Albert Kligman. JAMA Dermatol. 2021;157(2):153–5.
104. MacLure J. Unnatural resources: the colonial logic of the Holmesburg prison experiments. J Med Hum. 2021;42:423–33.
105. Williams DR, Lawrence JA, Davis BA. Racism and health: evidence and needed research. Annu Rev Public Health. 2019;40(1):105–25.
106. Palomba S, Daolio J, Romeo S, Battaglia FA, Marci R, La Sala GB. Lifestyle and fertility: the influence of stress and quality of life on female fertility. Reprod Biol Endocrinol. 2018;16(1):113.
107. Vigil P, Meléndez J, Soto H, Petkovic G, Bernal YA, Molina S. Chronic stress and ovulatory dysfunction: implications in times of COVID-19. Front Glob Womens Health. 2022;3:866104.
108. Ramya S, Poornima P, Jananisri A, Geofferina IP, Bavyataa V, Divya M, Priyanga P, Vadivukarasi J, Sujitha S, Elamathi S, Anand AV. Role of hormones and the potential impact of multiple stresses on infertility. Stress. 2023;3(2):454–74.
109. Carter RT. Racism and psychological and emotional injury: recognizing and assessing race-based traumatic stress. Couns Psychol. 2007;35(1):13–05.
110. Bryant-Davis T, Ocampo C. Racist incident–based trauma. Couns Psychol. 2005;33(4):479–500.
111. Mulligan CJ. Systemic racism can get under our skin and into our genes. Am J Phys Anthropol. 2021;175(2):399–405.
112. Harrell SP. A multidimensional conceptualization of racism-related stress: implications for the well-being of people of color. Am J Orthopsychiatry. 2000;70(1):42–57.
113. Kirmayer LJ, Gone JP, Moses J. Rethinking historical trauma. Transcult Psychiatry. 2014;51(3):299–319.
114. Brave Heart MY. The return to the sacred path: healing the historical trauma and historical unresolved grief response among the Lakota through a psychoeducational group intervention. Smith Coll Stud Soc Work. 1998;68(3):287–305.
115. Degruy-Leary J. Post-traumatic slave syndrome: America's legacy of enduring injury. Portland: Joy DeGruy Publications Inc.; 2017.
116. Sotero M. A conceptual model of historical trauma: implications for public health practice and research. J Health Disparities Res Pract. 2006;1(1):93–108.
117. Yehuda R, Daskalakis NP, Bierer LM, Bader HN, Klengel T, Holsboer F, Binder EB. Holocaust exposure induced intergenerational effects on FKBP5 methylation. Biol Psychiatry. 2016;80(5):372–80.
118. Lieberman AF, Chu A, Van Horn P, Harris WW. Trauma in early childhood: empirical evidence and clinical implications. Dev Psychopathol. 2011;23(2):397–410.
119. Williams DR, Mohammed SA. Discrimination and racial disparities in health: evidence and needed research. J Behav Med. 2009;32:20–47.
120. Danieli Y, editor. International handbook of multigenerational legacies of trauma. Springer Science & Business Media; 1998.
121. Mohatt NV, Thompson AB, Thai ND, Tebes JK. Historical trauma as public narrative: a conceptual review of how history impacts present-day health. Soc Sci Med. 2014;106:128–36.
122. Nelson A. Unequal treatment: confronting racial and ethnic disparities in health care. J Natl Med Assoc. 2002;94(8):666.
123. Betancourt JR, Green AR, Carrillo JE, Owusu Ananeh-Firempong II. Defining cultural competence: a practical framework for addressing racial/ethnic disparities in health and health care. Public Health Rep. 2003;118(4):293–302.

Chapter 14
Cultural Competence and Cultural Humility in Working with Latinx-Assisted Reproductive Patients

Ariadna Cymet-Lanski

Introduction

This chapter is the cross-section of the personal and professional. I grew up in Mexico and learned English when I was very young; my school was called "The Mexican American School". I traveled with my family to the USA frequently and was an exchange student in upstate New York in my teen years. Moving to the USA in my late 20s to complete a PsyD program seemed like an "easy next step" in my professional career. As it turns out, it was not that easy. My move in early 2000 brought some challenges, as I underestimated the impact that being Hispanic in the United States can have. It took a while to adjust in both my personal and professional life, as I navigated achieving success as a member of a minority population.

Suddenly, I was "the other." I had to take classes on cultural diversity and quickly became the teaching assistant for those classes. In doing so, I learned about acculturation, bias, prejudice, racism, cultural competence, and the treatment of minorities. Since then, the terms we use to describe these phenomena have evolved. Nowadays we talk about diversity and inclusion, cultural humility, and patient-centered care; I find myself more comfortable with these terms. I am also more comfortable with how others see me and how I see myself as part of the cultural fabric in which I live and work.

You are reading this book because you care about diverse patients' experiences in treatment and want to help them navigate a challenging phase of their lives. You want to understand and meet them where they are and provide the needed support to traverse the complicated waters of Assisted Reproductive Treatment. I hope you find this chapter useful as you work with Latinx patients.

A. Cymet-Lanski (✉)
ASRM Mental Health Group, Chicago, IL, USA

D. A. Kaplan (ed.), *Cultural Responsiveness in Assisted Reproductive Technology*, https://doi.org/10.1007/978-3-031-76204-8_14

Background

Sub-fertility is a life-changing experience with deep psychological repercussions. Anxiety, depression, and low self-esteem run through the infertility experience. Even though infertility is highly medicalized, the cultural and social contexts in which it occurs are what ultimately determine the psychological impact of infertility for any given patient [1]. With the expansion of globalization, immigration, and intercultural relationships, it is imperative to acknowledge cultural aspects and values inherent to patients' cultural experience of ART and unique cultural barriers to their care. Incorporating these aspects into clinical practice and developing cultural competence and cultural humility are essential elements of developing an ART practice that attracts, retains, and provides high-quality care to a diverse patient population.

According to the US Census Bureau, the U.S. Hispanic population reached 65 million in 2024, accounting for 19.5% of all Americans. As of 2024, Hispanics were the nation's second-largest racial or ethnic group, behind White Americans and ahead of Black Americans [2]. However, even these categories are reductive and misleading; the label "Hispanic" comprises diverse, heterogeneous, and culturally rich communities, each with its own history, beliefs, socioeconomic characteristics, and experiences in the United States.

The Hispanic human response to key life cycle events, including birth, death, marriage, divorce and changes in health status, is shaped by the individual's culture. Therefore, it is through understanding the culture that a provider can best understand and meet the patient's needs. This chapter will briefly cover historical content, family structure, education, and mental health perspectives that may inform infertility clinicians' work with Hispanic patients.

What's in a Name?

In this chapter, people will be referred to alternately as Hispanic or Latin/a/o/e/x. The United States Census Bureau primarily uses the term "Hispanic,"while research and academic centers employ "Hispanic" and "Latino" interchangeably. The word "Hispanic" refers to individuals from Spain or Spanish-speaking countries, excluding Brazil, while "Latino/Latina" refers to male and female individuals from Central and South America. The nongendered term "Latinx" has emerged as an alternative term to Hispanic and Latino in recent years, gaining traction in various contexts such as news, corporations, local governments, and academia.

"Hispanic" and "Latino" are not universally embraced by the population they purport to label, even as they are widely used. A 2019 Pew Research Center survey of US Latino adults found that only 23% of US adults who self-identify as Hispanic or Latino have heard the term "Latinx" [3]. Individuals aged 18 to 29 are most likely to have heard of the term: even among this group, only 42% are familiar with this designation, compared with 7% of those 65 and older. Some of the most common use of Latinx is among Hispanic women ages 18 to 29; 14% of these women say they use it, compared with 1% of Hispanic men in the same age group. Findings from the same survey suggest that 47% of Hispanics most often describe themselves by their family's country of origin (e.g., I identify as Mexican, while someone else will identify as Colombian or Chilean) while 39% use the terms Latino or Hispanic and 14% most often describe themselves as American [3].

History of the People and Territory

Hispanic/Latinx history in the current US territory goes back to the first encounters between Europeans and Indigenous people of the New Continent. More than 100 years before the Mayflower arrived in Plymouth, Juan Ponce de León of Spain became the first European to arrive on the coast of Florida in 1513. In 1565, Pedro Menéndez de Avilés founded Saint Augustine, the oldest continuously inhabited European-established settlement in the USA. In 1598, Juan de Oñate established the first settlement in today's New Mexico. In 1680, Spanish Franciscan missions expanded from El Paso to East Texas, leading to the foundation of San Antonio in 1718. The Presidio of San Diego was founded in 1769, and another Franciscan missionary, Junípero Serra, is credited with founding 21 missions between San Diego and San Francisco. The Caminos Reales or Royal Roads connected these missions to the rest of the Southern Hispanic territories [4].

At the beginning of colonization, the Spanish crown was not concerned with race. Instead, the idea of spreading Catholicism dominated the thinking of the time. Indigenous inhabitants of the colonized territories were regularly baptized, leading to frequent mixing between Spaniards and indigenous people regardless of their social classes. This led to the formation of the mixed ethnic group (*mestizos*) that is prevalent among Hispanic/Latin Americans today [5].

According to the thought of the time, Christian people could not be enslaved. Therefore, natives who embraced Catholicism were technically protected. However, contrary to what the Catholic monarchs mandated, it was common for Spanish soldiers to prevent the Christianization of indigenous people in order to enslave them. With the efforts of Fray Bartolome de las Casas, who proactively converted indigenous people to Catholicism, many otherwise vulnerable people were made legal subjects of the Spanish crown and thus protected from slavery. These conversions protected the indigenous population from enslavement but resulted in an increased slavery trade from Africa to America that lasted for centuries. Under Spanish rule, African slaves had more rights than in the English colonies. For instance, they were allowed to marry, own property, or buy their freedom. This increased the rates of racial mixing; interracial marriage was tolerated in the Spanish colonies, and free Blacks could not be discriminated against as soon as they embraced Catholicism. As such, it became common for enslaved Africans to escape from British colonies to Florida in search of freedom and a better life. The first settlement of freed slaves in current US territory was Fort Mose in Hispanic Florida [4].

Following independence from the British crown, the USA commenced its expansion by buying Louisiana in 1803 and Florida in 1819. With the conquest of the West, the US militia encountered and fought several Native American tribes that had partially assimilated the Hispanic culture and tradition and lived in *pueblos* (a Spanish word meaning "towns"). These people, now called Native Americans, had embraced Catholicism, had Spanish names, spoke Spanish, and had learned from Spanish colonizers to use guns and horses. Many had also learned agriculture techniques from the Jesuits. The state of Texas declared independence from Mexico in 1836 and was annexed to the USA in 1845. Following the USA-Mexican war in 1848, Mexico ceded nearly half its territory including the present-day states of California, Nevada, Arizona, New Mexico, Colorado, Nevada, Utah, Oklahoma, Kansas, and Wyoming. Thus, nearly half of the current US territory has a Hispanic ancestry [6].

Over a century later, the US government passed the Immigration and Nationality Act of 1965. The act, also known as the Hart-Celler Act after its sponsors, Senator Philip Hart and Representative Emanuel Celler, put an end to long-standing national origin quotas, allowing an influx of immigrants with an emphasis on family reunification and skilled labor [7, 8]. This wave of immigration led to the next big increase in the US Latinx population. Common motives for immigration during this time included economic opportunities in the United States and political instability and social unrest in Latin American countries, which prompted individuals to seek better prospects in the United States.

Today, Spanish is the second most spoken language in the United States, with the largest number of native speakers and the highest enrollment in school foreign language classes [9].

Colorism

Latinos can have a variety of skin tones. A 2021 Pew Research Center survey of Latino adults [10] showed respondents a palette of ten skin colors and asked them to indicate which most closely matched their own. Individuals surveyed gave responses across the continuum of choices, reflecting the diversity within the group. Eight in ten Latinos selected one of the four lightest skin colors, with the second-lightest ranking most common (28%), followed by the third (21%) and fourth lightest colors (17%). By contrast, only 3% of Latino respondents selected one of the four darkest skin colors.

A majority of Latino adults (57%) say that their skin color shapes their daily life experiences to some degree. Most say that having a darker skin color hurts Latinos' ability to advance in the United States (62%), while having a lighter skin color helps Latinos get ahead (59%) [10]. There is also some evidence that colorism is associated with health outcomes. For Latinx children educated in schools on the US mainland, darker skin tone is associated with poorer mental health outcomes [11]. Among

Puerto Ricans on the island, it is a better predictor of general health than all other sociodemographic classifications [12].

Providers should be aware that common ways that Latinos may be identified and categorized by others, such as through surnames or skin color, may be misleading or inconsistent with the ways that any given individual views themself. Like any putative identifier, the meaning of race, skin tone, and cultural designation varies with context and geography.

Cultural Aspects of the Latinx Community

Each Latinx cultural subgroup is characterized by its own values and distinct cultural elements, and any given patient may differ in their adherence to common cultural beliefs and values. Notwithstanding, many Latinx patients are influenced to some degree by common Latinx cultural values and conceptions of health and illness.

A cultural element that has been largely implicated in positive health outcomes for Hispanics is *familismo* (familism). *Familismo* implies a strong allegiance and attachment toward family and respect for elders [13]. The needs of the family may take priority over those of the individual, a concept with implications for key developmental, financial, and social decision-making. *Familismo* has been shown to play a role in areas as diverse as an academic motivation among Latinx college students [14] and diabetes self-management in first and second-generation Latino senior citizens [15]. The central role of family should be considered in multiple aspects of Hispanic patient care, including decision-making, counseling, treatment selection, and communication. Be aware that older patients may expect their children to provide material and decisional support when the family is dealing with illness. Some traditional Latinx families will also prefer to hear bad medical news before the patient and to communicate the news to the patient through a family spokesperson [16].

At the patient's request, infertility care providers should be amenable to including the family as a resource of care. Connectedness and family cohesion can empower families to face the illness with less shame and more unity, as well as mitigate the distress associated with infertility [17].

The centrality of family often extends well outside of the immediate family and into the wider community. Latino culture encourages connecting, reaching out, and mutual support. It is not at all unusual for people to think of their community as comprising many "*tíos*" (uncles) and "*comadres*" (godmothers in either a formal or colloquial sense). For Latino families, these nonbiological communities of kinship may play a central role throughout the lifecycle; culturally aware providers should be mindful of inquiring about members of an extended community who may provide patients with emotional, material, and decisional support.

The concept of *personalismo* refers to an interactional style characterized by mutual respect, trust, and the expression of verbal or physical warmth. In informal social settings, *personalismo* may manifest in hugs and kisses between acquaintances when entering or leaving a social interaction. Latinx patients who value *personalismo* may desire friendliness and overt warmth in their interactions and offer it in return. Providers working with clients who are high in *personalismo* may find that their understanding of professional communication differs from that preferred by their clients; a nurse in one qualitative study described patients on one side of an emergency-room curtain who spontaneously offered to interpret for Spanish-monolingual patients on the other side of the curtain, a situation that both exemplifies *personalismo* and creates potential complications with respect to notions of medical privacy [18].

The physician–patient relationship can also be influenced by the value of *respeto* (respect). *Respeto* is manifested through agreement with authority figures, deference, decorum, and adherence to expected public behavior. Because a healthcare provider represents a figure of high authority for many Hispanic people, patients may view the relationship as vertical rather than horizontal, and their communication style is therefore likely to be deferential. In the context of a consultation with a Reproductive Endocrinologist and Infertility (REI) specialist, *respeto* may manifest in a Hispanic patient demonstrating deference towards the specialist's expertise and suggestions. Thus, the patient might avoid asking questions about treatment, feel shame if they do not know or understand the information provided, or have a hard time advocating for themselves and sharing their treatment preferences and constraints. This could lead to a breakdown in trust and compromise the patient's adherence to treatment. While a paternalistic provider-patient relationship can be detrimental to patient autonomy, it has been shown that for patients who adhere strongly to the value of *respeto,* the vertical nature of the relationship can serve as a protective factor and enhance positive outcomes. Therefore, a balance that protects the autonomy of the patient while incorporating treatment that honors the patient's preferred communication style should be implemented [19].

Gender Roles

Gender roles have also been shown to impact Hispanic mental health and participation in infertility care. *Machismo* refers to ideologies and values that promote manliness, hypermasculinity, and associated behaviors in Hispanic men. Men are not expected to display emotions and show vulnerabilities, a presumption that may challenge their ability to display or regulate emotions, influence the family environment, and limit their ability to use effective emotional coping mechanisms [20]. Machismo negatively impacts the willingness of Hispanic men to seek mental health care. Importantly, the dominance expected in Hispanic men's behaviors also plays a role in gender-associated disparities, domestic violence, and distress in LGBTQIA+ and gender-diverse persons [21–23].

Machismo in the context of infertility can significantly impact male behavior and attitudes toward seeking fertility treatment. Due to the perception that infertility is solely attributable to women, men may resist undergoing semen analysis or seeking medical evaluation, fearing that the findings may undermine their sense of masculinity. This belief may deter them from accepting responsibility for potential issues with conception and delayed diagnosis. Some men who are strongly influenced by machismo may avoid medical appointments altogether to avoid feeling emasculated. In the case of gay Latino couples, machismo-related anxieties and internalized homophobia may intensify concerns about seeking fertility treatment, increase fear of judgment from treatment providers, and cause them to question their right to be parents.

Marianismo is a concept that has its roots in Catholicism and literally refers to the expectation that Latina women will emulate the Virgin Mary. In communities adhering to the value of *marianismo,* women are idealized in some respects and oppressed in others. The woman is expected to be the primary force holding the family and home together through work and cultural wisdom, serve as the primary caregiver, and take responsibility for most parenting. Latinas high in *marianismo* have been shown to be more likely to suffer from depression, remain in relationships where there is intimate partner violence, and consent to engage in unsafe sexual practices [24]. However, some research also suggests that for some traditional Latina women, the concept that they are the spiritual and moral head of the family may be protective against depression and substance abuse.

The belief that it is the role of the woman to care for the family may impact traditional Latinas' reaction to infertility and pregnancy loss. For some women, adherence to the values of *marianismo* may compound feelings of shame and stigma. For others, it may provide an explanatory framework for suffering and help to make meaning out of adverse life events [25]. It should also be noted that contemporary concepts of *marianismo* have expanded the notion of women as the moral pillars of the family to encompass notions of advocacy, mutual aid, and support for abortion rights [26].

Religion

Spiritual and religious influences play a major role in Hispanic patients' health, illness, and daily life. However, as is true for members of many cultural and ethnic groups, Hispanics practice a variety of religions in a multitude of ways.

Latinos' relationship with the church is changing. A 2022 survey from the Pew Research Center [27] found that most US Latinos (65%) say they were raised Catholic, while far fewer say they were raised Protestant (18%), religiously unaffiliated (13%) or in some other religion (3%). Older Latinos and those who were born outside the United States are especially likely to say they were raised Catholic. But like Americans overall, many Latinos switch away from their childhood religion. As of 2022, one-third of Latino adults indicated that their current religion is different from their childhood religion. Catholicism has seen the greatest losses due to religious switching among Hispanics. Nearly a quarter of all US Hispanics are former Catholics; while about two-thirds of Hispanic adults (65%) say they were raised Catholic, only 43% say they are *currently* Catholic. Additionally, for every 23 Latinos who have left the Catholic Church, only one has converted to Catholicism [27].

By contrast, the religiously unaffiliated have experienced the biggest gains. Few Latinos say they were raised with no religious affiliation. However, for every Latino raised without a religious affiliation who has joined a religion in adulthood (totaling 3% of all Latino adults), about seven Latinos have left their childhood religion and become unaffiliated (20%). Disaffiliation from religion is more common among United States-born Hispanics; about a quarter of United States-born Hispanics (23%) say they were raised in a faith but are now religiously unaffiliated, compared with 16% of foreign-born Hispanics [27].

Protestantism has seen more modest growth due to religious switching among Latinos. For every two Latinos who were raised as Protestants before converting to another faith or becoming unaffiliated, about three have converted to Protestantism in adulthood. In all, 18% of US Latinos say they were raised Protestant, while 21% say they are currently Protestant. United States-born Hispanics are about as likely to become Protestants as to leave Protestantism (7% vs. 8%). Among foreign-born Hispanics, 4% were raised Protestant but have since left the religion, compared with 11% who were raised in another tradition and have since become Protestants [27].

These changes in religious affiliation impact Hispanics' use of contraception, openness to abortion, and uptake of fertility treatment, including intrauterine insemination (IUI) and especially in vitro fertilization (IVF). Religiosity also impacts Latino patient's openness to third-party reproduction, with both the specific denomination and the degree of adherence playing a role in the perceived acceptability of these treatments. Finally, religiosity may be associated with the concept of fatalism, a common belief among traditional Latinx people that attributes suffering and illness to God's will or divine punishment; Latinx patients high in fatalism may be less likely to seek out fertility care, conceptualizing their inability to conceive as a condition to be borne rather than treated and seeking out faith-based solutions to their distress rather than medicalized ones.

The Role of Saints

Regardless of their general religious practices, Latino Catholics may turn to saints for intercession, asking them to petition God on their behalf in asking for a specific outcome. Each saint has a specialized health and religious function, some of which are listed below:

Infertility: St. Anne
Cancer: St. Peregrine

Dying: St. Joseph
Bodily ills: Our Lady of Lourdes
Chronic Illness: St. Juliana Falconieri
AIDS Patients and Caregivers: St. Aloysius Gonzaga
Arthritis/Rheumatism: St. James the Greater
Blood Donation: St. Januarius
Diseases of the Breast: St. Agatha
Headaches: St. Teresa of Avila

Complementary and Traditional Medicine

Latinx patients may be inclined to use integrative medicine alongside traditional IVF treatments. It is not uncommon for Latinx patients familiar with indigenous and spiritual medical practices to use culturally based healing practices either alone or in combination with allopathic medicine to address a variety of physical and emotional conditions [28]. Depending on their culture of origin and adherence to cultural conceptions of health and illness, some Latinx patients may employ the services of *yerberos* (herbalists), *sobadores* (massage therapists), *espiritistas* (spiritualists) or *santeros* (faith healers) [29]. In a recent study, [30] infertility patients in Chicago were surveyed about their infertility-related health practices. The study revealed that a significant portion of infertility patients incorporate herbal supplements, yoga, meditation, and massage with IVF. These approaches may offer benefits such as stress reduction and improved well-being for patients undergoing infertility treatment. REIs should emphasize the importance of evidence-based medicine while being knowledgeable and respectful of the cultural beliefs and practices surrounding reproductive health and infertility care. This understanding can promote comprehensive and culturally sensitive care during the IVF process [31].

Infertility and Fertility Care

Latinx individuals face unique challenges stemming from cultural beliefs and societal pressures when it comes to infertility and fertility care. Both formal sex education and family discussions of issues related to sexuality and sexual health within Latinx communities are often limited, contributing to misconceptions and inadequate knowledge about reproductive health and contraception [32, 33]. Moreover, there exists a pervasive stigma surrounding infertility, fueled by the stereotype that Latinx women are naturally fertile [34]. This misconception can lead to feelings of inadequacy and shame for individuals experiencing infertility.

Furthermore, traditional views emphasizing the importance of procreation and the notion of pregnancy as a divine gift rather than a scientific process can exacerbate the emotional burden associated with infertility. Gender roles also have a significant influence, with women often feeling responsible for fertility issues regardless of the underlying diagnosis. This societal expectation can lead to heightened anxiety, sadness, and shame, particularly for women, who may internalize feelings of failure in fulfilling familial and cultural expectations [35].

LGBTQ+

Latinx individuals who identify as LGBTQ+ face intersecting challenges stemming from both their cultural identity and sexual orientation or gender identity. Within the Latinx community, traditional notions of masculinity such as machismo can contribute to distress and alienation for LGBTQ+ and gender-diverse individuals. This pressure to conform to rigid norms may result in feelings of isolation and rejection.

Additionally, Latinx individuals within the LGBTQ+ community are often marginalized and underrepresented, exacerbating feelings of invisibility. Latinx LGBTQ+ patients may be hindered in their access to culturally competent healthcare services, as individuals may fear discrimination or judgment from healthcare providers. Many Latinx LGBTQ+ youth also report that the information given to them about their sexual health tends to be heteronormative, depriving them of relevant information about safe sex and contraception practices. Consequently, Latinx LGBTQ+ individuals are less likely to seek medical care, further exacerbating health disparities within this population [36–38]. Moreover, Latinx transgender women face heightened vulnerability to hate-based violence, which adds an additional layer of fear and insecurity [39]. The fear of discrimination and violence, coupled with the lack of culturally competent physical and mental healthcare options, creates significant barriers to accessing essential medical services and support networks [40, 41]. In combination, these factors make it less likely that Latinx LGBTQ+ patients can and will access reproductive healthcare, in turn decreasing the likelihood of appropriate and timely referrals to infertility care.

Access to Infertility Care and Treatment Outcomes Among Latinx Populations

Across multiple settings and contexts, Hispanic women have lower rates of use of infertility services than non-Hispanic White women [42]. Hispanic women report infertility more often than Caucasian women. However, Hispanic women are underrepresented in the population receiving infertility treatment compared to the demographics of reproductive-age women in the United States [42–44].

Komorowski and Jain [35] conducted a literature review outlining disparities in reproductive medicine affecting Hispanic women. Evaluation of Society of Assisted Reproductive Technology data from 1999 to 2000 from over 80,000 patients revealed that Hispanic patients made up only 5.4% of the US-assisted reproductive technology (ART) population [45]. Based on data from the 2002 National Survey of Family Growth, 15% of White women between ages 25 and 44 in the United States have sought medical help to get pregnant compared to only 7.6% of Hispanic women [44]. This discrepancy may be due to several barriers including lack of insurance coverage, limited English language proficiency coupled with a dearth of Spanish-speaking providers, geography, financial barriers, social stigma, religious beliefs, and a cultural emphasis on privacy [46].

A cross-sectional survey of Midwestern infertility patients conducted from 2004 to 2005 attempted to identify cultural factors contributing to disparities [47]. In the population surveyed, Hispanic and African American women had been attempting to conceive for 20 months longer than White women and were significantly more likely to be nulliparous when presenting for infertility care. Hispanic and African American women were also significantly more likely to report difficulties finding a physician with whom they felt comfortable, getting appointments with a physician, taking time off work for their appointment, and paying for treatment. Importantly, Hispanic and African-American women reported that it was more difficult to get treatment because of their race or ethnicity. Hispanic women were also more likely than non-Hispanic White women to report significant concerns or worries related to needing to consider adoption as an alternative to treatment first, friends or family finding out about treatment, using science or technology to conceive, short and long-term side effects of infertility treatment, having a miscarriage, having an ectopic pregnancy, or conceiving higher-order multiples [47]. Similarly, a telephone survey of American women examining factors involved in reproductive choices and infertility found that Hispanic and Black women had higher infertility stigma scores and more ethical concerns surrounding infertility than non-Hispanic White women [48].

More recently, a cross-sectional survey of 1460 women seeking fertility care at an academic center in Illinois, a state with mandated insurance coverage for fertility testing and treatment, assessed racial and socioeconomic characteristics and access to care. Hispanic women in this population traveled twice as far as White and Black women to access infertility treatment. Additionally, Hispanic, and Black women were twice as likely to report their income level and weight as barriers to treatment compared to non-Hispanic White and Asian women [46]. Hispanic patients were significantly more likely than non-Hispanic White patients to report being very or extremely worried about the side effects of treatment, miscarriage, ectopic pregnancy, and birth defects. Compared to non-Hispanic White patients, Hispanic patients were twice as likely to report being very/extremely worried about using science and technology to conceive and were more likely to report worry about violating religious beliefs [46].

Additionally, 81% of Hispanic women reported a belief that emotional stress can reduce the success of fertility treatment compared to 67% of non-Hispanic White women, a statistically significant difference [49]. Hispanic women were also significantly more likely to report that emotional stress can cause a miscarriage than non-Hispanic White women [49]. Hispanic women were also significantly less likely to have undergone genetic carrier screening [50]. In this study, only 49.4% of Hispanic infertility patients had genetic carrier screening performed. Hispanic patients were also less likely than White and Asian patients to agree with the statement that using left-over embryos for research should be allowed [50].

Although Latina patients are more likely to be uninsured or on public insurance that does not cover infertility care, financial barriers alone are unlikely to be the major barrier to access to care in this population. In 2003, a survey of Massachusetts women was conducted as mandated and comprehensive insurance coverage for infertility services became available [51]. Based on Massachusetts Census data in 2000, 6.8% of the state population identified as Hispanic/Latino ethnicity as compared to 3.9% of patients who presented for care at a large infertility clinic; this difference reached statistical significance [51]. Similarly, Dupree et al. assessed changes in the rate of use of IVF among over 18,000 health plan enrollees after a large employer provided IVF coverage [52]. The absolute rate increases in IVF use among Hispanic women was the lowest of the racial groups studied at 27.5%, while the absolute rate significantly increased among White women at 64.9% [52]. Similarly, Correira et al. [53] found that racial and ethnic disparities in utilization of IVF and clinical outcomes for autologous cycles persist regardless of state health insurance mandates. The findings of these studies demonstrate that lower use of ART among Hispanic women is unlikely to be driven solely by economic factors and that social and cultural factors may be contributing to the low rates of uptake of fertility care for the Latinx population.

Strategies to Improve Access to Care

Improved insurance coverage for infertility evaluation and treatment may encourage more patients to seek care and eliminate some financial barriers. It is important to note that although improved coverage does not solve the problems discussed in the previous section, it is a necessary precondition for achieving health equity. Coverage for infertility care must also be accompanied by an understanding of how to access these benefits. Only 8.9% of participants in a study conducted in the greater Boston area were aware of their personal insurance coverage for fertility treatment, with Latina patients being less likely to know if their insurance covered this treatment than non-Hispanic White patients [54].

Additionally, improved access to primary care and general gynecologic care is crucial as many causes of infertility are preventable if diagnosed early. For example, prevention and early treatment of obesity and sexually transmitted infections could lead to reductions in general infertility and tubal factor infertility rates, respectively. Similarly, though the expansion of Medicaid coverage has helped more Hispanic women access cervical cancer screening, they continue to be screened at lower rates than non-Hispanic White women. This screening is a critical part of preventative reproductive care with implications for fertility preservation [55]. Since general gynecologists often refer patients to Reproductive Endocrinology and Infertility (REI) specialists for infertility evaluation and treatment, access to general gynecology care is critical to improving access to infertility care. Improved awareness among general gynecologists and infertility specialists of ovulatory dysfunction in women with obesity, polycystic ovary syndrome (PCOS), and tubal factor infertility will aid in the earlier identification of possible fertility problems. It is important to remember that socioeconomic status and English language fluency will influence whether, where, and how often Latina women access general reproductive healthcare [56]. Therefore, it is important for physicians in many healthcare settings, including emergency rooms, to be informed about these issues and to have linguistically, financially, and culturally appropriate methods of sharing information about these conditions with their Latina patients and referring them for additional testing as needed.

Educational programming for patients addressing the causes of infertility and destigmatizing infertility may also improve both access to care and utilization of ART treatments. As previously described, Hispanic women may perceive more social stigma surrounding infertility and may have more ethical and religious concerns about ART treatment. Serou and Quintero [57] hypothesized that a major factor in reduced ART utilization rates among Hispanic patients is the lack of fertility information in commonly used Spanish media and social networks. Educational materials for patients should emphasize that infertility is a medical condition, that evaluation and treatment are available, and that IVF is not the only treatment option.

Physician education on implicit bias, cultural competency, and providing care to multicultural populations is key to improving the patient experience. Physicians who care for diverse populations of patients may provide different levels of care to different racial and ethnic groups. It is imperative that providers become aware of their implicit biases and the role they play in perpetuating health disparities in their fields. Patient satisfaction, adherence to treatment, and health outcomes can be optimized by effective patient–physician communication; however, patients of minority backgrounds have worse satisfaction with physician communication than White patients [58, 59]. Providers who receive education on the barriers in access to care and common fears regarding ethical and religious concerns about ART treatment may be better able to communicate with and advise minority patients on treatment options.

Finally, there remains a significant lack of minority representation in the physician population, which is not reflective of the general US population. The majority of active physicians identify as White (56.2%), followed by Asian (17.1%) with much lower proportions identifying as Hispanic (5.8%) and Black or African American (5.0%) [60]. Within obstetrics and gynecology, minorities remain underrepresented with 9.6% identifying as Black or African American and only 6.7% as Hispanic [60]. Within REI, a survey of members of the professional society for specialty-trained physicians practicing reproductive medicine found that most REI) physicians identified as Caucasian (76%) with only 6% identifying as Hispanic and

3% as African American [61]. To improve these disparities, residency programs should seek to actively recruit underrepresented minority applicants and consider offering second visits to these applicants [60]. Institutions should address diversity in hiring practices and seek to advance women and underrepresented minorities into leadership roles [62]. Diversifying the reproductive healthcare field has particular benefits for patients whose English proficiency is limited; research has demonstrated that treatment adherence across multiple specialties is enhanced by the availability of healthcare workers who can provide linguistically concordant care, over and above the presence of a medical interpreter [63].

Future research efforts should focus on better understanding access to care and ART outcomes in the Hispanic population. For this research to accurately capture the nature and extent of disparities, more complete reporting of race data across clinics will be needed.

Cultural Humility and Responsive Care in Reproductive Medicine

Provider cultural humility is fundamental to ensuring that reproductive care is sensitive to the diverse cultural backgrounds and experiences of patients. It involves continuous self-reflection, acknowledgment of the patient's expertise, sharing of power, and ongoing learning from patients [64]. Engaging in reflective practice is essential to recognizing how clinicians' personal values may influence patient care. By forming genuine partnerships with patients in their reproductive health journeys, clinicians can ensure that care is tailored to patients' identities, lived experiences, and values in a culturally appropriate manner.

ATR patients often experience profound losses, physical and emotional exhaustion, and heightened vulnerability. Recognizing and addressing these vulnerabilities are crucial in delivering services that effectively meet their needs. To do so in a culturally appropriate manner requires providers to take culture into consideration while not losing focus on resolution.

Cultural Considerations in Fertility Counseling

Mental Health Support

Particularly among Latinos who adhere to more traditional cultural views of mental health and illness, the decision to seek mental health support for psychological distress can be complex. For example, research has shown that Latinx patients suffering from depression report higher levels of shame about their illness than do non-Latinx Whites [65]. In consequence, Latino patients suffering from mental health conditions may be less likely to seek out psychological support out of fear of both internalized and public stigma [66]. A recent survey by NAMI bears this out; among members of the Latinx community who experience symptoms of a psychological disorder, 20% report talking to a doctor about their symptoms, and only 10% contact a mental health professional [67].

Internalized and community stigma are far from the only barriers to receiving mental health support for Latinx patients. Disparities in access to and quality of mental health care result in reduced help-seeking behaviors for Latinx patients experiencing psychological distress [68]. Across all groups of individuals experiencing mental health challenges, affordability of care is cited as the single greatest barrier to accessing treatment. Among those who can afford care, racial and ethnic minority patients have less access to evidence-based mental health treatments [69].

Latinx patients experiencing infertility may therefore face significant obstacles to seeking mental health support. The stigma associated with infertility and that associated with psychological distress may collude to prevent patients from accessing care. The limited availability and affordability of mental health providers with specialized training in both infertility counseling and the cultural aspects of care may further limit the uptake of mental health support for some patients, an issue that is compounded for those with limited English fluency. Meeting the mental health needs of Latinx infertility patients will therefore require both an improvement in cultural competency among qualified fertility counselors and structural and systemic modifications aimed at increasing access to care.

Best Practices for Infertility Counseling with Latinx Patients

Out-of-session recommendations:

Providers must be aware of their cultural and religious biases and assumptions and be cognizant not to distort clients' experiences with infertility because of their own beliefs [70].

1. Be willing to engage in introspection

   Ask yourself:

   What are my privileges? What are my implicit and explicit biases?

   How does my background help or hinder my work? What is my first reaction when I think of or see a person from a different background?

   How do my cultural identity and privilege limit my ability to see or understand lack of privilege and marginalization? What are my gut reactions to clients who have different cultural backgrounds than my own? How do I create space for clients to explore their cultural identities?

   How open am I to my clients' feedback about my level of cultural competence and cultural responsiveness?
2. Build community

   Seek out relationships with others in your profession, affiliated providers, and members of the communities you aim to serve. These trusted professionals can serve as a sounding board.

3. Review your forms and written materials

   Simplify your language. If there is an easier way to say something, do it.

   Provide documents in a language that your client can read and understand. Offer easy-to-follow visuals.
4. Bring in translators and interpreters

   When communicating with people who don't use English as their first language, we often revert to speaking slower or louder, which can be disrespectful. Hire a translator for your clients and translate important documents. Consider the accessibility of your services for people who are visually and hearing impaired, in addition to those whose language of greatest fluency is not English.
5. Build diverse and inclusive teams

   Hire intentionally and cultivate inclusive workplaces.

   Inclusivity means providing equal access to opportunities and resources for all people, no matter their race, culture, gender, sex, sexuality, ability, class, or other characteristics. Inclusivity also includes things like considering family, work, and caregiver responsibilities. For example, it can be hard for people with full-time jobs to attend meetings during regular business hours. How can you be more inclusive and offer some after-hours services?
6. Continue to seek education in culturally responsive care

   Educate yourself about microaggressions. Don't conflate biases or committing microaggressions with being a bad person or a bad counselor. Accepting your own imperfection around cultural biases is essential to maintaining a growth mindset, developing cultural humility, and developing increased awareness. Denying your own biases and microaggressions will cause them to persist.
7. Continue to seek education in reproductive medicine

   Qualified fertility counselors must be knowledgeable about the biomedical model of reproduction. Clients who are experiencing infertility may have varying degrees of knowledge—and at times, misinformation—regarding human sexuality, reproduction, and fertility options.

Although not within the scope of this chapter, providers must seek training in the best modalities for working with individuals and couples coping with infertility [71].

In-session recommendations:

1. Encourage Latinx patients to talk openly about sex and infertility. Ask directly about their sexual and reproductive concerns

   Providers can guide patients to express their thoughts through a series of prompting questions. Consider asking, "What questions do you have about…?" "Do any of your friends talk about …? What do they say?"
2. Provide needed psychoeducation

   Reproductive information and treatment information that is considered relevant may differ by patient experience. To determine what kinds of information would benefit a Latinx patient most, counselors should ask what they already know and which topics they would like to learn more about. Be aware that not all patients know what they do not know.

3. Be aware of privilege and power in relationships, especially regarding their effects on the therapeutic relationship

   Latinx patients who perceive the doctor-patient relationship as hierarchical may be hesitant to express confusion, disagree, or ask for clarification. Providers should also be aware that the power imbalance between themselves and the patient may enable, and at times, require them to serve as advocates for their patients with infertility care providers and affiliated clinic staff.

4. Acknowledge the cultural differences between you and the client

   Be explicit about the potential lack of awareness of the client's cultural experiences. Ask the patient about background, practices, religion, and culture to avoid stereotyping. Get comfortable saying "Can you tell me why this is important to you?". Invite the client to share their perspective on therapy, infertility, spirituality, or racism so you can get a better idea of who they are and what this process means to them.

   For example, clinicians may volunteer the following:

   "You shared today that you identify as Latinx, and I know that many Latinx people experience discrimination. If this is your experience, I really want to ensure that I am aware and sensitive to the effects of this. Even though I try to understand clients' experiences, I may unintentionally miss something in this area. As a person who is not Latinx, I may have blind spots about your experience, but I will work hard to overcome these. If at any point it seems that I am missing or misunderstanding something about your experience in this regard, I really welcome your comments on this."

   Latinx therapists working with Latinx clients may also differ in their experiences. A therapist born in New Jersey whose parents emigrated from El Salvador to escape gang violence may have many, some, or few commonalities with a second-generation Cuban American patient whose parents relocated to Miami with the support of the US government. Do not assume that a shared Census designation automatically confers a shared history or life experiences.

5. Develop a culture of feedback

   Providers cannot possibly have a complete understanding of how culture influences a particular client. Check on the therapeutic alliance routinely. Make a habit of asking patients how they think therapy is progressing and whether they feel understood in session. Set the stage for soliciting client feedback early in the relationship. For example, you might say the following as part of the intake process:

   "It is important for me to make sure that I understand your perspective. For instance, although I know some things about your cultural background, I may not fully understand at times how this impacts your life and relates to challenges that have brought you to counseling. I welcome your thoughts about anything you think I may not be getting in our sessions about you, your values, or your cultural experiences."

6. Practice nondefensiveness around a lack of awareness or demonstrations of cultural encapsulation.

   Acknowledge your biases or the microaggressions you commit in session. If you have a concern about something you said or did, check with the patient about how it was received. When appropriate, apologize for your lack of awareness and commit to educating yourself on the issue rather than putting the burden on the patient.

Case Examples

Working with a Latinx Couple

Veronica and Miguel have been married for 3 years. Veronica is a third-generation Mexican-American woman who attended Catholic schools throughout her childhood and attends Mass regularly. She is very close to her three sisters, her parents, and her aunts, all of whom live nearby. Veronica has a master's degree in social work; she lived with her parents while completing her education and moved to her own apartment only after she had been working for several years. Miguel came to the United States at age 6 with his mother and older brother. The rest of his family of origin lives in a small town in Central Mexico. Miguel is employed as a paralegal at a large law firm. Both he and his brother routinely send money to their mother to help with her household expenses. Veronica and Miguel have been trying to conceive since their marriage. Relatives in both the United States and Mexico are aware of their struggles and the couple is often told that their families and communities are praying for them to have a child. After years of trying to conceive without success, the couple attends an infertility workup. Veronica is diagnosed with primary ovarian insufficiency and is told that she is unlikely to conceive without the assistance of an egg donor. Veronica is asked whether she has any female relatives who might be willing to serve as directed donors. Her younger sister is 28 and has two children of her own.

Children are valued across cultures; however, the meaning of children, and thus, of childlessness, varies. The Latinx community is a collectivist culture and places high importance on family. Therefore, childlessness will not only be a crisis for the couple, who may stand to lose social standing and face being stigmatized but also a heartbreak for the whole family. Additionally, Latinx people who are high in the value of fatalism may view themselves as having less control over whether and how to address the crisis of infertility, believing that having children must occur the "natural" way and that it must be part of "God's will." As a result, some sub-fertile couples are more likely to experience infertility as a punishment or feel defeated, rather than taking action. Because the consequences of being childless are painful due to the strong expectations to meet social roles, some sub-fertile couples may be more willing to defy their religious and cultural beliefs to pursue various avenues for treatment.

With some unease and cognitive dissonance, some Latinx patients are opting for alternative reproductive choices such as third-party reproduction and are disclosing this to their communities. Directed gamete donation from a friend or relative becomes a possibility and disclosure to children and others is an important area of discussion.

While religion and spirituality can help Latinx couples maintain a sense of hope for a "miracle," this belief may also potentially hinder their ability to work towards a resolution, thus leaving them in chronic distress. Therefore, it is critical that providers be attuned to the dual role of religion and spirituality in their patients' lives as both a source of solace and a potential barrier to resolution. It is important not to offer false hope, knowing that many couples who seek medical treatment are ultimately unable to conceive.

With this basic cultural knowledge in the background, we also want to understand the individual perspective of the client or couple. We want to know their level of education, whether fertility and sexuality were openly discussed in their families, and what messages they received about these topics. Family values and communication patterns in the family are also important to understand, as is the degree to which traditional gender roles may have been internalized. This information will help providers determine the level of responsibility a woman may be unwittingly taking on for her infertility and the well-being of both her partner and her extended family.

Some of our goals for Veronica and Miguel would include:

- Normalizing the couple's experience and feelings.
- Externalizing the infertility experience, thus helping Veronica to move away from self-blame, guilt, or punishment to a more experiential perspective.
- Helping the couple gain control over their life decisions in light of their loss of control over their fertility.
- Aiding in communication skills with family members and other loved ones.

The counselor working with Veronica and Miguel must also be comfortable exploring the possibility of nonresolution to infertility. Veronica and Miguel may ultimately be uncomfortable with the option of donor gametes and may choose not to pursue treatment, even with the possibility that Veronica's sister would be willing to act as an egg donor. A culturally responsive approach to working with this couple would allow for the possibility that the medically recommended treatment may not be one that they choose to pursue. The counselor should be open to helping the couple explore options other than ongoing treatment and allow for the exploration of available alternatives to having a biologically linked child.

Working with a Gay Latinx Couple

Francisco is a 39 year-old attorney from Spain. His partner, Ricardo, is a 27 year-old man from the Dominican Republic who has a degree in hospitality and works in the wine and beverage industry. Although they have been together for 4 years, the couple is not legally married. Francisco has always wanted to be a father; early in their relationship, he was relieved and delighted to find that Ricardo also viewed children as part of his future. Ricardo has no family in the United States. Ricardo's family is aware of and supportive of his relationship, but he vividly recalls his parents making homophobic references to a cousin when he was a child. Francisco and Ricardo have attempted to conceive using Francisco's sperm, donor eggs from an egg bank, and the aid of a gestational carrier. Unfortunately, the gestational carrier has miscarried twice. Francisco and Ricardo are now faced with the decision of whether to attempt to conceive with their remaining embryos and the same gestational carrier or try another path to parenthood. They come to you for decisional support.

On intake, it becomes clear that Ricardo is showing signs of depression that he attributes to the couple's recent losses. He reports feeling marked sadness, low energy, and decreased ability to enjoy his work. Ricardo states that his family has made comments including "It's sad, but it wasn't really your baby anyway." and "Maybe this is a sign that you shouldn't try to have children." Although Francisco is eager to continue trying to grow their family, Ricardo has become increasingly ambivalent. It is also clear that Ricardo is skeptical about the benefits of therapy. He volunteers little information spontaneously and asks you about your experience working with "people like us."

Because of the well-defined cultural roles and the marked machismo in some Latinx communities, Latinx LGBTQ+ patients may walk through our doors with some level of distrust. These patients might have experienced healthcare-related trauma having to do with their sexual orientation and might not be as open with providers about their fears about engaging in treatment. LGBTQ+ Latinx patients might also delay treatment due to their own internalized homophobia, asking themselves if they "really deserve to be parents" and refraining from self-advocacy due to this fear.

Patients can also fear discrimination and lack of care from their providers. They might hold the expectation that a fertility clinic will not use appropriate language or have adequate paperwork that reflects their relationship. For example, Francisco and Ricardo are not legally married; clinics whose intake forms include only the words "spouse," or "husband and wife" do not have an option that reflects the nature of their partnership.

Reflection Questions:

- What is your existing knowledge base for providing reproductive counseling to LGBTQ people?
- What assumptions might you make about LGBTQ people and their desire for parenthood?
- How might you offer routine preventive healthcare to patients from a trauma-informed approach?

Counseling Considerations:

- LGBTQ people have the same range of reproductive intentions and desires as heterosexual individuals.

- Male gender does not preclude a desire for parenthood.
- The pain of infertility and loss is not limited to the intended parent whose gametes are used in conception.
- LGBTQ people may avoid healthcare facilities due to history of trauma as well as clinicians' lack of understanding of their health concerns.
- LGBTQ people report the need for more supportive resources and to educate their clinicians on their reproductive health.

Considerations for working with Ricardo and Francisco:

- Ask the couple about their reproductive desires and intentions in an open non-judgmental dialogue.
- Inquire as to the couple's preferred reproductive terms and build a trusting relationship. Understand their hopes, fears, and concerns about treatment.
- Don't assume that LGBTQ patients know and understand the multiple steps needed to have a child. Spend time talking about egg donation, embryo creation, pregnancy, delivery, and early parenthood.
- Acknowledge the disenfranchised grief that often accompanies infertility care and pregnancy loss for LGBTQ+ intended parents.

Conclusion

The disparities in access to infertility care faced by Hispanic women, along with the potential for worse IVF outcomes compared to non-Hispanic women, underscore the urgent need for a comprehensive and multifaceted approach to address these inequities. This approach should include expanded insurance coverage, enhanced education initiatives targeting both patients and healthcare providers, and further research to identify and mitigate barriers to care within the Hispanic population.

Cultural competency and cultural humility offer an extended framework for centering patient values, experiences, expectations, and goals. As healthcare professionals, we have a responsibility to identify and examine our assumptions, values, and biases, as well as to actively work to provide patient-centered reproductive services that support the human right to reproductive justice. By working within a culturally responsive framework, professionals hold the opportunity and honor of empowering all patients in their health.

Central to cultural humility is the recognition of our own cultural bias and the importance of comprehending our clients' subjective cultural experiences. This interpersonal stance not only empowers providers to improve client outcomes but also honors the cultural richness of our clients while fostering awareness of the effects of our privilege as counselors.

The best care is inclusive and respectful care! Despite progress, a shortage of medical and psychological research on the Latinx population and reproductive medicine remains. There is a tremendous opportunity for professional counselors to participate in infertility advocacy to bring greater awareness and acceptance of infertility and its treatments to marginalized communities. It is also essential that the mental health field furthers its understanding of the emotional complexities of the infertility experience for diverse populations to develop more tailored treatments.

In embracing these principles, we not only fulfill our professional obligations but also have the opportunity to positively impact the lives of all patients, regardless of their cultural background. By prioritizing cultural humility and cultural competency in our practice, we can contribute to a more equitable, inclusive, and respectful healthcare system.

Acknowledgment Assistant: Jordan Margolis Chomstein, Second-semester student at Bachelor of Science in Psychology, Department of Psychology, School of Arts and Sciences, Loyola University Chicago, Jor.margolis@hotmail.com, jmargolis2@luc.edu

References

1. Greil AL, Slauson-Blevins K, McQuillan J. The experience of infertility: a review of recent literature. Sociol Health Illn. 2010;32(1):140–62.
2. U.S. Census Bureau. New estimates highlight differences in growth between the U.S. Hispanic and non-Hispanic Populations [Internet]. Census.gov. https://www.census.gov/newsroom/press-releases/2024/population-estimates-characteristics.html#:~:text=The%20Hispanic%20population%20surpassed%2065,a%20total%20population%20of%2065%2C219%2C145.
3. Lopez LNB, Mora L, Hugo M. About one-in-four U.S. Hispanics have heard of Latinx but just 3% use it [Internet]. Pew Research Center. 2020. https://www.pewresearch.org/race-and-ethnicity/2020/08/11/about-one-in-four-u-s-hispanics-have-heard-of-latinx-but-just-3-use-it/.
4. Fernández-Armesto F. Our America: a Hispanic history of the United States. W. W. Norton; 2014.
5. Torres Martínez R. Sobre el concepto de América Latina¿ Invención francesa? Cahiers d'études romanes. Revue du CAER. 2016;5(32):89–98.
6. Leal DL, Limón JE, editors. Immigration and the border: politics and policy in the new Latino century. University of Notre Dame Press; 2013.
7. Wolgin PE. Re-forming the gates: Postwar immigration policy in the United States through the Hart-Celler Act of 1965. In: Wanted and welcome? Policies for highly skilled immigrants in comparative perspective. New York: Springer; 2013. p. 61–81.
8. Kammer J. The Hart-Celler immigration act of 1965. Center for Immigration Studies; 2015.
9. Dietrich S, Hernandez E. What languages do we speak in the United States? [Internet]. Census.gov. https://www.census.gov/library/stories/2022/12/languages-we-speak-in-united-states.html.
10. Lopez LNB, Gonzalez-Barrera A, Edwards K, Mora L, Hugo M. Majority of Latinos say skin color impacts opportunity in America and shapes daily life [Internet]. Pew Research Center. 2021. https://www.pewresearch.org/race-and-ethnicity/2021/11/04/majority-of-latinos-say-skin-color-impacts-opportunity-in-america-and-shapes-daily-life/.
11. Crutchfield J, Keyes L, Williams M, Eugene DR. A scoping review of colorism in schools: academic, social, and emotional experiences of students of color. Soc Sci. 2022;11(1):15.
12. Caraballo-Cueto J, Godreau IP. Colorism and health disparities in home countries: the case of Puerto Rico. J Immigr Minor Health. 2021;23(5):926–35.
13. Katiria Perez G, Cruess D. The impact of familism on physical and mental health among Hispanics in the United States. Health Psychol Rev. 2014;8(1):95–127.
14. Azpeitia J, Bacio GA. "Dedicado a Mi Familia": the role of familismo on academic outcomes among Latinx college students. Emerg Adulthood. 2022;10(4):923–37.

15. Reyes JA. Exploring the role of Familismo in diabetes self-management among first-and second-generation Latino elders with diabetes mellitus type 2 (Doctoral dissertation). Concordia University Chicago; 2023.
16. Kreling B, Selsky C, Perret-Gentil M, Huerta EE, Mandelblatt JS, Latin American Cancer Research Coalition. 'The worst thing about hospice is that they talk about death': contrasting hospice decisions and experience among immigrant Central and South American Latinos with US-born White, non-Latino cancer caregivers. Palliat Med. 2010;24(4):427–34.
17. Cano MÁ, Castro FG, De La Rosa M, Amaro H, Vega WA, Sánchez M, Rojas P, Ramírez-Ortiz D, Taskin T, Prado G, Schwartz SJ. Depressive symptoms and resilience among Hispanic emerging adults: examining the moderating effects of mindfulness, distress tolerance, emotion regulation, family cohesion, and social support. Behav Med. 2020;46(3–4):245–57.
18. Floríndez LI, Floríndez DC, Como DH, Secola R, Duker LI. Differing interpretations of health care encounters: a qualitative study of non-Latinx health care providers' perceptions of Latinx patient behaviors. PLoS One. 2020;15(8):e0236706.
19. Juckett G. Caring for Latino patients. Am Fam Physician. 2013;87(1):48–54.
20. Nuñez A, González P, Talavera GA, Sanchez-Johnsen L, Roesch SC, Davis SM, Arguelles W, Womack VY, Ostrovsky NW, Ojeda L, Penedo FJ. Machismo, marianismo, and negative cognitive-emotional factors: findings from the hispanic community health study/study of Latinos sociocultural ancillary study. J Latina/o Psychol. 2016;4(4):202.
21. Rosenberg BA, Dillon FR, Eklund A, Ebersole R. Traditional machismo, caballerismo, and sexual identity development among Latino sexual minority men. J Latinx Psychol. 2024; https://doi.org/10.1037/lat0000259.
22. McGlew SJ. Association of childhood sexual abuse and cultural machismo values with internalized homonegativity for Latino gay men (Doctoral dissertation). Adler School of Professional Psychology; 2015.
23. Ornelas LR, Miner CL, García RR, Mandujano JL. Need of belonging, Mexican men's normative socialization, and machismo as the root of couple problems, the role of alcohol use, and intimate partner violence. Revista iberoamericana de psicología. 2023;16(2):123–35.
24. Cano MÁ, Rojas P, Ramírez-Ortiz D, Sánchez M, De La Rosa M. Depression and gender roles among Hispanic immigrant women: examining associations of gender egalitarianism, marianismo, and self-silencing. J Health Care Poor Underserved. 2020;31(2):713–23.
25. Jones MK, Briones M. The impact of marianismo on the association between intersectional discrimination and depressive symptoms among Latina women: a profile analysis. J Latinx Psychol. 2022;10(4):304.
26. García R. "We're not all anti-choices": how controlling images shape Latina/x feminist abortion advocacy. Soc Perspect. 2022;65(6):1208–27.
27. Nadeem R. Among U.S. Latinos, Catholicism continues to decline but is still the largest faith [Internet]. Pew Research Center's Religion and Public Life Project. 2023. https://www.pewresearch.org/religion/2023/04/13/among-u-s-latinos-catholicism-continues-to-decline-but-is-still-the-largest-faith/.
28. Sorrell TR. Mexican traditional medicine: application of a traditional and complementary medicine system to improve opioid use treatment in Latinos. J Holist Nurs. 2020;38(4):384–99.
29. Ludwick A, Corey K, Meghani S. Racial and socioeconomic factors associated with the use of complementary and alternative modalities for pain in cancer outpatients: an integrative review. Pain Manag Nurs. 2020;21(2):142–50.
30. Sehgal S, Dyer A, Warren C, Galic I, Jain T. Integrative medicine utilization among infertility patients. Reprod Biol Endocrinol. 2023;21(1):71.
31. Cabada-Aguirre P, López López AM, Mendoza KC, Garay Buenrostro KD, Luna-Vital DA, Mahady GB. Mexican traditional medicines for women's reproductive health. Sci Rep. 2023;13(1):2807.
32. Barral RL, Cartujano B, Perales J, Ramirez M, Cowden JD, Trent ME, Ramaswamy M, Kessler SF. Knowledge, beliefs, and attitudes about contraception among rural Latino adolescents and young adults. J Rural Health. 2020;36(1):38–47.

33. Batek LM, Leblanc NM, Alio AP, Stein KF, McMahon JM. Facilitators and barriers to contraception access and use for Hispanic American adolescent women: an integrative literature review. PLOS Global Public Health. 2024;4(7):e0003169.
34. Portugal A, Kosturakis AK, Onyewuenyi TL, Rivera-Cruz G, Jimenez PT. Breaking down barriers: advancing toward health equity in fertility care for Black and Hispanic patients. Obstet Gynecol Clin. 2023;50(4):735–46.
35. Komorowski AS, Jain T. A review of disparities in access to infertility care and treatment outcomes among Hispanic women. Reprod Biol Endocrinol. 2022;20(1):1.
36. Brener S, Jiang S, Hazenberg E, Herrera D. A cyclical model of barriers to healthcare for the Hispanic/Latinx population. J Racial Ethn Health Disparities. 2024;11(2):1077–88.
37. Cerezo A, Ching S, Ramirez A. Healthcare access and health-related cultural norms in a community sample of Black and Latinx sexual minority gender expansive women. J Homosex. 2023;70(5):782–805.
38. Schmitz RM, Robinson BA, Tabler J. Navigating risk discourses: sexual and reproductive health and care among LBQ+ Latina young adults. Sex Res Soc Policy. 2020;17(1):61–74.
39. Ries BV. Looking backward to move forward: ending the 'history and tradition' of gun violence against the LGBTQ community. Duke Law J Online. 2023;73:119–58.
40. Garcia-Perez J. Lesbian, gay, bisexual, transgender, queer+ Latinx youth mental health disparities: a systematic review. J Gay Lesbian Soc Serv. 2020;32(4):440–78.
41. Schmitz RM, Tabler J. Health services and intersections of care: promises and pitfalls experienced by LGBTQ+ Latino/a emerging adults. J LGBT Youth. 2021;18(1):1–22.
42. Kelley AS, Qin Y, Marsh EE, Dupree JM. Disparities in accessing infertility care in the United States: results from the National Health and Nutrition Examination Survey, 2013–16. Fertil Steril. 2019;112(3):562–8.
43. Chandra A, Copen CE, Stephen EH. Infertility service use in the United States: data from the National Survey of Family Growth, 1982–2010. US Department of Health and Human Services, Centers for Disease Control and Prevention, National Center for Health Statistics; 2014.
44. Chandra A, Martinez GM, Mosher WD, Abma JC, Jones J. Fertility, family planning, and reproductive health of US women; data from the 2002 National Survey of Family Growth. U.S. Department of Health and Human Services; 2005.
45. Grainger DA, Seifer DB, Frazier LM, Rall MJ, Tjaden BL, Merrill JC. Racial disparity in clinical outcomes from women using advanced reproductive technologies (ART): analysis of 80,196 ART cycles from the SART database 1999 and 2000. Fertil Steril. 2004;82:S37–S8.
46. Galic I, Negris O, Warren C, Brown D, Bozen A, Jain T. Disparities in access to fertility care: who's in and who's out. F S Rep. 2021;2(1):109–17.
47. Missmer SA, Seifer DB, Jain T. Cultural factors contributing to health care disparities among patients with infertility in Midwestern United States. Fertil Steril. 2011;95(6):1943–9.
48. Greil AL, McQuillan J, Shreffler KM, Johnson KM, Slauson-Blevins KS. Race-ethnicity and medical services for infertility: stratified reproduction in a population-based sample of U.S. women. J Health Soc Behav. 2011;52(4):493–509.
49. Negris O, Lawson A, Brown D, Warren C, Galic I, Bozen A, et al. Emotional stress and reproduction: what do fertility patients believe? J Assist Reprod Genet. 2021;38(4):877–87.
50. McQueen DB, Warren CM, Xiao AH, Shulman LP, Jain T. Disparities among infertility patients regarding genetic carrier screening, sex selection, and gene editing. J Assist Reprod Genet. 2021;38:2319–25.
51. Jain T, Hornstein MD. Disparities in access to infertility services in a state with mandated insurance coverage. Fertil Steril. 2005;84(1):221–3.
52. Dupree JM, Levinson Z, Kelley AS, Manning M, Dalton VK, Levy H, et al. Provision of insurance coverage for IVF by a large employer and changes in IVF rates among health plan enrollees. JAMA. 2019;322(19):1920–1.
53. Correia KF, Kraschel K, Seifer DB. State insurance mandates for in vitro fertilization are not associated with improving racial and ethnic disparities in utilization and treatment outcomes. Am J Obstet Gynecol. 2023;228(3):313–e1.

54. Insogna IG, Lanes A, Hariton E, Blake-Lamb T, Schilling S, Hornstein MD. Self-reported barriers to accessing infertility care: patient perspectives from urban gynecology clinics. J Assist Reprod Genet. 2020;37:3007–14.
55. Sabik LM, Tarazi WW, Hochhalter S, Dahman B, Bradley CJ. Medicaid expansions and cervical cancer screening for low-income women. Health Serv Res. 2018;53:2870.
56. Guerra-Reyes L, Palacios I, Ferstead A. Managing precarity: understanding Latinas' sexual and reproductive care-seeking in a Midwest emergent Latino community. Qual Health Res. 2021;31(5):871–86.
57. Serou A, Quintero R. Media influence on awareness and utilization of assisted reproduction technology in Hispanic populations. Fertil Steril. 2011;95(3):e15.
58. Shen MJ, Peterson EB, Costas-Muñiz R, Hernandez MH, Jewell ST, Matsoukas K, et al. The effects of race and racial concordance on patient-physician communication: a systematic review of the literature. J Racial Ethn Health Disparities. 2018;5(1):117–40.
59. Stewart M, Brown JB, Boon H, Galajda J, Meredith L, Sangster M. Evidence on patient-doctor communication. Cancer Prev Control. 1999;3(1):25–30.
60. Mendiola M, Modest AM, Huang GC. Striving for diversity: National Survey of OB-GYN program directors reporting residency recruitment strategies for underrepresented minorities. J Surg Educ. 2021;78(5):1476–82.
61. Barnhart KT, Nakajima ST, Puscheck E, Price TM, Baker VL, Segars J. Practice patterns, satisfaction, and demographics of reproductive endocrinologists: results of the 2014 Society for Reproductive Endocrinology and Infertility Workforce Survey. Fertil Steril. 2016;105(5):1281–6.
62. Coe C, Piggott C, Davis A, Hall MN, Goodell K, Joo P, et al. Leadership pathways in academic family medicine: focus on underrepresented minorities and women. Fam Med. 2020;52(2):104–11.
63. Escobedo LE, Cervantes L, Havranek E. Barriers in healthcare for Latinx patients with limited English proficiency—a narrative review. J Gen Intern Med. 2023pr;38(5):1264–71.
64. Lekas HM, Pahl K, Fuller LC. Rethinking cultural competence: shifting to cultural humility. Health Serv Insights. 2020;13:1178632920970580.
65. Lopez V, Sanchez K, Killian MO, Eghaneyan BH. Depression screening and education: an examination of mental health literacy and stigma in a sample of Hispanic women. BMC Public Health. 2018;18:1–8.
66. Pérez-Flores NJ, Cabassa LJ. Effectiveness of mental health literacy and stigma interventions for Latino/a adults in the United States: a systematic review. Stigma Health. 2021;6(4):430.
67. National Alliance on Mental Ilness: Hispanic/Latinx. National Alliance on Mental Illness [Internet]. 2018. https://www.nami.org/Your-Journey/Identity-and-Cultural-Dimensions/Hispanic-Latinx.
68. Coombs NC, Meriwether WE, Caringi J, Newcomer SR. Barriers to healthcare access among US adults with mental health challenges: a population-based study. SSM Populat Health. 2021;15:100847.
69. Mongelli F, Georgakopoulos P, Pato MT. Challenges and opportunities to meet the mental health needs of underserved and disenfranchised populations in the United States. Focus. 2020;18(1):16–24.
70. Sue DW, Arredondo P, McDavis RJ. Multicultural counseling competencies and standards: a call to the profession. J Multicultural Counsel Dev. 1992;20(2):64–88.
71. Burns LH, Covington SN. Psychology of infertility. In: Infertility counseling: a comprehensive handbook for clinicians. Cambridge University Press; 2006. p. 1–9.

Part IV
Addressing the Issues

Chapter 15
Best Practices for Recruiting and Retaining Racially and Ethnically Diverse Populations in Reproductive Endocrinology Research

Morine Cebert

Section One

Why Diversity in Research Is Needed

Women and people from non-White racial and ethnic groups have long been underrepresented in empirical and clinical research in the United States [1]. Diversity in research samples in clinical and social science research is important to improving outcomes and experiences for those not currently represented in scientific inquiry. Diversity is a key element in improving health outcomes for racial and ethnic minorities as it enhances the generalizability of epidemiological, exploratory, or interventional research. This results in findings that can be applied and tailored to affected groups of all genders, ages, sexual orientations, ethnicities, and socioeconomic backgrounds. It is well documented in the literature that when clinical trials or social research studies include racial and ethnic minorities, the quality of care can be improved for those groups. For example, in the clinical research areas of eating disorders [2], cardiometabolic disease [3–5], and oncology [6], there have been calls to increase the inclusion of racially and ethnically diverse groups to meet the needs of those populations affected by the disease. Researchers note that tailored and targeted interventions cannot be developed with efficacy and efficiency if there is a lack of understanding of the populations of interest. However, most articles do not provide a comprehensive and practical understanding of the many challenges with recruiting racial and ethnic minorities or results oriented, actionable steps for researchers to overcome these challenges. In this chapter, I will first explore why

M. Cebert (✉)
Fertility Goals; Rory Meyers College of Nursing, New York University,
New York, NY, USA

D. A. Kaplan (ed.), *Cultural Responsiveness in Assisted Reproductive Technology*, https://doi.org/10.1007/978-3-031-76204-8_15

these disparities exist, primarily in the context of reproductive health research, and then discuss the steps that researchers can take to improve their recruitment and retention of diverse research participants.

Why Are There Diversity Disparities in Research Studies?

Prior to exploring practical tips for improving the inclusion of diverse groups in reproductive endocrinology research, it is important to understand both historical and current barriers to recruitment. These factors influence the terrain that investigators are attempting to navigate when building research studies. The historical misuse and exploitation of diverse participants in women's health research is extensive; however, it is by no means an all-encompassing description of the numerous grievances that racial and ethnic minority groups may have with the research community. Researchers should note that prior to embarking on a research project that includes historically unrepresented groups, it is critical to understand the history of why these groups were unstudied in the first place.

Current Context of Clinical Research Challenges in Reproductive Endocrinology

Research participation across racial and ethnic groups varies widely and reasons for nonparticipation are multi-factorial and nonlinear. They vary from group to group and according to the issue being studied. These factors can be attributed both to the investigators and the participants. Investigators may not adequately solicit participation from certain groups, rely on previous data sets that are not diverse, or not set targeted sample size goals with diversity in mind. Participants may face language barriers, knowledge deficits, or transportation barriers, or have mistrust of the research investigators or affiliated institutions [7, 8]. In the field of reproductive endocrinology, however, there are numerous social and psychological factors that researchers must contend with. Secrecy, shame, and other negative consequences of infertility may influence patients' interest or motivation to participate in research. It is well documented that certain groups may not disclose their infertility to their peers and/or family members [9–11]. For example, in Rosario Ceballo's study of 50 Black women experiencing infertility [11], all but one of her participants described a pervasive level of intense secrecy; these women reported that they did not share their fertility challenges even with close friends and family members. These factors can undoubtedly influence patients' participation in clinical and medical research, making it nearly impossible to recruit diverse samples who have their own experiences with the diagnosis and treatment of infertility.

Historical Barriers

Current barriers to the recruitment of minoritized patients are compounded by historical events that continue to have pervasive effects on the low rate of participation by members of diverse populations that we see in research studies. There are numerous historical events within the United States alone that have led to the mistrust that racial and ethnic minorities have in scientific research. However, for this chapter, we will explore three seminal events of medical injustice that have undoubtedly influenced these groups' participation in women's health-related projects. Prior to the establishment of the National Commission for the Protection of Human Subjects of Biomedical and Behavioral Research in 1974 and its development of the Belmont Report on ethical principles and guidelines for the protection of research participants [12], there were numerous and notably unethical research experiments conducted on vulnerable populations, namely racial, gender, and class minorities. Within the field of obstetrics and gynecological research, there are no other events that have built the foundation of medical mistrust like those of the work of Dr. J. Marion Sims, the experiences of Henrietta Lacks, and the forced sterilization of patients from marginalized communities.

Dr. J. Marion Sims

Perhaps the most notable contribution to challenges faced in engaging marginalized groups in reproductive endocrinology research is the life and work of Dr. J. Marion Sims, deemed the "father of gynecology". Prior to Dr. Sims's somewhat stumbling entry into the field of surgical gynecology in the nineteenth century, women's reproductive health issues were not taught in medical schools at the time; this was due to the mainly male medical student population of the time and the resultant concerns about the modesty and appropriateness of males examining female anatomy [13]. Dr. Sims was known as the first physician to perfect a technique to correct vesicovaginal fistulas, which he developed primarily between 1845 and 1849. However, his experimentation on enslaved African American women who experienced these fistulas to develop his technique raised massive concerns about the ethics of the manner in which he made his novel discoveries.

Vesicovaginal fistulas are an abnormal connection between the bladder and the vagina [14]. They are most commonly a result of crush injuries to the pelvic wall due to the prolonged or traumatic force of a fetus passing through the pelvic canal. Vesicovaginal fistulas can present numerous symptoms but an overwhelming majority of patients experience uncontrolled urinary or fecal leaking, leading to secondary infertility or social isolation. While the first record of vesicovaginal fistulas dates back to 1550 BC in Egypt, the treatment developed by Dr. Sims along with improvements to obstetrical care helped in eradicating vesicovaginal fistulas from industrialized nations [15].

While Dr. Sims corrected an issue that for centuries was seen as incurable, improving the quality of life for birthing women for centuries to come, his method of advancing medical science is largely criticized today. In his search for an effective treatment for the condition, Dr. Sims conducted experimental surgeries dozens of times on enslaved women, cruelly denying them the option of anesthesia for pain control.

Some ethicists and scientists argue, based on Dr. Sims' notes, that consent was obtained from his subjects [16]. However, many medical ethicist scholars refute the validity of this claim. Because enslaved Americans at this time were viewed as property, any and all decisions related to consent were given by the enslavers who permitted Dr. Sims to carry out his experiments rather than by the women on whom the experiments took place. In the present day, concerns about exploitation continue to impact the willingness of racial and ethnic minorities to participate in medical research. The importance of emphasizing participants' autonomy and obtaining thorough informed consent prior to participation cannot be underscored enough and is a critical element in enhancing participation.

Henrietta Lacks

In 1951, a mother of five children visited Dr. Howard Jones, a gynecologist at The Johns Hopkins Hospital [17]. Henrietta Lacks was 31 years old and complained of persistent vaginal bleeding. Following a diagnosis of cancer, Lacks was prescribed radium treatment. Dr. Jones also obtained a biopsy of her cells and sent the cells to Dr. George Gey, a cancer and virus researcher who commonly obtained samples from patients treated at the Baltimore hospital without the patients' consent to their use in research.

While the cells of patients often died within 24 h, Henrietta Lacks' cells proliferated in ways that had not been seen before, doubling in number every 24 h. Estimates suggest that HeLa cells (a shortened version of Lacks' name) have been replicated enough to weigh 50 million tons and have been included in over 100,000 publications for scientific research on polio and COVID-19 vaccine development, HIV/AIDS research, and groundbreaking cancer and infertility treatments [18]. While the benefits of these cells being replicated are widely appreciated, their use without the Lacks family's knowledge or consent has indeed contributed to the negative perception that marginalized populations have when considering biomedical research. The Johns Hopkins Hospital asserts that they have never experienced any financial gain from the HeLa cell line. They do acknowledge, however, that they should have informed Lacks and her family that her cells had been used due to the long-term consequences of having their family's genetic cell line made available to the public. Here, too, the absence of transparency and informed consent has added to the skepticism and mistrust that many minoritized patients feel about the collection and use of their personal medical information for research purposes.

Forced Sterilization

Forced sterilization refers to the permanent surgical or pharmacological removal of one's ability to reproduce that is involuntary, coercive, or forced. The process of sterilization originated in England in the nineteenth century; however, it was the United States that was first to introduce sterilization into law. As discussed at length elsewhere in this volume, the use of forced sterilization in the United States was an outgrowth of the eugenics movement, which asserted that progressives should do whatever was necessary to protect the "superior" gene pool. Americans who identified with the Progressive movement embraced eugenic ideas, leading them to limit immigration of "undesirable" groups and forcing the sterilization of those who they deemed intellectually or morally inferior [19]. Indiana was the first state to enact eugenic sterilization in 1907, a practice upheld by the US Supreme Court in 1927. Prior to the end of World War II, eugenic sterilizations were conducted almost exclusively inside inpatient psychiatric institutions or departments of corrections.

Following World War II, although rates of forced sterilization declined, its victims expanded to include young Native American women, poor rural women, and others. Research estimates report that in the 1960s and 1970s, of the 150,000 Native American women of childbearing age in the United States, nearly 3500 were involuntarily sterilized. While there are no states in the United States that currently operate a sterilization program, each year there are a few petitions in state courts to approve the sterilization of young women with limited mental capacity [19]. According to the World Health Organization's interagency report on forced sterilization [20], there are numerous countries in the current modern era that continue to sterilize groups without full, free, and informed consent, including those with HIV, people with varying physical and mental disabilities, indigenous groups and ethnic minorities, and transgender persons. Having government-sanctioned practices that threaten the reproduction of marginalized groups continues to be a real concern for many as they consider participation in research whose ultimate aim may be to curtail, rather than enhance, their reproductive potential.

Why It Matters Today

While many of these events occurred in the early centuries of the United States and have seemingly been addressed by interventions to completely transform the medical ethics guiding studies, their effects continue to loom today. In 2019 [21], Lee et al. examined the perspectives of 122 participants who identified as a racial or ethnic minority on participating in biospecimen collection research. They note, "several participants referenced the case of Henrietta Lacks to underscore their fears and their limited ability to conceive of risks in the present given the potential for change in the future" (p. 110). Many racial and ethnic minority groups experience significant medical mistrust related to the long-rooted history of unethical and dangerous experimental practices that were often sanctioned and approved by the United States government. Overcoming this mistrust is necessary for researchers interested in conducting ethical and equitable research in reproductive endocrinology and related fields.

Section Two

Practical Tips for Reproductive Endocrinology Research: From Conceptualization to Dissemination

In this section, I will detail practical tips to enhance the participation of racial and ethnic minority groups from the conceptualization stage to the final dissemination of a completed study's findings. These tips should optimize the experience of recruiting racial and ethnic minority individuals into studies that focus on issues in reproductive endocrinology. To provide the context for these practical tips, I will base these lessons on my own experiences conducting a study that involved Black women experiencing infertility, supported by recent evidence-based literature examining these essential elements.

In the Fall of 2019, I conducted a study titled, "Psychobiological, Clinical, and Sociocultural Factors that Influence Black Women to Seek, Initiate, and Complete Treatment for Infertility: A Mixed Methods Study." One portion of the data is published in the F&S Reports article titled, "Psychobiological, clinical, and sociocultural factors that influence Black women seeking treatment for infertility: a mixed-methods study" [22]. The purpose of this study was to conduct in an in-depth examination of the multidimensional reasons why Black women decide to seek care to address their inability to conceive or achieve a live pregnancy.

The study, a mixed methods study including chart review data and participants who were patients at a fertility clinic in the Washington DC metropolitan area, examined the barriers and facilitators that influenced Black women seeking treatment for their infertility. In this process, I recruited 13 Black women who had sought treatment for infertility between January 2015 and September 2019, the time at which I conducted the study. While ultimately the study was successfully completed and valid and trustworthy data were collected, there were many lessons learned that will undoubtedly shape and structure future research that I conduct involving Black women.

Step 1. Conceptualization: Frameworks and Teamwork

Conceptualization

The first step to improving recruitment for racial and ethnic minorities is to use theories, theoretical frameworks, or conceptual frameworks that consider varying groups' perspectives, experiences, and outcomes. Using Varpio, Paradis, Uijtdehaage, and Young's 2020 paper [23] we define these three similar but unique concepts. Theory is an abstract description of the relationships between concepts to help us to understand the world. A theoretical framework results from research in which investigators have engaged to show logical connections between theories and concepts. A conceptual framework, however, provides an understanding of the phenomenon at hand and outlines why this contribution to research is necessary to explore. When attending talks at reproductive medicine conferences, reading through journals centered on reproductive medicine and infertility care, or reviewing abstracts for submissions, I often find that discussions of theory and/or frameworks are left out of the majority of quantitative inquiry papers. Theory and frameworks provide not only context for the research methods but also the essential methodological philosophy to design and carry out our scientific research endeavors. Leaving out these theories in research practices often leads to research questions or procedures not being effective in identifying or addressing concerns that matter to groups who are often underrepresented. In the absence of a clear theoretical framework, researchers run the risk of asking research questions that are of questionable relevance to the population they hope to understand or, conversely, of neglecting to gather data that provide critical information.

There is therefore a need for theory and frameworks that position researchers to center and explore the voices of all people affected by the specific disease or experience of interest. Researchers interested in including more diverse participants in their work require the use of more critical lenses that highlight the historical and present systems that cause there to be multiple disparate realities in patients' experiences of healthcare. While critical race theory or feminist theory have been deeply politicized, they have practical uses that enable researchers to effectively explore the relationships among concepts that are unique to varying groups. Prior to developing protocols, researchers need to consider the lens through which they intend to explore their research questions and ideas. For example, in Harrison & Pinkney's 2024 paper that explored the counseling needs of Black women with infertility, the authors used feminist theory and intersectionality to develop interview questions and analyze data that recognize the role of history, society, race, and gender that impact Black women experiencing infertility [24].

In my parent study examining infertility treatment-seeking behaviors among Black women, I used Chrisman's Health Seeking Process Model [25]. The model itself has five conceptual domains that explore how patterns of health beliefs and practices vary in different sociocultural contexts. The domains include factors that may influence behaviors along a continuum of symptom definition, illness-related shifts in role behavior, lay consultation and referral, treatment actions, and treatment completion. Within each of these domains, qualitative and quantitative variables were formed and developed to ensure a comprehensive understanding of factors that influence decision-making. This comprehensive model allowed me to consider a broad range of perspectives and reasons why someone would or would not choose to navigate treatment for their fertility challenges beyond the most typically considered factors influencing treatment uptake.

Practical Tips

- Attend trainings on various theories, theoretical frameworks, and conceptual frameworks.
- Employ the use of research experts who have used frameworks that you may be unfamiliar with.
- Spend intentional time in assessing whether current frameworks create space for racial and ethnic minorities through their concepts, key components, and how data are operationalized and collected.

Step 2. Develop Culturally Competent Research Teams

The second step to improving recruitment for racial and ethnic minorities is to recruit and employ culturally competent research teams. After defining the aims and objectives of a study, it is important to include research associates, assistants, and other consultants who can possibly speak to the nuance and diversity of the group of interest. Perhaps most important is the leadership of a core set of culturally competent researchers who not only implement research recruitment and data collection but are actively involved in the development of the entire research approach. Race concordance is a long-studied theory in clinical research. In a study that examined Black patient's preferences for medical providers, participants stated that they strongly preferred race concordance because it provided a sense of safety and rapport with the medical team [26]. This may prove equally true for clinical research development and implementation.

For example, in understanding the cultural nuance of Black women sharing their fertility experiences, it was important for me to be the face of recruitment and discussion throughout the study. While I have never experienced infertility, I have intimate knowledge and experience of navigating clinical encounters as a Black woman in the United States. Many of the participants verbalized that they were more open to participating when they knew that a Black woman was leading the study. There were numerous aspects of the study that required participants' trust and care in the research team; having a Black woman at the helm of this project increased the participants' willingness to engage in the discussions that ensued.

Practical Tips

- Intentionally collaborate with diverse researchers.
- If you have interested collaborators who are not proficient in research, partner with a local school. Invest in research courses for new hires. It is known that underrepresented communities have lower exposure to clinical research development [27].
- Create internships or research experiences for diverse undergraduate or graduate students to participate in your studies as research assistants and co-authors.

Step 3. It's Not Just Sample Size Calculations: Stratify to Diversify

There are numerous resources in quantitative and qualitative inquiry that help in determining the overall sample size of research studies. In quantitative research, there are calculators that help in determining effective sample sizes based on the statistical approach being used. In qualitative research, there are similar systemized approaches to understanding when thematic saturation has been achieved. However, there is not much discussion on how to properly determine sample sizes when considering culturally diverse populations and the overall need for stratification.

In developing the research design for the qualitative arm of my study, I proposed to interview at least 20 Black women who experienced infertility and sought treatment at a specific clinic. I used a strategy called purposive sampling that further stratified the type of Black women I would need to include in this study. Due to the secondary aims that examined completion of infertility treatment, I stratified based on whether women initiated treatment for infertility as recommended by their provider or not. However, with my understanding of the many possible cultural identities of the women within this group, I knew that I needed to examine a diversity of Black women. Therefore, my goal was to also purposively sample Black women to stratify based on known racial and ethnic variations, namely those who were mixed race, Afro-Caribbean, and Afro-Latina. As the recruitment of the study went on, I began specifically asking for Black women who fit these sub-cultures. I wanted to understand if their experiences differed from each other.

It is crucial for investigators to establish goals for recruiting diverse samples within diverse groups. For example, if a participant sets a goal to have 20 Asian participants complete an interview for a qualitative study, there should be goals to also stratify based on regional or cultural ethnicities to ensure the generalizability of all findings. This would be stratified as 50% East Asian (Chinese, Japanese, Korean), 25% Southeast Asian (Filipino, Thai, Vietnamese, etc.), and 25% Hawai'i and Pacific Islands (Fijian, Native Hawaiians, Samoan, etc.) to reflect the proportion of each group represented in the overall Asian population of the United States. Breakdowns by ethnicity can be found using the Census Bureau's published data; researchers are encouraged to look beyond broad categories that may obscure the diversity within a given racial or ethnic group [28].

Practical Tips

- Using the support of knowledgeable statisticians or statistical software, conduct a power analysis needed for the entire study.
- Set a goal and strategy for recruiting various minoritized groups.
- Examine the variations of cultures and groups within the larger community you are examining. Consider stratifying by regions, languages, backgrounds, etc.
- Develop strategies to target these groups.

Step 4. Inclusive Marketing Recruitment

Recruitment into research studies requires the researcher and team to make all aspects of the project inclusive, especially in the ways investigators market recruitment. The first piece of this is developing engaging flyers that represent the wide array of people you hope to have involved in your study. This may require you to have multiple versions or iterations of the recruitment flyer that have visual representations of members of the target population you are trying to recruit. Further, the placement of the flyers is crucial. Using social media, societal organizations central to that group (for example, Black Greek Letter Organizations or cultural centers), churches, and community partners to direct where these flyers should go is essential to diverse recruitment.

Recruitment materials for my study included the face of a Black woman along with my face, identified as the primary investigator. This served as an additional point of interest to engage those who saw the flyer and hopefully provide some immediate feedback on who would be involved in the interview process. While there is not much research on whether the images on flyers attract certain groups to studies, evidence that racial concordance in clinical care can provide a more positive experience for patients suggests that concordance between the research team and the target population could similarly increase participants' comfort in joining a study. Further, there were several iterations of the flyer that ensured that the purpose and focus of the research study were clear. For placement of the flyers, I used Facebook, Instagram, GroupMe community group chats, and mass emails from the infertility clinic's database.

Practical Tips

- Design multiple flyers for each study. Have the population of your choice represented through stock images or even patients at your office who give written permission to have their likenesses used.
- If the primary investigator or co-investigators are of the same racial, ethnic, gender, sexual, or religious background as the study participants you are hoping to recruit, highlight their level of involvement in your recruitment materials.
- Use local people to translate the flyers using colloquial, yet professional language. Be wary of trying too hard and risking cultural appropriation (for exam-

ple, having a non-Native American person dressed in traditional Native American attire in an attempt to recruit from this group).
- Consider hiring a marketing strategist for your campaigns to help generate effective outreach strategies.

Step 5. Build Connections through Community Engagement

Community-based participatory research is a systemized approach that blends community wisdom with academic methodological approaches to conduct meaningful research. This type of research is designed to promote collaboration with representatives of communities affected by the issues being studied to improve health and well-being [29]. There are many components to community-based participatory research; perhaps the most important is to involve community liaisons in the design and implementation of all research projects that include marginalized racial and ethnic groups. Community members are seen as trusted gatekeepers to the populations to which they belong; therefore, their involvement should never be overlooked. In the realm of reproductive endocrinology, this is even more crucial to explore because the added layers of shame, grief, and mistrust associated with infertility may make people especially reluctant to discuss their experiences with researchers. Many of these factors are compounded due to the secrecy many marginalized groups experience surrounding infertility discussed in Section One. As younger generations may be shifting how they socialize and where they receive information, it will be crucial to partner with community members and organizations that have a sense of how to best reach their constituents.

Practical Tips

- Don't just use community groups to market projects; use them in the co-design process.
- Gather interested stakeholders to be leaders in recruitment and informing the community about the project.
- Understand how your communities convene; consider digital spaces such as Facebook groups, GroupMe groups, and other affinity groups.
- Always ask permission and solicit the input of community organizations before attempting to connect with their constituents.

Step 6. Ethical Considerations

The importance of ethical considerations when recruiting racial and ethnic minorities into research studies cannot be overstated. Providing proper informed consent along with proper safeguards to privacy and confidentiality are essential to not only gaining trust but also getting repeat participation from individuals or groups. Having consent forms developed using plain language and representative of the study's actual data collection procedures is essential. Making clear where data will be stored and who has access to this data is crucial to building trust. Transparency is key when sharing this information, ensuring that the participant is well aware of all processes of the research project. Obtaining informed consent can also be an opportunity to educate and expound upon the institutional review board process with your participants so they can understand the several layers of safeguards the research team employed to reduce harm and promote confidentiality.

When recruiting for my study, when patients were screened or had general inquiries about the study, I immediately provided the informed consent form for their review. I also read the consent form verbatim out loud to the participants and gave ample opportunity for questions. As required by the institution that oversaw my project, participants were also given the contact information of my institutional review board's hotline. However, my institution had a policy that proved to be an added barrier to participation; it required Social Security numbers for participants to be paid their incentives. In a population that already carried added levels of mistrust, this proved to be a point of contention; participants felt like they didn't know where this information was stored and feared unintended data breaches (which were growing in frequency at the time). Thankfully, my institution had a process for requesting special exemptions from the requirement to collect Social Security numbers that was originally put in place for studies that centered on immigrant population voices. After I was granted a special exemption, the process of incentivizing and therefore recruiting became much less complex.

Practical Tips

- Provide numerous opportunities for questions to be asked.
- Use the repeat back strategy to ensure that the participant knows what they are agreeing to participate in.
- Avoid having to collect highly sensitive information such as Social Security numbers. Request exemptions early in the IRB application process.

Step 7. Data Collection Strategies

While the type of data variables collected in a study is contingent on the actual research question and may not be able to be changed, the way that data collection occurs can be easily tailored to the needs of your communities. The literature does not endorse one specific method as superior in terms of increasing accessibility and reducing the burden of participating in studies. However, many agree that a combination of data-collection methods to enhance accessibility for participants may prove to be successful. First, ensure that those who are collecting the data are fluent in the language of those they are interested in, especially those with varying dialects. For example, Spanish speakers are not a monolith and there are variations based on region, class, and immigrant status. Spanish spoken in Mexico is different than Spanish spoken in Puerto Rico and Spain. Second, leverage the use of technology on various platforms to engage participants and make participation convenient for them. Online communication platforms vary in ease and accessibility and often require high-speed Internet connections to work. This may be a challenge for certain populations. Telephone conversations may be the most convenient for some participants. Lastly, offer numerous in-person options. Paying for participants' public transportation or ride share, or going to their homes to conduct the study may be advantageous in helping your participants feel relaxed enough to provide the information you need.

When conducting my study, I offered all participants the opportunity to do a one-time demographic survey and interview via the medium and in the location of their choice. Out of the 13 women who completed the study, one asked for the interview to occur in person at her home. Two asked for the interview to be over the phone, mainly because they had over an hour commute, and speaking during that time would be advantageous for timing and privacy. The remaining participants recorded their interviews over Zoom and asked that my camera be on to ensure that I was who I said I was. Interviews were recorded as early as 6:00 am and as late as 9:30 pm. I found great success in accommodating the participants' schedules.

Practical Tips

- Understand the various platforms for digital communication and the pros/cons of each. Ensure that the encryption level is aligned with institutional review board requirements.
- Be aware that not all participants may have access to high-speed internet connections and offer alternative platforms for communication.
- Make scheduling flexible and offer numerous opportunities during and after typical business hours.
- Ensure that all questions in questionnaires or interview guides are at a fourth-grade level of comprehension. Avoid medical jargon when developing these guides.

Step 8. Corroborate and Disseminate Findings to the Participants First

The final step of the process that will help in recruiting and retaining racially and ethnically diverse participants in clinical research involves invitations to corroborate findings and include the participants in disseminating this information. Corroboration in research is typically referred to as a process of triangulation. Triangulation is used heavily in qualitative research. However, there are areas in quantitative research in which this strategy can be used as well. Triangulation is defined as a strategy to test validity through the convergence of information from different sources [30]. A type of triangulation is member checking. Member checking involves returning to a portion of participants who completed the study, sharing the findings of the study with them, and asking if the themes or results truly reflect what they said or meant to say. Member checking allows participants to feel involved in ensuring that findings are an accurate portrayal of their views and beliefs [31].

Next, disseminate the findings with the participants in mind. Maintain communication throughout the study to ensure that the participants are aware of the study's progress. Collecting data and then never reaching back out to the participants can seem one-sided and may not foster the trust and relationship needed for them to participate in future studies. Also, offer that the research team is open to making future presentations to community groups or organizations of their choice to disseminate findings. While it may be ideal for the investigators to publish their material in high-impact journals, the highest impact for retaining participant interest would be to return to the communities who helped build the research.

When conducting my study, I did not use a formal process to conduct member checking. However, I would often reach back out to participants to inform them of the study's progress and share early ideas of themes and findings. These updates were communicated through email. Upon the completion of my dissertation, I actually sent all the participants my final written product (yes, all 200 pages!) and invited them to my final dissertation defense which was presented virtually in March 2020. Due to privacy rules through my institutional review board, I could not contact them after the study closed and I left my institution. However, I sent all the participants my contact information and many have remained connected and followed my work on LinkedIn. While I have not needed to reach back out to them to participate again, I have found that they are ready and willing to participate if need be.

Practical Tips

- Consider ways to keep the participants abreast of the study progress. Keep them looped in on various milestones.
- Provide an invitation to review the study's findings.
- Discuss what the results mean to the participant.
- Don't only make promises, but actually keep them. Send reports of the study—make sure to share that these are unpublished findings that should not be shared with anyone who is not involved in the research.
- Ask if they have any community events that they would like this information presented to when the study has wrapped up.

Conclusion

Recruiting racially and ethnically diverse groups in research can be a process that proves challenging for many researchers unfamiliar with these groups. The exclusion and maltreatment of minoritized groups from clinical research has led to stark disparities and inequitable access to care. The reasons have been multi-factorial and trace back to early eras of clinical research in the United States. While the eight steps shared are not a comprehensive listing of all that can be done to attract and retain diverse groups, they are a starting point to equip investigators to improve their research to finally improve healthcare for all. Research in reproductive endocrinology has added layers of challenges due to the sensitivity of the disease and its social implications. However, investigators interested and committed to doing the work can find great success in their future research endeavors.

References

1. Corneli A, Hanlen-Rosado E, McKenna K, Araojo R, Corbett D, Vasisht K, Siddiqi B, Johnson T, Clark LT, Calvert SB. Enhancing diversity and inclusion in clinical trials. Clin Pharmacol Ther. 2023;113(3):489–99.
2. Halbeisen G, Brandt G, Paslakis G. A plea for diversity in eating disorders research. Front Psych. 2022;13:820043.
3. Michos ED, Reddy TK, Gulati M, Brewer LC, Bond RM, Velarde GP, Bailey AL, Echols MR, Nasser SA, Bays HE, Navar AM. Improving the enrollment of women and racially/ethnically diverse populations in cardiovascular clinical trials: an ASPC practice statement. Am J Prevent Cardiol. 2021;8:100250.
4. Azzopardi R, Nicholls SJ, Nerlekar N, Scherer DJ, Chandramouli C, Lam CS, Muthalaly R, Tan S, Wong CX, Chew DP, Zoungas S. Asia-Pacific investigators and Asian enrollment in cardiometabolic trials: insights from publications between 2011 and 2020. JACC Asia. 2023;3(5):724–35.
5. Addison S, Yang Y, Metlock F, King M, McKoy A, Williams A, Gregory J, Gray DM, Joseph JJ, Nolan TS. The role of social support in cardiovascular clinical trial participation among Black men: Black impact. Int J Environ Res Public Health. 2022;19(19):12041.
6. Oyer RA, Hurley P, Boehmer L, Bruinooge SS, Levit K, Barrett N, Benson A, Bernick LA, Byatt L, Charlot M, Crews J. Increasing racial and ethnic diversity in cancer clinical trials: an American Society of Clinical Oncology and Association of Community Cancer Centers Joint Research Statement. J Clin Oncol. 2022;40(19):2163–71.
7. Luebbert R, Perez A. Barriers to clinical research participation among African Americans. J Transcult Nurs. 2016;27(5):456–63.
8. Safdari R, Ehtesham H, Robiaty M, Ziaee N. Barriers to participation in medical research from the perspective of researchers. J Educ Health Promotion. 2018;7(1):22.
9. Taebi M, Kariman N, Montazeri A, Majd HA. Infertility stigma: a qualitative study on feelings and experiences of infertile women. Int J Fertil Steril. 2021;15(3):189.
10. Miall CE. The stigma of involuntary childlessness. Soc Probl. 1986;33(4):268–82.
11. Ceballo R, Graham ET, Hart J. Silent and infertile: an intersectional analysis of the experiences of socioeconomically diverse African American women with infertility. Psychol Women Q. 2015;39(4):497–511.
12. Nagai H, Nakazawa E, Akabayashi A. The creation of the Belmont report and its effect on ethical principles: a historical study. Monash Bioeth Rev. 2022;40(2):157–70.
13. Ojanuga D. The medical ethics of the 'father of gynaecology', Dr J Marion Sims. J Med Ethics. 1993;19(1):28–31.
14. Shrestha DB, Budhathoki P, Karki P, Jha P, Mainali G, Dangal G, Baral G, Shrestha M, Gyawali P. Vesico-vaginal fistula in females in 2010–2020: a systemic review and meta-analysis. Reprod Sci. 2022;29(12):3346–64.
15. Chinthakanan O, Sirisreetreerux P, Saraluck A. Vesicovaginal fistulas: prevalence, impact, and management challenges. Medicina. 2023;59(11):1947.

16. Wall LL. The medical ethics of Dr J Marion Sims: a fresh look at the historical record. J Med Ethics. 2006;32(6):346–50.
17. Johns Hopkins Medicine. The legacy of Henrietta Lacks [Internet]. www.hopkinsmedicine.org. 2024. https://www.hopkinsmedicine.org/henrietta-lacks.
18. National Institutes of Health. HeLa cells: a lasting contribution to biomedical research [Internet]. Office of Science Policy. 2022. https://osp.od.nih.gov/hela-cells/.
19. Reilly PR. Eugenics and involuntary sterilization: 1907–2015. Annu Rev Genomics Hum Genet. 2015;16(1):351–68.
20. World Health Organization. Eliminating forced, coercive and otherwise involuntary sterilization: an interagency statement, OHCHR, UN Women, UNAIDS, UNDP, UNFPA, UNICEF and WHO. 2014.
21. Lee SS, Cho MK, Kraft SA, Varsava N, Gillespie K, Ormond KE, Wilfond BS, Magnus D. "I don't want to be Henrietta Lacks": diverse patient perspectives on donating biospecimens for precision medicine research. Genet Med. 2019;21(1):107–13.
22. Cebert-Gaitors M, Shannon-Baker PA, Silva SG, Hart RE, Jahandideh S, Gonzalez-Guarda R, Stevenson EL. Psychobiological, clinical, and sociocultural factors that influence Black women seeking treatment for infertility: a mixed-methods study. F&S Rep. 2022;3(2):29–39.
23. Varpio L, Paradis E, Uijtdehaage S, Young M. The distinctions between theory, theoretical framework, and conceptual framework. Acad Med. 2020;95(7):989–94.
24. Harrison A, Pinkney KE. Understanding the experiences and counseling needs of Black women with infertility. J Feminist Family Ther. 2024;36(1–2):21–42.
25. Chrisman NJ. The health seeking process: an approach to the natural history of illness. Cult Med Psychiatry. 1977;1(4):351–77.
26. Moore C, Coates E, Watson AR, de Heer R, McLeod A, Prudhomme A. "It's important to work with people that look like me": Black patients' preferences for patient-provider race concordance. J Racial Ethn Health Disparities. 2023;10(5):2552–64.
27. Richard-Davis G. The pipeline problem: barriers to access of Black patients and providers in reproductive medicine. Fertil Steril. 2021;116(2):292–5.
28. Broad Diversity of Asian, Native Hawaiian, Pacific Islander Population. United States Census Bureau [Internet]. United States Census Bureau. 2022. Available from: https://www.census.gov/library/stories/2022/05/aanhpi-population-diverse-geographically-dispersed.html.
29. Shalowitz MU, Isacco A, Barquin N, Clark-Kauffman E, Delger P, Nelson D, Quinn A, Wagenaar KA. Community-based participatory research: a review of the literature with strategies for community engagement. J Dev Behav Pediatr. 2009;30(4):350–61.
30. Carter N, Bryant-Lukosius D, DiCenso A, Blythe J, Neville A. The use of triangulation in qualitative research. Oncol Nurs Forum. 2014;41(5):545–7.
31. Candela AG. Exploring the function of member checking. Qual Rep. 2019;24(3):619–28.

Chapter 16
Strategies for Culturally Responsive Practice Management

Jennifer Matta Wood

Introduction

Fertility services have historically been a White person's privilege to access due to higher levels of fertility education, employment, and income. Although discussions around infertility have always been hampered by some degree of stigma, providers have been more likely to recommend fertility services to White patients struggling with family building than to non-White patients. People of color have received fewer referrals to specialists due to unconscious bias related to race and ethnicity as well as assumptions regarding their financial stability and ability to afford infertility care [1].

Improvements in access to reproductive health services have changed the landscape for patients entering treatment. Although they have not completely eliminated disparities in the uptake of infertility care across racial and ethnic groups, state insurance mandates have had a positive impact on decreasing racial inequities in access to care [1, 2]. An increase in grant-based financial support and insurance coverage for family-building efforts has resulted in a more diversified patient population; large fertility clinics can now expect to see more patients from marginalized racial, ethnic, and social groups than ever before.

The idea that only married, heterosexual men and women can build families is a notion of the past. Family dynamics and building have changed dramatically over the last decade, with an increase in families that are blended with respect to race and religion, increased acceptance of LGBTQIA+ family building, and the legality of same-sex marriage. Polyamory has risen, as have the rates of patients engaging in coparenting outside of marriage. These changes challenge IVF practices and clinical staff to become more inclusive in their approach to patient care; fertility practices must do their due diligence to provide training in culturally responsive care to

J. M. Wood (✉)
Shady Grove Fertility, Rockville, MD, USA
e-mail: jennifer.wood@sgfertility.com

D. A. Kaplan (ed.), *Cultural Responsiveness in Assisted Reproductive Technology*, https://doi.org/10.1007/978-3-031-76204-8_16

all staff while administering early course correction should an untoward patient interaction occur.

Culturally responsive care is not an all-or-nothing phenomenon: it is impossible to get it right with every encounter. However, consistent, small, incremental changes create a positive impact over time. The aggregate of those changes will present subtly in staff language, practice culture, patient adherence to treatment, patient satisfaction, and in the arena of public opinion.

The ideas presented in this chapter are based on research about the factors that impede or facilitate organizational change. They are also based on my decades of experience as a Clinical Nurse Educator and education specialist who has overseen the implementation of new standards of care across a multisite infertility clinic. It is my hope that the reader will come away with an understanding of why integrating initiatives to promote cultural responsiveness in infertility clinics can be challenging—and of action steps for taking on that challenge. This chapter focuses on both concrete and attitudinal changes that infertility clinics can implement to improve cultural responsiveness in infertility care.

Why Does Cultural Responsiveness Matter? Legal, Ethical, and Financial Implications

Lack of inclusion or cultural sensitivity comes with a cost to the clinical practice. An immediate financial implication is the loss of one of the largest referral sources—patient-to-patient recommendations. Patients searching for support often read blogs, engage in exhaustive online research, speak with friends, and participate in online support groups and message boards, looking for encouragement and guidance from peers experiencing the same loss and frustration in their own family building journeys. Given how easy it is to find reviews and opinions about infertility clinics on Yelp, Google, and a host of social media platforms, patients' assessment of a practice's cultural responsiveness can drive referrals to the clinic; a lack of cultural responsiveness can just as easily drive them away.

In addition to patient dissatisfaction with the lack of inclusion and culturally competent care, inattention to creating a culturally responsive practice may also result in a decrease in morale among clinic staff due to the negative or insensitive behaviors of their colleagues. Staff who are themselves members of marginalized communities may have suffered both personally and professionally from cultural insensitivity or outright acts of racism [3]. Some may have been repeatedly passed over for promotion while watching less experienced colleagues enter into leadership roles. Others may have experienced microaggressions by patients, such as the look of surprise or discomfort from a patient who, expecting to be given medication instructions from a White nurse, is instead greeted by a Black one. For these staff, there can be an internal struggle about whether to discuss insensitive care or acts of bias for fear of company retaliation. As valid concerns are brought to the attention of leadership, the employee may be ignored, or the complaint dismissed as a "misunderstanding" due to the lack of resources for managing such grievances. Employees whose concerns are minimized or dismissed may experience threats to their own self-esteem and a decline in their work performance and focus. Ultimately, they may seek employment elsewhere rather than remain in a company that does not support sensitivity to LBGTQIA+ or BIPOC patients, or patients' cultural or religious needs [4]. This may lead in turn to a lack of diverse representation within the clinic—and to patients simply leaving the practice to seek care elsewhere. In contrast, a diverse staffing model speaks volumes to patients and staff alike, as they feel a connectedness in healthcare settings where they are represented.

Clinics that fail to address the needs of diverse populations in infertility care also risk placing themselves at odds with legal mandates for the delivery of healthcare. In 2000, President Clinton signed Executive Order 13166, mandating that federal agencies and those that receive federal funding examine their policies for providing services to people with Limited English Proficiency [5]. The Order further mandates that these entities revise their services as needed to provide equal access to all patients regardless of English language fluency. The failure to do so places healthcare providers in violation of Title VI of the Civil Rights Act of 1964 [6]. This is not just a legal violation; it places IVF clinics that are housed within any institution that receives federal funding—for instance, a university at which research is supported by NIH grants—at risk of disqualification for financial support.

Modifying clinic policies and practices requires providers to understand the difference between equity and equality. Shel Silverstein's book *The Giving Tree*, later adapted and illustrated by Tony Ruth, provides a simple visual tool to understand the difference between these concepts [7]. In the book, a tree full of apples leans to one side, providing easy access to the fruit for those standing on the correct side of the tree. The other side of the tree does not have an equal number of apples and leans away, making it more difficult to reach the fruit. This uncomplicated visual illustrates the concept of inequality. To solve this issue, a ladder is provided at different heights to make access to the tree equal; however, most of the fruit remains on one side of the tree, a visual representation of inequity. To further correct this disparity in access and achieve equity, the tree is tethered to stand up straight, with ladders of equal height and equal amounts of fruit placed on all sides of the tree. Awareness of the difference between equity and equality is crucial when completing a review of current practice gaps and strategic improvement planning, as providing "equal" treatment to all patients does not guarantee equity in infertility care.

Stages of Change

Change is not as simple as it appears even when presented to clinical staff in the clearest and most comprehensive terms. Awareness of the necessity for adjustments to existing patient care is the first step; for clinics with the goal of providing more culturally responsive care, this involves recognizing gaps in inclusion and cultural sensitivity. But where and how does one begin to implement changes within the practice without causing clinical staff to feel overwhelmed with change? Strategic planning, implementation, and evaluation within the practice in slow, small increments will assist in staff acceptance of critical culture changes necessary to elevate the practice's reputation and increase patient satisfaction [8].

The psychology of change, popularized by Prochaska, Norcross, and DiClemente [9, 10] posits that changing a behavior comprises six stages: pre-contemplation, contemplation, preparation, action, maintenance, and relapse [11]. In the *pre-contemplation* stage, a person or system has no intention of changing an existing behavior. There may be an unawareness of the necessity for adjustment or that the behavior has problematic consequences. A person or system in pre-contemplation with respect to cultural responsiveness may exhibit repeated negative behaviors or engage in ineffective verbal communications with diverse patient populations. For example, front-desk staff in the precontemplation stage may routinely refer to patients by the pronouns associated with their natal sex rather than those consistent with their gender identity. They may defend their behavior, viewing change as an inconvenience rather than considering the positive impact changes bring to personal and professional development.

In the *contemplation* stage, providers may have some awareness that a problem exists but are not yet committed to making needed changes. Clinic staff in the contemplation stage may notice that patient satisfaction scores for their clinic are routinely lower among patients of color but be unconvinced that this requires changes in clinic policies and procedures. This is also the stage in which many people become ambivalent or "stuck," recognizing a problem without knowing how to progress to the next stage [11]. The change in problematic behavior may not be perceived as worthwhile relative to the sustained efforts that are required to bring change about. The contemplation stage may last from several days to several months or longer. In the setting of a clinical practice, administrative oversight and a timeline for concrete steps toward change may be necessary to promote forward movement toward positive change.

Moving into the *preparation* stage demonstrates a commitment to the creation of procedures to execute and evaluate behavioral changes [10]. In the clinical setting, a period of discovery and careful review of practice gaps will shape the resources necessary for the implementation of change. Gathering information from trusted resources may seem a daunting task; however credible resources exist to aid in and successfully support inclusive and culturally sensitive patient care. Consider diversity and inclusion consulting companies, certification courses, self-help books, and community leaders to assist in creating a learning pathway for leadership and staff. These resources can provide an organized approach to training while providing a means for ongoing support as practices begin the behavioral work of implementing change.

The action and maintenance stages follow preparation. The *action* stage involves forward motion toward behavior modification [11]. Taking concrete steps to begin the journey of change is the primary focus. An IVF practice in the action stage may commit to an extensive review of its forms and paperwork to ensure that they are inclusive of patients of all genders or are available in more than one language. Continued encouragement is necessary to promote behavior change. Working with support systems within and outside the clinic motivates individuals to continue in this stage and diminishes the likelihood of behavioral relapse [11]. In the *maintenance* stage, the focus is on the reinforcement of changed behavior, increasing the likelihood that new standards and systems are cultivated. During this stage, new discoveries can occur as individuals begin to reevaluate actions or workflows for better engagement. Individuals within the larger system are independently encouraged to be mindful of factors that could result in relapse, such as fatigue or a heavier-than-usual volume of patients, making staff more vulnerable to snap judgments and resorting to overlearned responses. In a group setting, the team will hold each other accountable and should work cohesively to correct course when necessary.

Relapse may occur when old triggers result in resumption of previous behaviors [12]. For example, patient or staff concerns regarding lack of inclusion or equity may be met with skepticism and a delay in the leadership's investigation into claims. The once-enthusiastic employee may begin to withdraw from the practice outreach program for LGBTQ+ or BIPOC educational opportunities. An uptick in patient dissatisfaction regarding staff interactions and patient care may become more commonplace. Diversity in eligible staff candidates may begin to decrease. Whether conscious or unconscious in nature, behaviors indicating that a relapse has occurred need to be identified and corrected. Recidivism should not be seen as a total undoing of previously made progress but rather an opportunity to re-educate new and existing members of the team [10, 11]. Recognizing a regression in behavior and providing course correction or reevaluation is essential to the evolution of improved behaviors. Within the clinic, teams should meet to discuss triggers or barriers that caused a relapse in behavior. Reengagement of members who may have felt undervalued may bolster staff retention as well as patient satisfaction. Ongoing objective reevaluation of current coaching plans also serves to create robust resources and better educated clinical staff.

The stages of organizational change closely mirror those related to individual behavioral change. Organizational psychologist Kurt Lewin refers to organizations as being in one of three stages with respect to change [13]. The "unfreezing" stage can be seen as comprising contemplation and preparation. In this stage, the organization is required to develop a sense of urgency around the need for change, create guidelines for bringing change about, and communicate the desired changes to key stakeholders [14]. According to Lewin, organizations then enter the "moving" phase; at this stage, it is the task of the organization to implement small behavioral changes, evaluate their effects, and consolidate gains. "Refreezing" is akin to maintenance; organizations in the refreezing stage of change contemplate any new actions through the lens of the desired cultural shift and evaluate their success according to the new paradigm that they have worked to implement [15].

Resistance to Change

Unfortunately, most efforts at organizational change fail; some studies estimate that between 60% and 70% of organizational change initiatives do not result in sustained improvements [16]. Resistance to change is common for both people and organizations. The need for change suggests that a person's current beliefs are misguided, or that something is amiss with their lifelong concepts or ideology. Whether the belief that was challenged was political or romantic, each of us has had the experience of holding an initial set of assumptions only to later realize that what we believed was untrue. Initially, there was a sense of disappointment or even grief, both of which can hamper the ability to engage in the reflection needed to change our beliefs and behavior. The same applies to revising or eliminating practices that have not been inclusive or culturally respectful. The process of evaluating, acknowledging, and correcting bias may be accompanied by anger, fear, or resistance. The requirement to change behavior to correspond to a new way of thinking can cause systems and the individuals within them to fear retribution or a loss of control. It is not unusual, then, for requests for change to be met with fear or defiance. This may be particularly true when an organization or individual is confronted with evidence that bias has impacted their patient care; the responses of healthcare providers who are given evidence of their own biases may include shame, self-justification, or even disagreement that the evidence pointing to their biases is valid [17]. Eventual acceptance may occur but is not without its challenges.

Individual resistance to change can be compounded by an organization that fails to set the stage for understanding and acceptance of the changes being proposed. Employees are less likely to accept and implement proposed changes if they have difficulty seeing how these changes benefit them over the long term [18]. For example, a nurse who is asked to use interpreter services for limited English proficiency patients who need blood drawn may view this request as an unnecessary step that decreases efficiency. Staff acceptance of change may be enhanced by first providing the rationale and intended goal for anticipated modifications [8]. Dispelling myths and misconceptions and helping key stakeholders view the proposed changes as beneficial rather than burdensome helps alleviate a degree of anxiety related to the misunderstood or unknown and increases cooperation and collaboration. Patient care is a multidisciplinary endeavor in which all departments contribute to the culture of clinical practice. The use of actual patient examples of the impact of current practice gaps in culturally responsive care can also help to enlighten staff and promote empathy. These examples should be shared with both patient-facing and non-patient-facing staff to increase acceptance of proposed changes.

Change efforts can also be impeded by a failure to solicit input and information from key stakeholders within the clinic when proposing changes to longstanding policies and practices [15]. When developing and implementing modifications to increase a practice's cultural responsiveness, it is important to solicit active staff engagement [8]. A proposed change to clinic intake procedures, for example, is less likely to be accepted by front desk staff if they are not involved in the development of the new standards and evaluation of their impact. Allow a forum for open and honest discussion on feelings, perceptions, comfort levels, and frustration related to any changes that are under consideration. Staff members may provide a perspective on their own experiences regarding workflow, patient interactions, bias, or daily microaggressions. This meeting should include guidelines on conversation, language, respect for the opinions of others, and purpose. Individuals should not fear admonishment by their management for sharing an opinion in a safe setting. A third-party facilitator may also provide the audience with guidance and a deeper understanding of strong opinions. The facilitator can play the role of mediator, evaluating the discussion without bias and providing additional recommendations on assisting the team in making necessary changes [19]. The inclusion of key staff members in identifying areas for change and developing an action plan reassures staff that changes are not meant to be punitive but rather an opportunity for personal and professional growth.

In addition, presentations and discussions led by practice leadership regarding areas of weakness and plans for improvement can improve staff understanding of the business of inclusive and culturally sensitive patient care. Research demonstrates that trusted leaders who express a clear vision and promote a sense of shared enthusiasm about change are more likely to successfully shepherd their organizations and employees through the prolonged efforts needed to implement sustainable change [20, 21].

Effective change is not forced but rather, as appropriate, phased into place over time. As previously discussed, movement through the stages of change takes time. Sudden or unexpected adjustments to clinic routines and structure can be incredibly difficult and disruptive to staff morale [22]. Staff members' resistance to change may present in body language, microaggressions, tone, volume, and cadence when speaking with patients, or passive-aggressive language between staff or with patients in patient-facing areas. In most cases, this behavior is unintentional but in need of correction. Maladaptive behaviors are often subjective and difficult to document for corrective action. Nonetheless, poor behaviors must be addressed while providing education on empathy and inclusion. In some cases, staff resistance to change manifests as attrition; staff who are unhappy with proposed changes may leave the clinic altogether, leading to high turnover [23].

Organizational Self-Examination

For those charged with evaluating and modifying the culture and practice model of an infertility clinic, the exhortation to "become more culturally responsive" is both daunting and ill-defined. Organizations seeking to identify the root cause of an issue in need of attention have often used a version of the "Five Whys" technique. First developed by Toyota as a way of identifying the root causes of manufacturing errors or inefficiencies, the technique involves identifying a problem and recursively asking why the problem occurs until the factors that need to be changed are identified [24]. In infertility care, a Five Whys analysis might take the following form:

Problem: Patient satisfaction scores are low among transgender patients
Why? Patient ratings indicate a lack of clinic sensitivity
Why? Patients indicate that their providers do not show sensitivity to patients' gender identity

Why? Providers routinely misgender patients on first meeting
Why? Providers see incorrect information about the patient's gender in the EMR before meeting the patient
Why? Check-in requires patient to have a government-issued ID, many of which identify patients by natal sex
Proposed Solution: Allow patients to waive the use of an ID at check-in

Proponents of the Five Whys approach in healthcare management invoke its simplicity and its wide acceptance across multiple industries and fields of study. Its critics caution that the approach is observational rather than empirical, and that different groups of observers can easily arrive at wholly different root causes for the same issue [25]. Therefore, the Five Whys are best used as a tool for brainstorming; the root causes identified as a result of the exercise can then be used as the starting point for experimenting with changing clinic policies and procedures and gathering data as to the results of the change.

Improving Staff Cultural Responsiveness

The primary focus of diversity, equity, and inclusion initiatives in fertility care should be working with all staff, patient facing or otherwise, to understand the basics of inclusive language, systemic inequities, and conscious and unconscious bias and how these can affect the fertility patient's experience. Transparent addressing of these issues is part of the learning process. Over time, the discomfort around discussions of bias or inequity should decline as clinic staff and leadership invest in diversity, equity, and inclusion (DEI) improvements.

Formal training sessions are helpful in the implementation of cultural sensitivity and inclusion initiatives in any practice. Robust diversity, equity, and inclusion discussions should be led by specially trained individuals who have completed a formal training program and can help practice leaders with the development of an inclusive model of infertility care [26, 27]. Trained diversity consultants and educators have the tools for facilitating often difficult and emotional conversations, fostering an emotionally safe climate in which opinions and experiences can be shared respectfully. Consultants can also collaborate with practice leadership on strategic planning for implementation of inclusion initiatives and strategies for maintaining positive modified behaviors. Training should comprise attention to inclusive language in written and verbal communication, with a focus on identifying and modifying language suggestive of bias.

Training for practice leaders and staff should also comprise a discussion of microaggressions. Sue and colleagues define microaggressions as "brief, everyday exchanges that send denigrating messages to people of color because they belong to a racial minority group" [28, p. 273]. However, a member of any marginalized group is likely to have experienced recurrent identity-based microaggressions both inside and outside the fertility clinic. A same-sex female couple seeking fertility care, for example, might be told that their fertility work-up was normal and that it's unfortunate they can't get pregnant "the old-fashioned way." If they are successful in achieving a pregnancy, the non-carrying partner might then attend prenatal appointments and be told that "it's so nice of you to come and support your sister". Training on the impact of microaggressions in healthcare is particularly important as this behavior is more common in daily patient interactions than acts of overt discrimination [29]. Team members may be unaware of the microaggressions to which patients are exposed in the practice. Supplying staff with examples of microaggressions will raise awareness and enable individuals to reflect on their intent and impact when speaking with patients or peers.

Training sessions can be tailored to the needs of the practice with a focus on the populations most served. For example, centers with a larger population of Muslim or Orthodox Jewish patients may require educational sessions related to religious restrictions during treatment and respecting holidays or days of prayer. Practices with a larger number of transgender or non-binary patients benefit from education on inclusive language and the patient journey through gender identity confirmation. Understanding the struggles that many LGBTQIA+ patients face in getting adequate medical care helps to dispel myths and misunderstandings about those patients seeking care. Staff may volunteer to share their personal accounts related to inclusion and discuss how others succeeded or were ineffective in their interactions. Staff offering their own narratives promotes camaraderie and a positive practice culture within their team.

Sympathy Versus Empathy in Infertility Care

Effective training should include discussions on empathy and bias in addition to DEI and cultural sensitivity. There is a benefit to understanding the difference between empathy and sympathy as they apply to patient care in infertility. As described by Morse, sympathy "is an expression of the caregiver's own sorrow at another's plight" [30, p. 78]. Although having an emotional reaction to the misfortune of another may be warranted, sympathy without the ability to imagine a remedy can result in caregiver distress; taken to an extreme, it can impede rather than enhance the ability to act effectively on patients' behalf. Empathy, in contrast, comprises both cognitive and emotional components, requiring us to both understand an event or situation from the perspective of another and have an emotional response to the other's experience. These components in combination help caregivers move from a position that centers their own distress to one in which effectively addressing the distress of their patients becomes possible.

Understanding how someone feels and showing effective empathy is simpler than one would imagine. For example, nonverbal communication such as making eye contact and providing someone with your full attention in conversation shows empathy. Connecting with a person's emotions while providing concrete support also requires a change in both words and behavior. According to author Brené Brown, meeting a person in an emotional crisis where they are requires not just caring from a distance but demonstrating an understanding of their experience and offering help [31]. Fertility patients have heard multiple apologies and expressions of sympathy during their family-building journey. These condolences can be perceived as a dismissal, or a formality used in order to quickly move through an uncomfortable conversation and on to the next topic on the agenda. Marginalized patients have also heard performative apologies all too often in their daily lives without corresponding efforts to improve the situation. Apologies for the inability to accommodate seating in the waiting room due to body habitus, lack of robust resources for the hearing impaired or non- English-speaking patients, or lack of diverse healthcare providers and support staff have for too long replaced concrete action. The reproductive healthcare setting is mandated to provide support and empathy without bias to all patients seeking fertility services. Providing vetted resources for language translation services for all educational materials (including closed captioning for video education for hearing impaired) should be among the simplest changes a practice makes to demonstrate empathy for and meet the needs of more patients. Similarly, it is inappropriate to assume that all patients presenting to the clinic are of the same weight and that waiting rooms, office chairs and exam tables need not accommodate patients with markedly elevated BMI. Empathy by way of making concrete changes to clinic waiting and exam rooms assists overweight patients in accessing care.

Intake Procedures

Review the practice through the lens of hypothetical patients belonging to various marginalized groups and observe areas where bias or cultural blindness can adversely affect the patient experience. Beginning with the patient check-in and intake process, review the types of questions asked for inclusive language and for the need to ask each question at all. For example, forms that ask patients to identify themselves as "husband" and "wife" should be revised to include the word "partner." Similarly, front desk staff who are used to asking patients if they will be joined for the consultation by their husband should practice using neutral language such as "Is anyone joining you for the consultation today? Who is it?". Forms should also ask patients to specify their pronouns and preferred salutation as an alternative to gathering this information from patients' legal identification; for example, legal forms of identification may often display transgender patients' "dead name" rather than the name that they currently use.

Intake forms should also provide an opportunity for patients to explain any religious or cultural restrictions they must adhere to in their daily living that need special accommodation during their care in the clinic. Providers, leadership, and staff should periodically review all intake paperwork and procedures to formulate a plan for providing a culturally responsive and respectful point of entry into care for the patient and their partner.

Physical Environment

Sitting in the waiting room for the first appointment can be anxiety-provoking for most patients. They must overcome fear of the unknown and may be dealing with the emotional aftermath of silent losses. There are cases where patients are presenting to the offices without the support of their immediate family or in fear of ridicule from their community [32]. For members of marginalized communities, presenting for fertility care at all may be accompanied by a heightened sense of shame and apprehension both due to cultural stigmas around infertility and concern that they will be met by providers who fail to understand their experiences. The waiting area and consult rooms should be a welcoming, serene, safe space for patients and their partners. The design of the space sets the tone for the culture of patient care. Review your public areas for inclusive and sensitive décor. Art and reading materials displaying LGBTQIA+ faces, people of color, single parents, and non-pregnant people are more inclusive than those portraying exclusively White couples and families. If there are photographs or marketing materials throughout patient-facing areas, review them for inclusion as well. Do the faces in the pictures and language of these promotional materials reflect the patients being served?

Holidays present another opportunity to show allyship with diverse patients and staff [26]. The United States celebrates holidays based on longstanding tradition. From New Year's Day to Christmas and all months in between, holidays are promoted everywhere; traditionally, however, these holidays are those celebrated primarily by US-born, Christian populations. Recognizing special religious or cultural holidays by placing tasteful embellishments in the waiting areas may be an option for the office. Include a positive historical fact related to the holiday for all to become better informed. A small display at the front desk or signage for Kwanzaa, Native American Heritage Day, Chanukah or the beginning of Ramadan can be valued by patients; be aware that many religious holidays fall on different dates on the Julian (secular) calendar each year. Commemorating the heritage months dedicated to acknowledging the contributions of people from a variety of racial and ethnic backgrounds provides a further opportunity to feature diverse pioneers in science, education, or civil rights. Seek volunteers from the clinic staff to find interesting facts about unknown trailblazers to build conviviality.

Be aware that displaying a single photo of a biracial family or placing a Chanukah menorah on the front desk may well be read by patients as performative rather than as a demonstration of a true commitment to equitable care. Office décor should be considered in conjunction with other facets of the patient experience to ensure that diverse patient populations are welcomed at all points of contact with the clinic.

Modification to Workflow

Established practice workflows are created based on staffing models, practice guidelines, and standard operating procedures set forth by administration, physician leadership, and risk management. These trusted systems are typically simple to train in and follow but not necessarily equitable in practice. The prospect of changing existing systems and workflow may lead to apprehension and fear that changes may lead to risk in gamete or embryo care. Strict guidelines stand in place to protect the patient and practice; however, there are often safe alternatives in structured workflow to promote inclusivity. Careful examination of workflow practices for inclusion and cultural sensitivity should be considered.

Reproductive health management allows for a degree of flexibility with monitoring and medication dosing. For religious Jewish patients, for example, medically realistic adjustments in a treatment cycle to avoid a weekend or high holiday are a reasonable proposal that does not compromise treatment outcomes. In addition, in cases where patient identification is needed for a procedure and the patient is restricted from carrying the identification because of prohibitions on what can be carried on Shabbat or on major religious holidays, adjustments can be made in workflow to allow a copy of the identification to be provided several days prior to the anticipated procedure date. These modifications will be the exception and not routine in practice; therefore, clear and detailed communication to employees in all relevant departments will allow the patient and partner to receive care without the need for elaborate explanations in the moment. Collaboration with relevant clinic staff regarding such scenarios provides an opportunity for input, education, and constructive dialogue within the patient care teams, promoting staff engagement with the practice.

Partnership with Community Stakeholders

Partnership with key stakeholders and community leaders in improving cultural responsiveness can take many forms. Outside the walls of the IVF clinic, it might entail a visible partnership between a religious leader who is a member of a minoritized group and a reproductive educator to provide sex education for young couples planning to marry or those considering family building. Community-based spiritual leaders can also provide education for clinic staff about the religious directives that may inform patients' choices in infertility care. Such collaboration fosters a sense of community between the fertility center and diverse patient populations and better prepares providers to meet the needs of these patients in treatment. Within the clinic, community leaders can provide monthly or quarterly town hall meetings to discuss the significance of inclusion and equity initiatives for patients and support staff. Proposed changes to clinic policies, procedures, and forms meant to promote cultural responsiveness should be reviewed not only by clinic staff and legal experts but by the patient populations they are meant to serve. Taking feedback from patients and staff on their experiences in the clinic to aid in assessing the gaps in inclusion is key to the success of all DEI initiatives. Implementation and evaluation are an ongoing process in which patients and DEI specialists alike can support the success of the practice.

Soliciting stakeholder feedback is also critical to evaluating the impact of newly implemented changes [8]. Much patient feedback is delivered informally, either through direct communication with healthcare workers or through social media platforms and online forums. However, practices have the opportunity to capture patient feedback in a more systematic way. Providing all patients with an anonymous survey is one of the simplest options for assessing patients' reactions to initiatives meant to improve culturally responsive care. There are multiple surveys that can be completed either in person or online that can aid practices in understanding patients' experiences of care [33]. They comprise questions about aspects of the patient experience ranging from wait time and the medical staff's communication skills to the quality of written and educational materials provided. These surveys can easily be adapted to include questions about a practice's commitment to cultural responsiveness.

Promoting survey completion should begin with the provider and end with the last staff person to be in contact with the patient during the visit or following the completion of a treatment cycle. The invitation to complete a survey can be introduced with empathic language, such as "We know family building or fertility preservation can be challenging. We would appreciate your feedback on your patient experience today. Your opinion is important to us as we are constantly seeking ways to improve the patient experience and celebrate positive experiences." This type of phrasing encourages patients to provide constructive feedback versus solely providing negative commentary. Managers and leadership can review scores and comments to look for positive or negative trends, then enlist the assistance of staff for corrective action. Some studies have demonstrated that patient feedback has the greatest impact on intake procedures and the nature and quality of patient education materials [33], the two areas in which clinics have perhaps the most concrete opportunity to make changes that demonstrate cultural responsiveness.

Community Collaboration

A commitment to partnering with diverse communities as a visible and active ally should be the goal of all reproductive health practices. This speaks to the core values of the practice and communicates to prospective patients that the practice is committed to providing inclusive and respectful care. For example, showing allyship with LGBTQIA+ communities goes beyond including a graphic of a rainbow or intersex flag on a practice website. Rather, a clinic can demonstrate commitment to meeting the family-building needs of the community by posting information on the practice website celebrating and providing information about options for

LGBTQIA+ family building or participating in local Pride festivals. Collaborating with specialty service partners to develop a list of additional resources for same-sex family building is another avenue to demonstrate inclusion. Clinics can work with referring providers or patients to create resource lists of infertility and pregnancy loss support groups, qualified reproductive mental health professionals, and OB/GYNs who have specialized understanding of the community's unique mental health and pregnancy management needs.

Similarly, a clinic can demonstrate active allyship and collaboration with the BIPOC community via participation in cultural festivals, partnership with religious men and women's group meetings, and providing reproductive health information at health fairs specific to marginalized populations. These actions not only increase visibility for the fertility clinic but provide BIPOC patients with critical education on fertility literacy and the importance of overall health prior to family building.

Summary and Conclusions

Systemic inequities in healthcare persist; this is equally true in reproductive healthcare for marginalized populations. Increasing inclusivity and cultural sensitivity in infertility care requires a careful systematic approach. Changes to current workflows and patient care can be challenging for staff. However effective communication surrounding the rationale for modification promotes staff buy-in and decreases anxiety [8]. Change is not an effortless process for individuals or the systems in which they work. Transparency into practice gaps in inclusive care for the increasingly diverse population seeking fertility services is key. A close objective review may cause ambivalence in providers or staff and eliciting staff buy-in is crucial to the successful and enduring implementation of any proposed changes. Proper training, implementation and evaluation provide the practice with opportunities to foster relationships with underserved communities. A gradual increase in patient or physician referrals will occur in time as a clinic's reputation for inclusivity and cultural sensitivity spreads. The benefits of making needed changes to improve a practice's cultural responsiveness cannot be quantified in referrals alone. Fertility clinics have a duty to provide additional support for marginalized patient populations seeking care. Respectful family building is everyone's human right, and every patient interaction provides all staff members with the space to make a positive impact on the patients they endeavor to serve.

References

1. Sutton MY, Anachebe NF, Lee R, Skanes H. Racial and ethnic disparities in reproductive health services and outcomes, 2020. Obstet Gynecol. 2021;137(2):225–33.
2. Korkidakis A, DeSantis CE, Kissin DM, Hacker MR, Koniares K, Yartel A, et al. State insurance mandates and racial and ethnic inequities in assisted reproductive technology utilization. Fertil Steril. 2024;121(1):54–62.

3. Smith IA, Griffiths A. Microaggressions, everyday discrimination, workplace incivilities, and other subtle slights at work: a meta-synthesis. Hum Resour Dev Rev. 2022;21(3):275–99.
4. Metinyurt T, Haynes-Baratz MC, Bond MA. A systematic review of interventions to address workplace bias: what we know, what we don't, and lessons learned. New Ideas Psychol. 2021;63:100879.
5. Improving access to services for persons with limited English proficiency, Executive Order 13166. Federal Register. 2000; 65(159).
6. Office for Civil Rights, Office of the Secretary, U.S. Department of Health and Human Services. Nondiscrimination in health programs and activities: final rule. Federal Register. 2016;81(96):Part IV.
7. Silverstein S. The giving tree. Harper Collins; 2014.
8. Brecher J. 5 keys to effective change management. 2023. https://www.asisonline.org/security-management-magazine/articles/2023/01/5-keys-to-effective-change-management/.
9. Prochaska JO, Norcross JC. Stages of change. Psychother Theory Res Pract Train. 2001;38(4):443.
10. Prochaska JO, Norcross JC, DiClemente CC. Applying the stages of change. Psychother Austr. 2013;19(2):10–5.
11. Raihan N, Cogburn M. Stages of change theory. Treasure Island: StatPearls Publishing; 2023.
12. Oyebode O, Ndulue C, Mulchandani D, Zamil Adib A, Alhasani M, Orji R. Tailoring persuasive and behaviour change systems based on stages of change and motivation. In: Proceedings of the 2021 CHI conference on human factors in computing systems. CHI; 2021. p. 1–19.
13. Burnes B. The origins of Lewin's three-step model of change. J Appl Behav Sci. 2020;56(1):32–59.
14. Hussain ST, Lei S, Akram T, Haider MJ, Hussain SH, Ali M. Kurt Lewin's change model: a critical review of the role of leadership and employee involvement in organizational change. J Innov Knowl. 2018;3(3):123–7.
15. Errida A, Lotfi B. The determinants of organizational change management success: literature review and case study. Int J Eng Bus Manage. 2021;13:1–15. https://doi.org/10.1177/18479790211016273.
16. Jones J, Firth J, Hannibal C, Ogunseyin M. Factors contributing to organizational change success or failure: a qualitative meta-analysis of 200 reflective case studies. In: Research anthology on digital transformation, organizational change, and the impact of remote work. IGI Global; 2021. p. 1427–50.
17. Sukhera J, Milne A, Teunissen PW, Lingard L, Watling C. The actual versus idealized self: exploring responses to feedback about implicit bias in health professionals. Acad Med. 2018;93(4):623–9.
18. Alasadi R, Askary S. Employee involvement and the barriers to organizational change. Int J Inform Bus Manage. 2014;6(1):29.
19. Devine PG, Ash TL. Diversity training goals, limitations, and promise: a review of multidisciplinary literature. Ann Rev Psychol. 2021;73(1):403–29.
20. Peng J, Li M, Wang Z, Lin Y. Transformational leadership and employees' reactions to organizational change: evidence from a meta-analysis. J Appl Behav Sci. 2021;57(3):369–97.
21. Islam MN, Furuoka F, Idris A. Mapping the relationship between transformational leadership, trust in leadership and employee championing behavior during organizational change. Asia Pacific Manage Rev. 2021;26(2):95–102.
22. Mento A, Jones R, Dirndorfer W. A change management process: grounded in both theory and practice. J Change Manage. 2002;3(1):45–59.
23. Khaw KW, Alnoor A, Al-Abrrow H, Tiberius V, Ganesan Y, Atshan NA. Reactions towards organizational change: a systematic literature review. Curr Psychol. 2023;42(22):19137–60.
24. Francis DM. Using root cause analysis to help students examine social problems. Teach J Mass Commun. 2021;11(1):61–4.
25. Card AJ. The problem with '5 whys'. BMJ Qual Saf. 2017;26(8):671–7.
26. Marjadi B, Flavel J, Baker K, Glenister K, Morns M, Triantafyllou M, et al. Twelve tips for inclusive practice in healthcare settings. Int J Environ Res Public Health. 2023;20(5):4657.

27. Sukhera J, Watling C. A framework for integrating implicit bias recognition into health professions education. Acad Med. 2018;93(1):35–40.
28. Sue DW, Capodilupo CM, Torino GC, Bucceri JM, Holder A, Nadal KL, Esquilin M. Racial microaggressions in everyday life: implications for clinical practice. Am Psychol. 2007;62(4):271.
29. Ehie O, Muse I, Hill L, Bastien A. Professionalism: microaggression in the healthcare setting. Curr Opin Anaesthesiol. 2021;34(2):131–6.
30. Morse JM, Bottorff J, Anderson G, O'Brien B, Solberg S. Beyond empathy: expanding expressions of caring. J Adv Nursing. 1992;17(7):809–21.
31. Brown B. Atlas of the heart: mapping meaningful connection and the language of human experience. New York: Random House; 2021.
32. The Ethics Committee of the American Society for Reproductive Medicine. Disparities in access to effective treatment for infertility in the United States: an Ethics Committee opinion. Fertil Steril. 2021;116(1):54–63.
33. Lloyd R, Munro J, Evans K, Gaskin-Williams A, Hui A, Pearson M, Slade M, Kotera Y, Day G, Loughlin-Ridley J, Enston C. Health service improvement using positive patient feedback: systematic scoping review. PLoS One. 2023;18(10):e0275045.

Chapter 17
Culturally Responsive Reproductive Mental Health Practice: Pitfalls and Possibilities

Danielle A. Kaplan

1. *Amy and Paul are a married couple who are interested in pursuing couples counseling while they undergo fertility treatment. 18 months ago, they experienced an unexplained pregnancy loss at 17 weeks and have not been able to conceive since. The couple attempted two rounds of* in vitro *fertilization (IVF) but did not obtain any embryos even after using intracytoplasmic sperm injection (ICSI). It has been recommended that the couple consider using donor sperm. Amy and Paul are both still grieving their pregnancy loss and Amy is becoming increasingly depressed and anxious with each new unsuccessful round of treatment. Both members of the couple are uncertain about their willingness to proceed to a gamete donor. They are seeking therapy both for support around decision-making and to address their different styles of dealing with their pregnancy loss and coping with the stress of infertility treatment.*

   Where do you begin with Amy and Paul?

   How does your answer change if the couple is Muslim? If Amy is from Africa and Paul from Canada? If Paul is first-generation Chinese-American?
2. *A single 39 year-old woman presents to your office for psychological support around involuntary childlessness and decision-making around pursuing parenthood without a partner. How does your approach to treatment change if this patient:*

   Is male? Also use a wheelchair? Did not complete high school?

D. A. Kaplan (✉)
Department of Psychiatry, NYU Langone Medical Center, New York, NY, USA

D. A. Kaplan (ed.), *Cultural Responsiveness in Assisted Reproductive Technology*, https://doi.org/10.1007/978-3-031-76204-8_17

Introduction

ASRM guidelines recognize that qualified fertility counselors interact with infertility patients at many stages of their treatment. They provide ongoing therapeutic support to individuals, groups, and couples, engage in crisis counseling, provide psychoeducation and counseling around reproductive decision-making, and interface with reproductive endocrinology and infertility staff. When third-party collaborators are involved in pregnancy, fertility counselors engage in the psychological evaluation of gamete donors and gestational carriers, administer and interpret psychological tests, and meet with intended parents considering the use of a gamete donor for psychoeducation and implications counseling. In each of these roles, fertility counselors are exhorted to practice with cultural competency and to be aware of the cultural and religious factors involved in decision-making [1]. At every stage of the process, clinicians' comfort in dealing with issues of culture and diversity can enhance or impede the experience of minoritized patients. Mirroring the guidelines put forth by ASRM, this chapter will focus both on best practices in culturally responsive fertility counseling and on structural and clinician factors that can have a negative impact on minoritized patients' experience of care.

Like all infertility care professionals—and all members of the helping professions—mental health practitioners are as subject to implicit biases as members of the general population. Although data on implicit bias among mental health professionals are limited, what we do know is unsurprising. When measured by clinician self-report, levels of multicultural competency covary with years of training and education. Levels of implicit bias, however, remain unchanged. This finding is true irrespective of whether clinicians have taken coursework in multicultural awareness and competency [2–5].

Biases persist among mental healthcare providers for the same reasons that they persist among nurses, teachers, and grocery store owners. All of us are steeped in a culture in which we receive repeated messaging about the characteristics of groups other than and including our own. Such messages, repeated and internalized over a lifetime, are durable and difficult to overwrite with brief exposure to counter-stereotypical examples or a series of standalone courses in cultural competency [6]. However, bias among mental healthcare providers may also be reified by the nature and scope of mental health training itself.

Historically, psychotherapy has emphasized conceptualization and intervention at the level of the individual, at times widening the lens to focus on the couple, family, or small group. Even when cultural factors are explicitly considered, focusing on the smaller unit rather than on the larger system locates both pathology and its remedy in the individual. The emphasis on clinical and cultural competency over structural competency ignores upstream determinants of health and illness that place minoritized individuals at greater risk of mental illness, substance abuse, and other negative health effects [7, 8]. A clinician who focuses on the experience of the individual without considering the social determinants of health and illness—that is, whether clients have consistent access to healthy food, air, and water, stable housing, quality education, and a safe environment—risks overpathologizing clients' presentations and missing critical opportunities to serve as an advocate and an ally in the fight for more equitable systems of care [9, 10].

Bias and stereotyping in mental healthcare are also perpetuated by a system in which most mental health practitioners and the overwhelming majority of those who train them are cisgender, able bodied, and White. For example, although recent trends suggest that current doctoral candidates in psychology are more diverse than their predecessors, the psychology workforce is significantly less racially and ethnically diverse than the overall US population. This is particularly true of practitioners over 50, 92% of whom identify as White [11]. The scarcity of diverse teachers, mentors, and colleagues deprives mental health practitioners of the opportunity to challenge and ameliorate their biases and assumptions through prolonged and varied contact with a diverse workforce [6].

Bias and Mental Healthcare

Olivia is a 34 year-old Black woman. When she was 17, she presented to the ER with intense stomach pains and nausea. The ER doctor attributed her symptoms to gastritis and sent her home with a prescription for an antacid. Olivia returned to the ER 2 days later with a 102-degree fever and was diagnosed with a ruptured appendix. Olivia is now seeking a preconception consultation with a reproductive psychiatrist to address symptoms of OCD. The psychiatrist recommends that Olivia begin an SSRI, citing research that suggests that it is considered safe for pregnancy and breastfeeding. Olivia raises concerns about outcomes for a developing fetus, but the psychiatrist repeats her assertions and ascribes Olivia's concerns to her obsessional thinking. Olivia leaves with a prescription for an SSRI but does not fill it.

Even outside the realm of infertility counseling, holding one or more marginalized identities decreases the likelihood that a patient in need of mental health care will get accessible and effective therapeutic support. Limited insurance coverage, a lack of affordable providers, and difficulties finding a provider whose office is accessible in terms of linguistic competence, disability accommodations, geography, or scheduling can all serve as structural barriers to accessing mental health care [12, 13]. It is unsurprising, then, that marginalized patients are more likely to access mental health support through crisis settings rather than through an ongoing therapeutic relationship [14, 15].

If they are seen at all, minoritized patients are more likely to be offered medication rather than talk therapy as a first-line treatment [16]. This may be due in part to the settings in which treatment is accessed, an example of disparities in access to care leading to disparities in treatment and outcomes. However, the overreliance on psychotropic medication as a first-line treatment for minoritized patients' mental health issues also stems from the impact of provider bias on psychiatric diagnosis. Even when using standardized diagnostic criteria, Black patients are routinely overdiagnosed with psychotic disorders relative to White patients. Similarly, psychiatrists presented with images of Black faces are more likely to recall words associated with psychotic disorders, treatment noncompliance, and antipsychotic medication [17, 18].

Prior experiences of healthcare discrimination can also impact the likelihood that minoritized patients will seek mental health support. When struggling with depression, patients who have experienced healthcare discrimination are less likely to attempt to access therapeutic support and engage in shared treatment decision-making, a trend that can result in a delay in help-seeking and a concomitant worsening of symptoms [19]. Patients who have experienced discrimination in healthcare also demonstrate decreased levels of trust in their providers, which in turn is associated with decreased adherence to treatment with psychotropic medications [20]. Providers' tendency to view marginalized patients as less compliant with treatment recommendations can easily become a self-fulfilling prophecy; providers who expect their patients to be nonadherent to treatment recommendations are likely to interact with them in a way that compromises patients' faith in those recommendations and make them less likely to follow the proposed plan of care.

Among patients who do seek out ongoing psychotherapeutic support, holding one or more marginalized identities can impact the experience of treatment, beginning with the ease of obtaining an appointment at all. In private practice settings, for example, middle-class White women are more likely to get a call back when requesting an initial appointment with a therapist than are working-class Black men [4]. Once in the door, patients' perceptions of provider bias can impact their experience of the therapeutic relationship. Although the data suggest a weak association at best between client/therapist ethnic match and treatment outcomes [21], there is some evidence that racial or gender matching, which clients may use as a proxy for provider cultural responsiveness, can influence minoritized patients' decision to pursue treatment and the length of time that they remain in care [22, 23]. In contrast, perceptions of provider bias can impede patient self-disclosure and lead to higher rates of premature dropout from treatment [24].

Provider bias is often discussed in terms of race and ethnicity. However, the factors that interfere with BIPOC patients' experience of mental health treatment are equally relevant for patients holding other marginalized identities. Implicit and explicit bias and discrimination, structural inequities, and minority stress place LGBTQ+ patients at substantially higher risk of mental illness, substance abuse, and suicidality than heterosexual patients, with transgender patients and those holding multiple minoritized identities (for example, being Black and trans) at the highest risk of illness and distress [25]. Sadly, however, the anticipation of receiving care from a biased or ill-informed provider often interferes with LGBTQ+ patients seeking treatment when in distress. In a recent study of LGBTQ+ youth, more than half reported wanting mental healthcare but not receiving any. The discrepancy between their desire for treatment and their reluctance to seek it was due to prior negative experiences with healthcare and their belief that clinicians would not understand issues related to their sexuality or gender identity [26]. In a study of LGBTQ+ patients who did manage to engage in mental healthcare, sexual minority patients were more likely to report that their providers spent inadequate time with them or looked down on or judged them for their sexual orientation. Unsurprisingly, these patients experienced decreased trust in their providers. With such factors at play, LGBTQ+ clients felt less confident in their ability to seek out and receive mental healthcare should they need it in the future [27].

Patients seeking therapeutic support for infertility may therefore arrive with a lifetime of history and associations with mental and medical healthcare in tow. For minoritized patients facing infertility, the decision to seek mental health support at all may present a dual challenge. The difficulty of finding a counselor who is trained in the specific issues associated with infertility and its treatment may be compounded by reasonable doubts about finding a provider who is open to understanding their experiences of holding one or more minoritized identities. Like all providers, fertility counselors can either approach their work with cultural awareness and humility or risk creating a therapeutic environment that compounds stress for the patients we are endeavoring to support.

Infertility Counseling

Infertility happens to people with already existing and intersecting cultural identities, each of which may be more or less salient to the individual at different points in their treatment. As Bonds-Grocher and Gerrits remind us,

> "[in]fertility is not simply a medically-diagnosed reproductive impairment, but a socially-constructed reality where people's cultural background and their (marginalized) position may and do matter in how they view fertility problems, the treatment options they seek [and] have access to, and the care they need and receive." [28, p. 185]

Relatedly, the authors emphasize the importance of not "essentializing" race and culture in the counseling of a diverse patient population [28]. The cultural beliefs of a fourth-generation Mexican-American patient about the social acceptability of fertility treatment may differ widely from those of a Mexican-born patient who moved to the United States as an adult to pursue career opportunities. A Korean-American woman who attends Catholic mass regularly may choose to discontinue treatment at a different point from one who attends a Protestant church or no church at all.

Ultimately, any decisions that patients make around treatment are as informed by their access to accurate information, their access to care, and their prior experiences of feeling heard and understood by their care providers as they are by the cultures with which they identify [29]. Cultural responsiveness is a critical factor in determining patients' experience of infertility counseling. For it to be relevant at all, however, patients must be able to find and access providers who have availability at times when patients are not working, whose offices are located in a geographically accessible area, and whose services they can afford.

Guidance on providing mental health support to infertility patients from specific cultural backgrounds is discussed at length in other chapters throughout this volume. When working with a patient of any cultural background, however, fertility counselors should keep several guiding principles in mind.

Fertility Literacy

Patients vary widely in their awareness of their own fertility and its limitations and of the treatment options available to them. Community samples of adults generally have inaccurate assumptions about age-related changes in fertility, spontaneous pregnancy rates, and available treatment options [30]. Fertility literacy is further compromised among people with lower socioeconomic status and levels of education [31]. Although not all minoritized patients are poor or have low levels of educational attainment, the downstream effects of structural racism can place minoritized patients at disproportionate risk of decreased fertility literacy by virtue of their decreased access to high-quality education and healthcare [32].

Minoritized patients may be at additional risk of low fertility awareness for reasons that are culture specific. Patients who perceive cultural taboos around discussions of sexuality are deprived of valuable opportunities for informal information sharing about fertility within their families and communities. For some patients, perceived cultural or religious stigma around infertility may dissuade them from disclosing challenges with conception, which may in turn decrease the likelihood of being referred for timely care [33]. Notably, this stigma can be compounded for patients holding multiple cultural identities; for example, Latina Catholic patients may simultaneously hold the belief that childless marriages are a failure and adhere to a Church doctrine that prohibits most forms of fertility treatment [33, 34].

Competence in fertility counseling requires us to be able to provide accurate education to all patients about fertility myths and realities. It also requires us to be attuned to the cultural messaging that our clients might have received around their fertility and accessing care. Asking patients where their understanding of their fertility comes from and what messages they have received about procreation, childlessness, and treatment can help expose any misconceptions that patients may hold, laying the groundwork for timely referral for infertility care.

Helping a diverse patient population to understand their fertility also requires us to examine our biases around what a parent looks like. Single people, people with disabilities, and members of all racialized and minoritized groups desire children at comparable rates [35, 36]. However, they may receive disparate treatment when it comes to their access to reproductive healthcare; members of some minoritized groups report that their providers erroneously consider discussions of sexuality, contraception, and fertility to be irrelevant [36]. Fertility counselors whose vision of a parent comprises able-bodied women but not single men with disabilities or college-educated Asian-Americans but not Latinx immigrants who didn't complete high school run the risk of providing inequitable care by exploring issues of sexuality, fertility treatment, and access to care only with those patients who fit their image of a person who desires and "deserves" children.

Regardless of their income, education, or levels of fertility literacy, BIPOC patients are referred for infertility workups and subsequent care at lower rates than White patients. Although increased fertility literacy is helpful to patients in self-referring for care, the onus for receiving equitable care should not be on the patient.

Rather, it is the responsibility of the fertility counselor- along with primary care physicians, OB-GYNs, and REIs- to work towards a system of care that is unhampered by clinician bias and provides adequate information and treatment to all patients.

Decisional Support

Fertility counselors frequently work with patients who are at a crossroads when it comes to choosing the next steps in their treatment. Some patients may be faced with a decision about whether to begin infertility care. Others have exhausted options involving their gametes and have been advised to proceed with donor gametes or, in some cases, with a gestational carrier. For others, the decisions they face involve not how to proceed but whether to continue in treatment, pursue parenthood through other means, or contemplate child-free living.

Financial, logistical, and emotional constraints factor heavily in the decisions that patients make about fertility care; by definition, a salaried patient with flexible work hours and private insurance has more options for treatment than an hourly wage worker with public insurance whose shifts are scheduled by their employer [37, 38]. Culturally responsive decisional support for patients involves a willingness to discuss the structural constraints on treatment. For example, a patient who would like to proceed with IVF but lacks insurance coverage for the procedure would benefit from working with a counselor who is aware of fertility grants that are available to patients from a variety of backgrounds and circumstances.

However, even among patients whose social and financial circumstances facilitate treatment, cultural and religious beliefs about infertility care influence the acceptability of treatment options and the uptake of ART treatments. Culturally responsive fertility counselors support patients in choosing infertility care options that are consistent with their religious and cultural beliefs. This may involve collaboration with cultural brokers who are able to help all members of a patient's care team better understand the cultural implications of available care options or of choosing to discontinue treatment in the face of strong cultural messaging about the centrality of childbearing [39, 40].

Social Support and Grief

Jennifer and Shruti are a married lesbian couple. Jennifer considers herself to be "culturally Jewish"; Shruti is Hindu. They have been attempting to have a child with Jennifer's eggs and the collaboration of a known sperm donor. Unfortunately, Jennifer has experienced two miscarriages. The couple is now contemplating whether to continue trying to conceive with Jennifer's eggs and with her as the carrying partner or whether Shruti should now attempt to conceive and carry a pregnancy.

The couple tells you that they were originally quite aligned in their desire for a baby and decisions about fertility treatment. After the miscarriages, however, they began to notice themselves feeling more distant from each other. Shruti reports that "we always used to be so good at comforting each other; now it's like we're having two entirely different experiences." Jennifer has been very open about their challenges, seeking support from her family and participating in online message boards about pregnancy loss. In contrast, Shruti has not spoken to anyone but Jennifer about the miscarriages. They initiate therapy with you to improve their communication before deciding how to proceed with treatment.

Providing competent infertility counseling also requires us to be aware of the ways in which culture can inform clients' decisions around community support and mourning. Infertility and pregnancy loss can both engender feelings of disenfranchised grief, a term commonly used for the experience of a loss that may not be recognized by the larger community and for which there are no agreed-upon rituals [41, 42]. Patients' ways of coping with this grief can be heavily influenced by the cultures with which they identify and the messages that these cultures convey. For example, the ways that patients conceptualize pregnancy loss can be heavily influenced by cultural and religious conceptions of pregnancy [43]. Some Ultraorthodox Jewish women may find that their grief is complicated by a religious doctrine that does not endorse communal mourning rituals after miscarriage or stillbirth [44].[1] In contrast, some devout Islamic women experiencing pregnancy loss have been shown to benefit from counseling that incorporates verses from the Quran that deal directly with pregnancy, grief, and the loss of an infant or fetus [45].

Patients' ways of coping with the disenfranchised grief of infertility may similarly be influenced by the cultures with which they identify. For some, leaning heavily on family, friends, and religious community can serve as a buffer against the isolation of disenfranchised grief. For others, even the impact of family support can be heavily influenced by cultural messaging; in one study of Vietnamese women experiencing infertility, for example, social support by the husband's family counterintuitively increased distress and feelings of failure after a failed treatment cycle [46].

For the infertility counselor, helping patients to navigate disenfranchised grief around infertility and loss involves understanding what sources of connection are available and helpful to a diverse patient population. A fertility counselor who refers her same-sex patients to an infertility support group otherwise composed entirely of heterosexual couples may find that her patients' experiences of diagnosis and treatment may not be mirrored by others in the group. Similarly, patients whose religious community stigmatizes or explicitly prohibits most infertility treatments may find that a faith commitment that was previously a source of solace now engenders

[1] It should be noted, however, that grassroots religious organizations such as A Time have recognized the need for pregnancy loss support in the Orthodox community and responded with religiously-consonant support packets and assistance with burial preparation for a fetus that can be made available to observant Jews after a miscarriage or stillbirth (https://www.atime.org/services/hug/).

ambivalence or increased isolation. Culturally responsive fertility counselors should familiarize themselves with community and Internet-based resources that address the grief of infertility and loss in ways that are specific to a variety of cultural groups. They also have the opportunity to help patients create rituals around disenfranchised grief that reflect the patients' own cultural values and beliefs about what has been lost.

Recipient Consultations

Implications counseling with parents who intend to conceive using donor gametes involves considering the lifelong development of donor-conceived people. Fertility counselors working with intended parents are asked to discuss the implications of decisions made at all points in the donor conception process, from the selection of a donor to the series of conversations that will help donor-conceived people better understand their origins and identities.

Race and Ethnicity in Donor Gamete Selection

Although race and ethnicity are ill-defined concepts at best, they are often of great importance to patients considering building their families through donor conception. Egg and sperm banks generally ask donors to self-identify in terms of race or ethnicity [47], and recipient parents who are contemplating conception with donor gametes are often advised to choose a donor who is a close ethnic or racial match for their existing family to avoid intrusive questions about how a child fits in their family [48, 49].

This presents a particular conundrum for recipient families who are seeking a gamete donor of color. Relative to both the general population and the population of donor gamete recipients, there is a dearth of both egg and sperm donors of color, with the most notable scarcity existing among Black or African American donors [50, 51]. Thus, White recipient parents are often counseled to select a donor whose race or ethnicity mirrors their own to increase the likelihood of conceiving a child who resembles them. In contrast, BIPOC recipients of donor gametes are often informed that a donor who matches their own racial or ethnic self-identification is unlikely to be available and that they should consider broadening their search for a donor to select for other characteristics such as hair and eye color, or to focus on the donor's general health characteristics and forego any attempt at phenotypic similarity [52]. This discrepancy might result in decreased uptake of donor gametes among non-White patients; in a recent study, Black patients desiring a Black donor were both less likely to attempt to conceive with donor gametes than were White patients seeking a White donor and reported lower levels of satisfaction with the process of donor conception [53].

Scholars who argue in favor of racial or ethnic matching in donor conception suggest that recipient parents who share the identity of their offspring are best equipped to help their children navigate the complexities of living as a minoritized person [54, 55]. Some, however, argue that this process serves to reify the importance of race as a primary characteristic and prioritizes physical similarity over other commonalities and relational bonds [55, 56] as a marker of family and belonging.

Discussions of race and ethnicity are a critical part of recipient–parent psychoeducational consultations. For some recipient parents, the grief and loss that often accompany the decision to use donor gametes may be compounded by the anticipated loss of shared heritage with the child they conceive through third-party reproduction. Raising a donor-conceived child from a different ethnic or racial group also requires raising parents to meet their children's needs for cultural mirrors within their communities and tools for coping with racism and discrimination in society at large and within the family [57]. From the perspective of the donor-conceived person, ethnic, racial, or cultural details available about their genetic parent may inform their identity throughout their development and impact their sense of belonging in both their raising and genetic families. The culturally aware counselor should not hesitate to explore the meaning of racial concordance or discordance with gamete donor recipients and to anticipate the emotional consequences to both the recipient parent and the donor-conceived child if a racially or ethnically similar donor is not available. Fertility counselors should also be aware of the impact of being told to adopt a "close enough" mindset on diverse patients' comfort with conceiving with gametes from donors of a different ethnic or racial background from their own, and on their trust in the providers who propose this.

Disclosure

Current best practices in third-party assisted reproduction support early disclosure and ongoing dialogue about donor conception as supportive of the long-term mental health and well-being of donor-conceived people [58]. However, rates of disclosure vary widely as a function of culture and country of origin; for example, relatively low rates of disclosure have been documented in both China and Iran despite the increasing uptake of donor gametes in both countries [59, 60]. Some cultural groups may view disclosure as threatening the stability of familial and community relationships. For members of these groups, disclosure may risk decreased acceptance of the donor-conceived child and a loss of face for the rearing parent who required donor gametes [59]. This may lead parents to be selective in the nature of the information that they provide to their offspring or the family members to whom they disclose their reproductive history. Views on the desirability of disclosure may also be impacted by membership in a religious group, such as Orthodox Judaism or Sunni Islam, in which conception with donor gametes at times runs counter to religious laws and customs [61, 62].

Recipient parents must balance their cultural beliefs and the realities of the communities in which they intend to raise their children with current best practices around child-centered disclosure. Fertility counselors should be aware of the cultural influences on willingness to discuss donor conception. Respectfully and openly inquiring about patients' concerns about the cultural impact of disclosure can help intended parents find a synthesis among their cultural realities, the emotional well-being of their future children, and the impossibility of maintaining secrecy and anonymity in the current environment.

Psychological Evaluation of Third-Party Collaborators

Jordan is a 24 year-old sperm donor candidate from Chicago. On evaluation, he tells you that his father was raised in the Cabrini Green Homes, a now-demolished public housing project notorious for high rates of gang violence and substance abuse. Jordan's father and his uncles routinely witnessed violence in the hallways of their building and heard gunshots in the stairwells; Jordan recalls his father telling him that he was assaulted twice by gang members who mistakenly believed him to be a member of a rival gang. Two of Jordan's uncles have developed substance abuse problems. His father did not graduate from high school due to chronic absenteeism. Jordan's father also spent 18 months in prison on an assault charge after seriously injuring an acquaintance in a physical altercation. Based on Jordan's description, his father continues to exhibit symptoms consistent with PTSD. Jordan is slowly working toward a college degree while working shifts in a restaurant kitchen. He reports that he tried alcohol as a teenager but states that "I knew if I really started drinking, I'd never stop."

Does Jordan meet criteria for sperm donation? Why or why not?

ASRM best practice guidelines require the comprehensive medical and psychological evaluation of all third-party collaborators and, when relevant, their partners [63]. Psychological evaluation of sperm and oocyte donors and gestational carriers involves taking a throughout developmental, educational, legal, social, sexual, and psychiatric history and assessing for current life stressors [64, 65]. The intentions behind conducting an evaluation of this scope are beneficent; a comprehensive evaluation is meant to be protective for all parties involved in third-party reproduction. It decreases the likelihood of passing adverse heritable conditions to donor-conceived offspring and increases the chance that all parties have the emotional capacity and structural support needed to promote their well-being during the process of assisted reproduction and beyond. Each component of this evaluation process, however, requires fertility counselors to be mindful of the role of race and culture in both the lived experiences of third-party collaborators and the way interview and test data are understood.

The downstream effects of structural and systemic racism touch almost every aspect of the lived experience of racialized populations in the United States. Being a member of a marginalized group is associated with poorer mental and physical health outcomes, lower rates of home ownership and total household wealth, and lower educational attainment [66–69]. Black, Latinx, or Native American citizens continue to be incarcerated at rates higher than their representation in the US population or to have experienced the incarceration of a relative [70–72]. Unsurprisingly, then, Black, Native American, and Latinx patients are overrepresented among the poor and therefore disproportionately more likely to be enrolled in Medicaid or receive other public health benefits [73]. Applicants are generally excluded from third-party collaboration in situations of financial precarity or when financial need raises the possibility that their participation is coerced rather than voluntary [64, 65]. There is no indication that this exclusion criterion should be reevaluated for applicants from marginalized communities. It should be noted, however, that the downstream effects of systemic racism make it more likely that some potential third-party collaborators of color will be excluded from participation solely based on poverty and its associated instability.

Prospective gamete donors and gestational carriers who have passed initial screening criteria proceed to a clinical interview. As part of this process, they should be given standardized self-report measures to assess their psychological functioning and personality organization. Here again, the intention is to better understand an applicant's ability both to collaborate in the immediate process of reproduction and act in ways that are in the lifelong interests of donor-conceived people. Unfortunately, however, standardized psychological tests are as vulnerable to bias as the people who create, administer, and interpret them.

The Personality Assessment Inventory, generally thought to be the standard for evaluation in donor and gestational carrier screening, is available from its publisher only in English and Spanish versions translated for both Europe and Latin America [74]. The Minnesota Multiphasic Personality Inventory (MMPI), a recommended alternative to the PAI for practitioners who are trained in its use, has significantly more verified translations available, many of which include country-specific population norms [75]. However, the question remains of how to interpret test data for an applicant who was born in one country and educated in another, or whose reading level in a language that they speak with fluency is lower than what test completion requires.

Even for third-party candidates whose language fluency is not at issue, racial and cultural differences can influence response patterns to standardized measures. Data on differences in response patterns by self-reported race or ethnicity are inconsistent. However, many studies have pointed to a pattern of higher scores on the Schizophrenia, Infrequency, and Lie scales on the MMPI and MMPI-2 among Black and Latinx respondents in the absence of psychopathology [76], suggesting that the measure may lack the sensitivity to distinguish clinical paranoia from cultural mistrust [77]. Although later editions of the MMPI, including the MMPI-2RF and MMPI-3 demonstrate fewer instances of clinical elevation in the absence of clinical psychopathology among minoritized respondents, some evidence suggests that Latinx college students may still be more likely to produce invalid profiles than non-Latinx White students [78, 79]. Similar cultural differences have been found in response patterns to the PAI, with Latinx respondents and Asian-American respondents more likely to show elevations on scales reflecting paranoia and psychotic experiences [80] in the absence of true pathology.

None of these factors on its own may be automatically disqualifying for serving as a collaborator in third-party reproduction. Absent an understanding of the biases inherent in our clinical interview questions and assessment tools, however, they may lead to the unnecessary disqualification of potentially successful gestational carriers and gamete donors. Ethical evaluators act out of an abundance of caution and concern for the well-being of all parties involved. However, the evaluator who is unable to interpret a gamete donor or gestational carrier's history or test data in the context of sociocultural factors risks turning away potential collaborators who are otherwise well suited to the role they are being asked to play and perpetuating the scarcity of diverse donors for recipient parents who are interested in conceiving a racially or ethnically similar child.

Conclusions and Recommendations

For some readers, the exhortation to add cultural responsiveness to the already long list of requirements for infertility counseling may seem daunting. In a field that requires familiarity with reproductive anatomy, medical terminology and procedures, ongoing education in counseling and assessment, and significant peer consultation, the charge to consider issues of culture, bias, and equity may seem like an additional burdensome item on the to-do list. Approaching fertility counseling with cultural responsiveness and humility, however, draws on many skills and ethical principles that qualified fertility counselors have already incorporated into their practices. Culturally responsive care is patient-centered care: it requires us to be "receptive and responsive to the preferences, needs, and values of the patient and family" [81, p. 314]. Culturally responsive care is trauma-informed care: it recognizes that adverse experiences have significant impacts on health and can influence the ways that people experience and interact with systems of care [82]. Above all, culturally responsive care is ethical care, reminding us to approach our patients with an eye to justice, respect for their rights and dignity, and attitudes and behaviors that promote and safeguard the well-being of those in our care [83].

In interactions with fertility patients, cultural responsiveness requires us to maintain an attitude of respectful curiosity about our patients' choices in fertility care and the ways they cope with infertility-related distress. Awareness of our own biases about what a parent looks like and acceptable ways to build a family can keep us from providing one-size-fits-all psychoeducation and therapeutic intervention to patients whose beliefs differ from our own.

As evaluators of third-party collaborators, we have a responsibility to recognize the biases inherent in the tools we use for assessment. We may also be required to balance the current best practices in the field around criteria for participation as a gamete donor or gestational carrier with consideration of the ways in which the downstream effects of structural racism may decrease the pool of applicants of color who are accepted into these roles.

Outside our offices, cultural responsiveness involves acting as advocates and allies in the structures and systems in which we practice. For fertility counselors, this might mean being willing to interface with clients' medical teams to discuss ways in which their history with the medical system might impact their needs in treatment. It also means making an active commitment to diversifying the field of infertility counseling by actively recruiting, mentoring, and sharing power and influence with colleagues with a diversity of identities [10, 84].

Mental health professionals are uniquely positioned to provide holistic support to patients struggling with infertility [85]. As the patient population seeking infertility support continues to become more diverse, we have the responsibility to ensure that the care we provide is grounded in an awareness of structural inequities, our own biases, and the intersectional identities of people who seek our support.

References

1. Committee P. Guidance on qualifications for fertility counselors: a committee opinion. Fertil Steril. 2021;115(6):1411–5.
2. Boysen GA. A review of experimental studies of explicit and implicit bias among counselors. J Multicultural Counsel Dev. 2009;37(4):240–9.
3. Boysen GA, Vogel DL. The relationship between level of training, implicit bias, and multicultural competency among counselor trainees. Train Educ Prof Psychol. 2008;2(2):103.
4. Merino Y, Adams L, Hall WJ. Implicit bias and mental health professionals: priorities and directions for research. Psychiatr Serv. 2018;69(6):723–5.
5. Stevens FL, Abernethy AD. Neuroscience and racism: the power of groups for overcoming implicit bias. Int J Group Psychother. 2018;68(4):561–84.
6. Greenwald AG, Dasgupta N, Dovidio JF, Kang J, Moss-Racusin CA, Teachman BA. Implicit-bias remedies: treating discriminatory bias as a public-health problem. Psychol Sci Public Interest. 2022;23(1):7–40.
7. Metzl JM, Hansen H. Structural competency: theorizing a new medical engagement with stigma and inequality. Soc Sci Med. 2014;103:126–33.
8. Laynor G. Structural competency in mental health and medicine: a case-based approach to treating the social determinants of health. J Med Library Assoc. 2021;109(2):346.
9. Wilcox MM. Oppression is not "culture": the need to center systemic and structural determinants to address anti-Black racism and racial trauma in psychotherapy. Psychotherapy. 2023;60(1):76.
10. Williams MT, Faber SC, Duniya C. Being an anti-racist clinician. Cognitive Behav Ther. 2022;15:e19.
11. American Psychological Association. Psychology's workforce is becoming more diverse. APA Monitor Psychol. 2020;51:11–9.
12. Mongelli F, Georgakopoulos P, Pato MT. Challenges and opportunities to meet the mental health needs of underserved and disenfranchised populations in the United States. Focus. 2020;18(1):16–24.
13. Giusto A, Jack HE, Magidson JF, Ayuku D, Johnson SL, Lovero KL, Hankerson SH, Sweetland AC, Myers B, Fortunato dos Santos P, Puffer ES. Global is local: leveraging global mental-health methods to promote equity and address disparities in the United States. Clin Psychol Sci. 2024;12(2):270–89.

14. Bignall T, Jeraj S, Helsby E, Butt J. Racial disparities in mental health. Race Equality Foundation; 2019.
15. Progovac AM, Cortés DE, Chambers V, Delman J, Delman D, McCormick D, Lee E, De Castro S, Sánchez Román MJ, Kaushal NA, Creedon TB. Understanding the role of past health care discrimination in help-seeking and shared decision-making for depression treatment preferences. Qual Health Res. 2020;30(12):1833–50.
16. Tiwari D. "But I'm Not Racist": how implicit racial bias, feedback and racial affective states impact clinical judgment in mental health treatment (Doctoral dissertation). University of Denver; 2021.
17. Gara MA, Minsky S, Silverstein SM, Miskimen T, Strakowski SM. A naturalistic study of racial disparities in diagnoses at an outpatient behavioral health clinic. Psychiatr Serv. 2019;70(2):130–4.
18. Londono Tobon A, Flores JM, Taylor JH, Johnson I, Landeros-Weisenberger A, Aboiralor O, Avila-Quintero VJ, Bloch MH. Racial implicit associations in psychiatric diagnosis, treatment, and compliance expectations. Acad Psychiatry. 2021;45:23–33.
19. Sonik RA, Creedon TB, Progovac AM, Carson N, Delman J, Delman D, Lê Cook B, Soffer TF, Chambers V, Quinerly CR, Mann Z. Depression treatment preferences by race/ethnicity and gender and associations between past healthcare discrimination experiences and present preferences in a nationally representative sample. Soc Sci Med. 2020;253:112939.
20. Pugh M, Perrin PB, Rybarczyk B, Tan J. Racism, mental health, healthcare provider trust, and medication adherence among black patients in safety-net primary care. J Clin Psychol Med Settings. 2021;28:181–90.
21. Hung YH, Linville D, Janes E, Yee S. Race matching in predicting relational therapy outcome: a machine learning approach. Int J Syst Therapy. 2023;34(2):83–94.
22. Ilagan GS, Heatherington L. Advancing the understanding of factors that influence client preferences for race and gender matching in psychotherapy. Counsel Psychol Q. 2022;35(3):694–717.
23. Cheng AW, Nakash O, Cruz-Gonzalez M, Fillbrunn MK, Alegría M. The association between patient–provider racial/ethnic concordance, working alliance, and length of treatment in behavioral health settings. Psychol Serv. 2023;20(S1):145.
24. Stevens F, Shriver E. The shame of implicit racial bias. J Soc Psychol. 2024;164(2):258–72.
25. Fadus M. Mental health disparities and medical student education: teaching in psychiatry for LGBTQ care, communication, and advocacy. Acad Psychiatry. 2019;43(3):306–10.
26. Choi KR, Wisk LE, Zima BT. Availability of LGBTQ mental health services for US youth, 2014 to 2020. JAMA Pediatr. 2023;177(8):865–7.
27. Schuller KA, Crawford RP. Impact of interpersonal client–provider relationship on satisfaction with mental healthcare among the LGBTQ+ population. J Mental Health. 2022;31(5):634–41.
28. Grocher K, Gerrits T. A racially and culturally sensitive approach to fertility counseling. Fertil Counsel Clin Guide. 2022;8:183.
29. Weiss MS, Marsh EE. Navigating unequal paths: racial disparities in the infertility journey. Obstet Gynecol. 2022;5:10–97.
30. Meissner C, Schippert C, von Versen-Höynck F. Awareness, knowledge, and perceptions of infertility, fertility assessment, and assisted reproductive technologies in the era of oocyte freezing among female and male university students. J Assist Reprod Genet. 2016;33:719–29.
31. Hoffman JR, Delaney MA, Valdes CT, Herrera D, Washington SL, Aghajanova L, Smith JF, Herndon CN. Disparities in fertility knowledge among women from low and high resource settings presenting for fertility care in two United States metropolitan centers. Fertil Res Pract. 2020;6:1–9.
32. Schillinger D. The intersections between social determinants of health, health literacy, and health disparities. Stud Health Technol Inform. 2020;269:22.
33. Portugal A, Kosturakis AK, Onyewuenyi TL, Rivera-Cruz G, Jimenez PT. Breaking down barriers: advancing toward health equity in fertility care for Black and Hispanic patients. Obstet Gynecol Clin. 2023;50(4):735–46.
34. Donnenfeld SR, Mehta A. The urologist's guide to religion and male factor fertility treatment. Urology. 2022;167:128–31.

35. Ethics Committee of the American Society for Reproductive Medicine. Access to fertility treatment irrespective of marital status, sexual orientation, or gender identity: an Ethics Committee opinion. Fertil Steril. 2021;116(2):326–30.
36. Horner-Johnson W, Dissanayake M, Wu JP, Caughey AB, Darney BG. Pregnancy intendedness by maternal disability status and type in the United States. Perspect Sex Reprod Health. 2020;52(1):31–8.
37. Cebert-Gaitors M, Shannon-Baker PA, Silva SG, Hart RE, Jahandideh S, Gonzalez-Guarda R, Stevenson EL. Psychobiological, clinical, and sociocultural factors that influence Black women seeking treatment for infertility: a mixed-methods study. F&S Rep. 2022;3(2):29–39.
38. Cebert-Gaitors M, Abdelnalbi S, Mantell E, Woodward A, Gonzalez-Guarda R, Stevenson EL. Multidimensional barriers and facilitators to treatment seeking for infertility among women in the United States: a systematic review. F&S Rev. 2022;3(1):76–89.
39. Handtke O, Schilgen B, Mösko M. Culturally competent healthcare—a scoping review of strategies implemented in healthcare organizations and a model of culturally competent healthcare provision. PLoS One. 2019;14(7):e0219971.
40. Abramov M, Shalom-Paz E, Benyamini Y. Persevering in fertility treatments despite failures: unrealistic optimism and the reality of a pronatalist culture. Int J Behav Med. 2022;29(2):209–19.
41. Brigance CA, Cottone RR. Addressing infertility through family therapy: an emotionally-focused family therapy approach. Contemporary Family Therapy. 2023;45(4):437–49.
42. Cassidy PR. The disenfranchisement of perinatal grief: How silence, silencing and self-censorship complicate bereavement (a mixed methods study). OMEGA J Death Dying. 2023;88(2):709–31.
43. Crockett JE, Rogers JL, Binkley EE. Cultural dimensions of early pregnancy loss: spiritual and religious issues. Counsel Values. 2021;66(1):21–39.
44. Levitan F, Frei-Landau R, Sabar-Ben-Yehoshua NA. "I Just Needed a Hug": culturally-based disenfranchised grief of Jewish ultraorthodox women following pregnancy loss. OMEGA J Death Dying. 2022; https://doi.org/10.1177/00302228221133864.
45. Mahmoodi V, Akhavan A, Virk Z. Integration of Islamic spirituality in the treatment of grief for pregnancy loss: a case series of loss during early, mid-, and late pregnancy. Spiritual Clin Pract. 2023;10(1):52.
46. Lam TQ, Linh TT, Thuy LB. The impact of social support on infertility-related stress: a study in the vietnamese context. Open J Soc Sci. 2021;9(12):259–73.
47. Hudson N. Gamete donation and 'race'. eLS; 2015.
48. Nordqvist P. 'I don't want us to stand out more than we already do': Lesbian couples negotiating family connections in donor conception. Sexualities. 2012;15(5–6):644–61.
49. Wong KA. Donor conception and "passing," or; why Australian parents of donor-conceived children want donors who look like them. J Bioethical Inquiry. 2017;14(1):77–86.
50. Moreta LE, Simpson AE, Ghidei L, Wiltshire AM. Sperm donor availability and selection based on race and ethnicity. Fertil Steril. 2022;118(4):e383–4.
51. Tsai S, Chung EH, Truong T, Farrell AS, Wu J, Ohamadike O, Eaton JL. Racial and ethnic disparities among donor oocyte banks in the United States. Fertil Steril. 2022;117(3):622–8.
52. Schuman L, Leondires M. Building your family: the complete guide to donor conception. St. Martins Essentials; 2023.
53. Mebane S, Harris BS, Woodward JT, Brucker A, Erkanli A, Nagle CT, Steele D, Neal S. A survey study evaluating donor gamete utilization rates, patient satisfaction and fertility treatment outcomes according to desired race and ethnicity of the gamete donor. Fertil Steril. 2023;120(4):e261.
54. Tucker A. "You should be grateful": stories of race, identity, and transracial adoption. Beacon Press; 2023.
55. Maung HH. Ethical problems with ethnic matching in gamete donation. J Med Ethics. 2019;45(2):112–6.

56. Starza-Allen A. The racial matching of gamete donors in UK fertility clinics. University of Kent; 2021.
57. Mikkelsen M, Tang M. Navigating cross-racial matches of intended parents & gamete donors: a DCP-centered approach. Donor Conceived Community Webinar. 1 May 2024.
58. ESHRE Working Group on Reproductive Donation, Kirkman-Brown J, Calhaz-Jorge C, Dancet EA, Lundin K, Martins M, Tilleman K, Thorn P, Vermeulen N, Frith L. Good practice recommendations for information provision for those involved in reproductive donation. Hum Reprod Open. 2022;2022(1):hoac001.
59. Tsui EY, Cheng JO. The living experience of losing genetic continuity: concealment tendency in Chinese recipients of donor-assisted conception. J Health Psychol. 2021;26(4):525–42.
60. Hadizadeh-Talasaz F, Simbar M, Roudsari RL. Exploring infertile couples' decisions to disclose donor conception to the future child. Int J Fertil Steril. 2020;14(3):240.
61. Farid MS, Tasnim S. Assisted Reproductive Technologies: comparing abrahamic monotheistic religions. Asian Bioethics Rev. 2023;15(1):53–67.
62. Inhorn MC. Two 'quiet' reproductive revolutions: Islam, gender, and (in) fertility. In: The Routledge handbook of Islam and gender. Routledge; 2020. p. 343–57.
63. Practice Committee of the American Society for Reproductive Medicine, Practice Committee for the Society for Assisted Reproductive Technology. Guidance regarding gamete and embryo donation. Fertil Steril. 2021;115(6):1395–410.
64. Rosenquist S. Psychological evaluations for assisted reproductive intervention: guidelines for clinical practice. J Health Serv Psychol. 2020;46(1):21–8.
65. Simpson T, Riddle M. Special assessments considerations and arrangements in gestational surrogacy. Fertil Counsel Clin Guide. 2022;8:125.
66. Fink-Samnick E. The social determinants of mental health: definitions, distinctions, and dimensions for professional case management: part 1. Prof Case Manage. 2021;26(3):121–37.
67. Shrider EA, Creamer J. Poverty in the United States: 2022. US Census Bureau; 2023.
68. Kermani A, Wong F. Racial disparities in housing returns. National Bureau of Economic Research; 2021.
69. Carnevale AP, Peltier Campbell K, Cheah B, Fasules ML, Gulish A, Quinn MC, Sablan JR, Smith N, Strohl J, Barrese S. The cost of economic and racial injustice in postsecondary education. 2021.
70. Heimer K, Malone SE, De Coster S. Trends in women's incarceration rates in US prisons and jails: a tale of inequalities. Ann Rev Criminol. 2023;6:85–106.
71. Jeffers JL. Justice is not blind: disproportionate incarceration rate of people of color. In: Race and social policy. Routledge; 2022. p. 113–21.
72. Muller C, Roehrkasse AF. Racial and class inequality in US incarceration in the early twenty-first century. Soc Forces. 2022;101(2):803–28.
73. Michener JD. Politics, pandemic, and racial justice through the lens of Medicaid. Am J Public Health. 2021;111(4):643–6.
74. https://www.parinc.com/Products/Pkey/287.
75. https://www.upress.umn.edu/test-division/translations-permissions/available-translations.
76. Schapiro SJ, Ellis D, Golden C. MMPI: Black and White differences in the United States. Arch Assess Psychol. 2023;13(1):69–92.
77. Dixon JN, Caddell TM, Alexander AA, Burchett D, Anderson JL, Marek RJ, Glassmire DM. Adapting assessment processes to consider cultural mistrust in forensic practices: an example with the MMPI instruments. Law Hum Behav. 2023;47(1):292.
78. Shumaker NE. Exploring potential ethnic bias among MMPI-3 scales in assessing personality psychopathology (Doctoral dissertation). Sam Houston State University; 2022.
79. Benuto LT, Casas JB, Bennett NM, Leany BD. The MMPI-2-RF: a pilot study of Latinx vs. non-Latinx Whites profiles. Prof Psychol Res Pract. 2020;51(5):496.
80. Estrada AR, Smith SR. An exploration of Latina/o respondent scores on the Personality Assessment Inventory. Curr Psychol. 2019;38:782–91.

81. McGrady ME, Pai AL, Prosser LA. Using discrete choice experiments to develop and deliver patient-centered psychological interventions: a systematic review. Health Psychol Rev. 2021;15(2):314–32.
82. Ranjbar N, Erb M, Mohammad O, Moreno FA. Trauma-informed care and cultural humility in the mental health care of people from minoritized communities. Focus. 2020;18(1):8–15.
83. American Psychological Association. Ethical principles of psychologists and code of conduct. American Psychological Association; 2020. https://www.apa.org/ethics.code.
84. Fix RL, Silverstein MW, Nuhu N, Gray WN. Scholars committed to opportunities in psychological education: a training and mentoring program for future psychologists of color. Mentor Tutor Partnership Learn. 2020;28(1):44–59.
85. Sax MR, Lawson AK. Emotional support for infertility patients: integrating mental health professionals in the fertility care team. Women. 2022;2(1):68–75.

Chapter 18
Recognizing and Ameliorating Provider Implicit Bias

Danielle A. Kaplan

Introduction

As is true for all people, reproductive healthcare providers hold biases about those they consider to be the "other." These biases, whether implicit or explicit, negatively impact the diagnosis and clinical care of patients who hold marginalized identities. For example, implicit bias routinely causes healthcare providers to ascribe to the historically based myths about the hyperfertility of Black and Latina women [1]. Combined with the structural factors that decrease BIPOC women's access to regular, high-quality reproductive healthcare, this misapprehension can result in decreased or delayed rates of referral to infertility care—a healthcare disparity that is directly tied to a decreased likelihood of live birth among Black and Latina women in infertility treatment [2]. Women with disabilities are also significantly less likely to receive routine gynecological or preconception care, with studies as recent as 2014 suggesting that over 40% of gynecology practices are physically inaccessible to them [3]. In a striking parallel to the myth of Black women's hyperfertility, most research on the reproductive lives of women with disabilities has focused on preventing unintended pregnancies. In truth, however, women with disabilities are significantly more likely to experience infertility and significantly less likely to access infertility treatment [4]. Provider implicit biases have also been shown to impact the fertility care experiences of LGBTQIA+ individuals and couples [5], linguistic and religious minorities [6], and other non-White, nonaffluent users of infertility care.

The impact of provider bias on the infertility experiences of specific groups is covered at length elsewhere in this volume. It is clear, however, that recognizing and ameliorating provider biases that exist on both an implicit and explicit level is

D. A. Kaplan (✉)
Department of Psychiatry, NYU Langone Medical Center, New York, NY, USA

D. A. Kaplan (ed.), *Cultural Responsiveness in Assisted Reproductive Technology*, https://doi.org/10.1007/978-3-031-76204-8_18

integral to providing culturally responsive ART care. Addressing the existence and impact of bias on a diverse patient population involves intervention at the level of both the individual provider and the broader system of infertility care delivery. Effective efforts to decrease the impact of provider and clinic biases begin long before minoritized patients come face to face with their care providers, starting with the programs and institutions in which reproductive endocrinology and infertility (REI) clinic staff and affiliated providers are trained.

Experimental Interventions

Most efforts to address implicit bias have fallen into one of two categories. The first comprises several experimental interventions referred to collectively as "debiasing" interventions. Such interventions might involve exposing subjects to information that runs counter to their implicit biases [7]. For example, attempts to counter the implicit association between physical and intellectual disability might involve providing subjects with information about the pioneering disability-rights advocate Judy Heumann, who was instrumental in bringing about educational reform for students with disabilities and who subsequently served as an advisor to the World Bank. Some researchers have studied the impact of pairing cues related to the stereotyped group with words or concepts that evoke positive associations. Others have attempted to prime participants with explicit instructions meant to overcome bias, such as reminding them that some aspects of a narrative might be irrelevant before asking them to draw conclusions about its subject [8].

Debiasing interventions have two goals: the first is to reduce scores on measures of implicit bias such as the Implicit Associations Test. The second, of far greater importance for members of stereotyped groups, is to reduce the frequency of discriminatory practices that result from implicit biases and their impact in the workplace and healthcare settings.

Early studies [9, 10] suggested that debiasing interventions held promise for decreasing implicit bias among research subjects. However, a closer look at the literature suggests that these interventions show their greatest—and perhaps their only—effectiveness in the very short term. Recent findings suggest that the most significant impact of debiasing interventions occurs within the first 15 minutes of presenting information that runs counter to learned associations [11]. In the majority of studies, participant scores on measures of implicit bias administered as soon as a day after the information is presented have returned to baseline [12]. These findings raise the question of whether debiasing interventions outside a laboratory setting have any real-world impact. After all, it is impractical at best and impossible on a large scale for healthcare providers to be presented with debiasing information prior to seeing every patient about whom they might carry an unconscious negative association.

The rapidity with which implicit biases revert to baseline is unsurprising. In the words of one physician presented with his results on the Implicit Associations Test:

> "And part of the unconscious part of it is also, like personally like what you've grown up seeing, hearing, you know that kind of gets embedded in it, and I think to overcome that you have to be very active and diligent about it. I think it's very hard because, especially if you've had 25 years, right, from a physician's perspective before you start training, so to deconstruct all those stigmas, I mean that takes a while, and it has to be done, you have to actively seek it out and do it." [13, p. 4]

Debiasing interventions were based on the assumption that a single positive exposure to a member of a stereotyped group could undo a lifetime of conditioned associations developed through media exposure, parental and community messaging, and underrepresentation of stereotyped groups in positions of power and influence. The short-term impact of these interventions suggests that this assumption was unduly optimistic. With this understanding, subsequent efforts towards decreasing implicit bias relied less on a single-session intervention and more on helping participants become aware of the universal existence of implicit biases and providing tools to counter them [12].

The next generation of researchers and anti-bias educators turned increasingly to group-based interventions to aid in this goal. The specific components of these interventions vary across studies and contexts, making it difficult to study their impact as a whole. However, group-based bias reduction efforts are typically conducted by a facilitator whose professional focus is on Diversity, Equity, Inclusion, and Belonging (DEIB). The facilitator meets with a group to present interventions and engage in experiential exercises that broadly fall under the heading of "diversity training." These trainings often involve discussing the pervasiveness of implicit bias, helping group members to become aware of their biases through taking the Implicit Associations Test or game-based simulations, providing training in mindfulness to encourage participants to slow down their automatic responses, and providing counter-stereotypical exemplars of stereotyped groups [14–16].

Of these components, only providing examples that run counter to implicit biases and reminding participants to remember their intentions when interacting with members of stereotyped groups have been tested empirically [15]. Like individual debiasing interventions, group-based bias reduction training shows its greatest effects immediately after the intervention; data on the durability of changes in participant implicit biases are limited. Critics of group-based interventions have also correctly pointed out that increasing awareness of bias as it pertains to one stereotyped group might not translate into comparable awareness of the experiences of groups that are not specifically discussed [15]. Making group participants aware of the contributions of Latinx people to science, medicine, and the arts, for example, may have no impact on participants' biases about people with disabilities or even other people of color. The dearth of empirical research on the components of group-based interventions and the heterogeneity of these interventions and the training of those who conduct them suggest that any conclusions as to their efficacy are tentative at best [12].

Naturalistic Interventions

A common extension of the group-based interventions studied in experimental settings involves diversity training at the organizational level. Like laboratory interventions, organizational "diversity training" connotes a wide umbrella of interventions and is conducted by facilitators with a range of expertise and training. Components of organizational diversity training often mirror those used in laboratory settings. Participants might additionally be encouraged to reflect on their identities, explore the relative power and privilege these identities confer, or imagine the lived experiences of the diverse patient populations they serve. In medical settings, participants often receive additional information about the history of racism in medical care, with those who specialize in reproductive medicine learning about the coerced or involuntary contributions of enslaved, poor, and disenfranchised people to advances in the field [17–20].

Research suggests that these interventions have limited efficacy in improving diverse representation in the workplace and decreasing workplace bias. Disappointingly, they can also actually contribute to a worse climate for stereotyped and minoritized groups. Kaiser [21] suggests that diversity training in which trainer recommendations are unsubstantiated by data can create an "illusory sense of fairness." This results in a workplace culture in which training recipients "legitimize the status quo by becoming less sensitive to discrimination targeted at underrepresented groups and reacting more harshly toward underrepresented group members who claim discrimination" (p. 504). In other words, having participated in implicit bias training can lead participants to become overly confident in their own awareness and ability to act in a bias-free manner. This creates the danger that they will view subsequent discrimination and bias complaints as reflecting a problem with the complainant rather than with their own behavior, which they now judge to be bias-proof.

Although the research on diversity training interventions has been conducted primarily in organizational settings, untested DEIB interventions in medical and mental health training can have similarly unintended consequences. In a series of studies on implicit bias reduction in medicine, physicians were presented with evidence of their own biases as demonstrated on the Implicit Associations Test. Although some demonstrated acceptance and a stated commitment to change, many responded with disbelief in the accuracy of their results, criticism of the test as a valid measure of their attitudes, or justification for their biases based on their experiences with patients [13, 22].

Similarly, mental health practitioners with more years of training and those who have taken specific coursework in multicultural awareness and competency generally report that they feel more competent to work with diverse client populations. Unfortunately, however, neither years of training nor having taken standalone coursework in cultural responsiveness actually produces demonstrable change in measures of counselors' implicit biases [23–26]. The only notable exception to this finding occurs when classes in multicultural awareness are taught by instructors who are themselves members of stereotyped groups—a finding that is most likely due to the effect of prolonged contact with an admired instructor rather than to the content of the course itself.

Despite their pervasiveness and promise, standalone DEIB interventions run the risk of leaving participants with a false sense of security about their immunity to bias. This is particularly troubling for the field of reproductive medicine because these are the interventions to which current providers are most likely to have been exposed through medical school coursework, in-service trainings, or conference presentations. Given that these trainings will continue to be the most accessible to the current generation of reproductive endocrinologists and affiliated staff, more research is needed on how to improve the effectiveness of these interventions. Research should focus on identifying the components of training that lead to a durable reduction in provider biases, and which actually result in an improved experience of care for diverse populations seeking ART. It should be noted that standalone diversity trainings have their greatest efficacy when they occur within organizations that demonstrate an ongoing commitment to diversity at all levels [16], including hiring, retention, and promotion practices and investment in the culturally responsive treatment of staff and patients alike.

Prolonged Contact

Prolonged and repeated interaction with members of groups to which one does not belong has long been recommended as a key component of ameliorating implicit bias. Anti-racist educators stress the importance of cross-racial and cross-cultural friendship, work, and worship [27]. Unlike other face-valid interventions with limited empirical support, however, prolonged contact with members of stereotyped groups is the only intervention that has reliably been shown to decrease implicit biases in both experimental and naturalistic settings. For example, White college students who were randomly assigned to have Black roommates demonstrated decreased negative associations with Black faces at the end of the academic year [28]. Similarly, medical students whose required rotations involved providing care in clinics with large LGBTQIA+ populations and who had the opportunity to learn with and from colleagues of diverse sexual orientations demonstrated decreased implicit bias related to sexual orientation at the end of their medical training [29].

Geographic proximity to diverse groups alone has little effect on the automatic associations through which implicit biases emerge. However, a structured context is not required for people to benefit from prolonged contact with members of marginalized groups. Friendships that are formed through participation in shared activities, worship, and informal social gatherings provide opportunities for new input and can help to mitigate learned associations. There is some evidence to suggest that friendships formed earlier in life play a more direct role in mitigating implicit bias, likely through providing early and consistent input through which associations are formed. In contrast, friendships formed in adulthood appear to have a greater impact on stated attitudes about race, ethnicity, and ability status than they do on internally held biases [27, 30].

Historically, our opportunity to interact with those whose lived experiences differ from our own has been limited by the communities in which we live, work, and socialize. As the world becomes increasingly connected through virtual spaces, however, the opportunities to address our biases through exposure to information about others' experiences increases. Providers of infertility care now have access to a world of literature, blogs, social media feeds and podcasts produced by members of marginalized communities, including those that are specific to their experiences with reproductive health and infertility. Although learning about the experience of one patient does not automatically provide us with information about another, becoming familiar with common themes and experiences discussed by minoritized patients in reproductive healthcare provides us with an additional check on our own potential snap judgments and reactions.

Interventions at the Level of the Provider

There is an increasing recognition that implicit bias exists among providers of infertility care and impacts patient engagement and treatment outcomes [6, 31–33]. Although this recognition has been accompanied by conceptual recommendations for best practices, to date there is no direct research on ameliorating implicit bias among ART practitioners and affiliated staff. However, best-practice guidelines developed in general medical care can provide some guidance for the individual practitioner and serve as a possible road map for infertility care providers and clinics seeking to lessen the impact of provider implicit bias on the patients they serve.

Intentionality

Every interaction with a patient from a stereotyped or marginalized group is an opportunity for reproductive healthcare providers to combat the effects of their assumptions and biases. Since implicit biases involve repeatedly inculcated automatic beliefs about members of stereotyped groups, Byrne and his colleagues [34] propose that a process of "rehabituation" is required for healthcare providers to approach their interactions with minoritized patients through a new lens. They suggest that providers use each new interaction with patients who are members of underprivileged or stereotyped social groups as an opportunity to reinforce and act on their commitment to health equity and egalitarian social values. As this intention becomes "chronically accessible," it competes with providers' tendency to revert to stereotypes in their interactions with patients. Similarly, being reminded of which aspects of patient presentation to attend to and where implicit biases are most likely to impact clinical judgment has been shown to increase healthcare providers' diagnostic accuracy and improve their treatment recommendations [35, 36]. As previously noted, the impact of similar reminders in a laboratory setting is brief [12]. ART providers are therefore most likely to benefit from this intervention if discussions about the impact of biases on provider judgment become a regular and normalized part of team meetings and patient case consultations.

Mindfulness

Multiple studies have shown that provider implicit biases are likely to have more of an impact on their interactions with patients when providers are tired, stressed, overworked, or under time constraints when making decisions [37]. This finding has led researchers to suggest that engaging in a regular mindfulness practice can decrease provider vulnerability to making clinical decisions that are influenced by their automatic associations [38, 39].

Research supports the effectiveness of a 10-minute mindfulness intervention in decreasing the impact of implicit bias in cross-racial interactions. Like many single-session interventions, this intervention may have its greatest direct efficacy in the moments immediately following mindfulness practice [40]. More hopefully, however, meta-analyses support the effectiveness of prolonged mindfulness training in reducing burnout, workplace stress, and depersonalization among nurses and physicians. A regular mindfulness practice by physicians has also been shown to have moderate effects on improving patient treatment outcomes and increasing patient-centered care [41–44]. To the extent that decreasing burnout and stress levels improves providers' ability to think critically and creatively in their interactions with patients, regular mindfulness practice continues to hold promise as an adjunctive intervention for decreasing the impact of providers' implicit bias on their treatment of infertility patients.

Brief mindfulness meditations, including those that are specific to infertility patients, are readily available online and as downloadable apps. Many IVF clinics also offer mind–body groups as a part of their complement of services for patients. The content of these groups often comprises mindful breathing techniques, a body scan exercise, and instructions for noticing and coexisting with unwanted or painful thoughts and experiences as they arise. These techniques are easily modifiable for providers in reproductive medicine who are interested in incorporating a mindfulness practice into their personal and professional self-care.

Although mindfulness-based strategies used over time show promise in decreasing care providers' vulnerability to implicit bias, the work of combatting bias requires repeated action across multiple domains. The goal of decreasing implicit bias must therefore coexist with explicit procedures and systemic safeguards that decrease the likelihood that provider implicit bias will compromise the quality of care given to minoritized patients.

PLACE Strategy

Galiatsatos and his colleagues [45] suggest that the impact of provider implicit bias can be lessened when the provider is reminded to attend to the key components of a provider–patient alliance. They propose that providers use the PLACE strategy to help them focus on these components. The text box below outlines the PLACE strategy and provides examples of how providers can employ it in interactions with ART patients.

PAUSE: Use mindful grounding to decrease the impact of amygdala activity on the interaction

LISTEN: Has my patient shared all their concerns? Have I checked my own comprehension?

"Is there anything else about your history of receiving medical care that you think is important for me to know?"

"I'm hearing that it took a long time for anyone to take your concerns about your menstrual cycle seriously. Do you feel like I understand what you've been trying to tell me today?"

ALLY: Have I asked my patient if I have addressed all their questions? Have I engaged in advocacy with the other members of the care team?

"This patient needs an ASL interpreter for follow-up appointments and monitoring. They are next scheduled to come in on Wednesday morning. Can we please arrange to have an interpreter present?"

COLLABORATE: How is my tone? My body language? Have I asked for my patient's input on the plan of care?

"We've talked about a number of options today and I understand that you might need some time to weigh them all out. At the moment, are there any that seem like they are off the table for you?"

EMPOWER (and maintain humility): Have I given my patient the tools, resources, and information they need to be a full partner in the treatment?

"Here is the information for the sperm banks that we typically work with. Unfortunately, I've realized that we don't have up-to-date information on the ones that have more donors of color, in part because there isn't great information out there. Is that something that matters to you in choosing a donor? I'm going to bring this up at the next donor team meeting and will make sure that someone gets this information to you."

"Our clinic offers a mind-body group for fertility patients and I'm happy to provide you with information about that. Would you be interested in information about other types of support that are specific to the Orthodox Jewish community? Are there other kinds of support that feel more relevant to you?"

As the examples above demonstrate, empowering patients with the resources necessary to partner in their treatment requires fertility clinics and affiliated providers to be equipped with references, referrals, and information that are relevant to a diverse patient population.

Language and Talk Time

Recordings of physician–patient interactions have shown that physicians with high levels of implicit bias use more simplified and negative language when talking with minoritized patients than they do with White patients. Relatedly, studies of provider–patient talk time ratios show that these physicians also talk substantially more in their interactions with Black and Hispanic patients than do the patients themselves [46–48]. Speaking down to, over, or more than one's patient decreases trust in the patient–provider interaction [47], a factor associated with decreased rates of accessing fertility services among minoritized patients [6] and decreased satisfaction with fertility treatment among patients in general [49].

Similarly, reviews of medical student charting and clinic-based electronic health records demonstrate that providers who are higher in implicit bias use more negative language when documenting patient encounters with patients from marginalized communities [50–52]. Negative language enshrined in the medical record has implications for both how the provider recalls their interaction with the patient and how the patient is viewed by the rest of the medical team. Consider, for example, the impact of documenting a patient's discomfort with a treatment recommendation in the following ways:

> *"Ms. X is a 43 year-old single Black woman who needs donor sperm. Ms. X was resistant to my recommendation that she proceed directly to an embryo creation cycle instead of attempting IUI. She became agitated when presented with data about the likelihood of conceiving via IUI and repeatedly challenged my assertion that she was unlikely to conceive successfully with this procedure."*
>
> *"Ms. X is a 43 year-old Black woman. She does not currently have a partner and is interested in conceiving via sperm donation. I discussed with Ms. X the low likelihood of conceiving via IUI and suggested that she move directly to an embryo creation cycle. Ms. X became quite upset when presented with this recommendation, which she had not expected, and has many questions that she would like to address before she is comfortable proceeding."*

Interestingly, there is some suggestion that the impact of physician bias can also be ameliorated when minoritized patients are coached to be more active in interactions with their doctors. In a study of simulated patients, Black patients were coached to present with a list of questions, speak more, and advocate for themselves during the meeting with their physician. Blind raters rated the quality of physician–patient interactions as higher for patients who had been coached to take a more active role regardless of the level of implicit bias demonstrated by their physicians [53]. The authors hypothesize that when minoritized patients take a more active role in their treatment and provide their doctors with more information about their needs, wishes, and the context in which they present for care, their physicians are more likely to view them as whole people and not solely as members of a stereotyped group.

Importantly, the authors caution that "patients from minoritized groups are disproportionately burdened to handle discrimination within the health care system, and asking them to actively engage to reduce biases can exacerbate this burden. Thus, for both practical and ethical reasons, scholars and clinicians must also focus on developing and implementing health equity interventions that focus on changing clinician attitudes and behavior, as well as policies in health care systems." [53, p. 4].

Nevertheless, research on provider and patient language and talk time suggests useful in-the-moment guidelines for reducing the impact of provider implicit biases on marginalized patients' experiences in fertility care. Providers should be mindful of allowing ample time for patients to speak and encourage them to come to initial and follow-up meetings with a list of questions. As suggested by the "PLACE" strategy, providers should routinely ask patients if they have any concerns or discomfort with the treatment options being suggested and if there is anything in the patient's personal or medical history that is relevant to their selection of treatment options. Finally, providers should review their charting for use of potentially biasing language such as "challenging", "resistant", "argumentative," and "agitated" and make sure to use consistent terminology across patients when documenting patient encounters and describing patients' demeanor and affect.

Interventions at the Level of the Clinic

At a structural level, all clinics should ensure that their forms, policies, and procedures promote equitable access to care for all patients pursuing infertility treatment. For example, clinics should ensure that their referral list for mental health providers who specialize in infertility counseling includes culturally and linguistically diverse providers and those who have specific expertise in LGBTQIA+ family building. Clinics are also advised to generate resource lists that are relevant to a diverse patient population, such as a list of fertility grants that are available to specific populations to aid in financing their treatment. REIs and nurses who refer patients in distress for psychological support would be well served to familiarize themselves with both in-person and Internet-based resources for patients of color experiencing infertility.

Clinic forms should also reflect inclusive language and contain space for patients to self-identify with respect to their gender, race, or ethnicity, and any reasonable accommodations that they require to participate in and benefit from treatment. Relatedly, injection training videos and written information about treatment and medications should be available in the patient's language of greatest comfort and, optimally, at a variety of lexical levels.

Patients should also be asked proactively whether they require an interpreter for medical appointments or physical accommodations related to a disability. Multiple executive orders underscore the need for healthcare providers to provide linguistically appropriate services for patients with limited English proficiency. At the time of this writing, at least 43 states have enacted legislation addressing the issue of language access in healthcare settings [54]. Further, the provision of linguistically appropriate accommodations at the expense of the healthcare provider is a requirement of Title VI of the Civil Rights Act for all institutions receiving federal funding; requiring patients to assume the cost of an interpreter or asking them to bring a family member to appointments to interpret is therefore a civil rights violation and should be avoided. It should be noted that Title VI applies to any institution built in whole or part with federal funding and compliance with its tenets is required in all programs housed under the auspices of that institution, regardless of whether the specific program is funded through federal assistance [55].

Decision Blinding and Discretion Elimination

Decision blinding involves procedures that prevent a decision maker from knowing the demographic characteristics of a person being evaluated, making it functionally impossible for implicit biases to impact decision making. For example, a professor grading an essay from which the name of the student has been removed is able to attend only to the characteristics of the essay rather than those of its author. Relatedly, *discretion elimination* includes procedures that restrict the basis for making a decision to information that is relevant to the decision itself and requires the person making the decision to disregard irrelevant demographic information [12]. Discretion elimination would be at play if anyone able to run a mile in under 7 minutes were invited to join the high school track team, regardless of their gender.

The practice of ART and affiliated services involves an individualized approach to patient care in which patient demographics such as age, gender, and race are critical pieces of data that inform treatment and are essential to the delivery of patient-centered care. Nevertheless, providers interested in ameliorating the effects of implicit bias on patient care must balance individualized treatment planning with having standardized criteria in place for decisions about common treatment scenarios. For example, the stereotype of the "angry Black woman" (or, conversely, the possibility that women of color might refrain from overt expressions of distress during consultations out of concern that they will be judged too angry) could lead to infertility care providers referring patients of color for mental health support at differential rates [56]. Similarly, Kirubarajan [6] cautions against providers offering different treatment options to patients of color based on the provider's assumptions about what patients can afford. Having standardized criteria for treatment suggestions and referrals allows the infertility care provider to be aware of when they are deviating from their standard approach—a useful check on whether implicit biases might be impacting treatment decisions.

As the ART world increasingly explores ways of integrating Artificial Intelligence (AI) technology into clinical care, opportunities to employ decision blinding and discretion elimination in clinical decision-making might become more realistic. For example, the use of AI to assist in embryo grading and selection already holds promise as a means of decreasing provider bias in the laboratory. As similar algorithms are developed for reviewing patients' bloodwork, ultrasounds, and response to medication, there will be increasing opportunities to determine whether standardized criteria are useful in decreasing the impact of provider implicit bias while preserving the virtues of individualized care and decision making [57–59].

Structural Remedies and the Pipeline Problem

In 2019, the National Equity Project released a paper aptly entitled "Don't Talk About Implicit Bias Without Talking About Structural Racism" [60]. In it, the authors remind us that structural inequities in housing, education, policing practices, and healthcare produce differentially negative outcomes for racialized and minoritized people. These negative outcomes reinforce harmful stereotypes about members of these groups, and these stereotypes are in turn used as justification for perpetuating inequitable practices. For example, inequitable hiring practices can lead to a disproportionate number of Black and Latinx patients who are on public insurance rather than employer-subsidized plans. The medications prescribed by healthcare providers may not be in the formulary of approved medications for public insurance plans, making them prohibitively expensive for patients. Patients who cannot afford medication cannot take it regularly; these patients may therefore be viewed by their providers as nonadherent to treatment recommendations and the provider–patient relationship may be compromised as a result.

The impact of structural racism on the lived experiences and fertility outcomes of marginalized patients is discussed at length throughout this volume, as are the components of its remedies. For true equity in healthcare to exist, however, it is necessary to examine the root causes and structural determinants of inequities in reproductive and infertility healthcare across multiple levels. This includes the recognition that attempts to address provider biases at the individual level must be coupled with an attempt to remedy the structural inequities that exist within the field of reproductive healthcare itself.

Among the most obvious structural inequities in reproductive healthcare is the fact that REIs, clinic staff, and affiliated healthcare providers rarely mirror the demographics of the general population. In the 2020–2021 training year, 63.5% of REI fellows were White, 10% were Asian, 3% were Hispanic/Latinx, and 6.5% were Black [61]. Recent data about the demographic characteristics of nurses suggest a similar trend, with 80% of nurses self-identifying as White, 6.3% as Black, 7.4% as Asian/Pacific Islander, and 6.9% as Hispanic/Latinx [62]. Similar patterns hold among embryologists [63] and psychologists, an overwhelming 84% of whom identify as White [64]. Across all these fields, Native American and Pacific Islander representation remains vanishingly small. In contrast, the most recent US census data suggest that the percentage of the population identifying as Hispanic or Latino approaches 20%, and over 13.5% of the population identifies as Black or African American [65]. Any true effort to address biases in reproductive healthcare must therefore include active efforts to diversify the population of REIs and affiliated care providers.

Increasing representation of BIPOC reproductive endocrinologists, nurses, and affiliated staff is an intervention with multiple virtues. Diversifying the REI workplace increases the opportunity for providers themselves to interact in prolonged and meaningful ways with colleagues who hold multiple identities, providing them with ongoing opportunities to combat long-held associations and stereotypes about members of groups to which they do not belong. In this situation, benefits accrue both to the fertility care provider, who has the opportunity to interact with and learn from a more diverse group of colleagues, and to the infertility patient, who has the opportunity to receive care from a provider who is less susceptible to acting on implicit biases.

From a patient-centered perspective, diversifying the REI clinic and affiliated services also has multiple advantages. Patients who see their own multiple identities mirrored in the REI clinic staff are more likely to seek reproductive care and feel welcomed into the clinic when they do so. Data suggest that racial concordance between patients and providers may improve reproductive health outcomes for birthing people and neonates alike; there is some evidence suggesting that patients in infertility care would similarly benefit from racially and culturally concordant care [66–69].

Among patients who seek mental health support, racial or ethnic concordance between the therapist and patient predicts increased time in therapy and a stronger working alliance among patients who remain with their therapists for more than 3 months [70]. The stressors associated with infertility and its treatment are generally ongoing; mental health support for patients facing these stressors has been shown to reduce the odds of premature patient dropout from infertility treatment [71]. A more racially and culturally diverse therapist population with specialized training in reproductive mental health might increase the likelihood of marginalized patients in infertility care seeking out and remaining in mental health treatment, thereby increasing their odds of persisting in the face of adverse treatment outcomes.

Increasing diverse representation across the full spectrum of infertility care requires multiple structural interventions that begin long before the hiring process. It begins with the recruitment and retention of a diverse student population in medical, nursing, and mental health graduate training programs. Richard-Davis [72] has suggested multiple strategies for increasing the diversity of the medical student population, with the eventual aim of diversifying the REI workforce. Partnering with organizations involved in promoting STEM education in racialized and minoritized communities and engaging in outreach to colleges and universities with high BIPOC enrollment allows for the early introduction of reproductive endocrinology as a possible field of interest for young students who are beginning to contemplate possible career paths. Similarly, introducing reproductive and perinatal mental health into the curricula of undergraduate psychology courses and graduate programs in mental health can expose a more diverse group of students to this area of specialization.

Creating a more diverse REI workforce also involves employing more holistic criteria for medical school admissions. For example, admitting students with a wider range of MCAT scores has been demonstrated to diversify medical school enrollment without compromising student success [73]. Notably, parallel recommendations have been made for increasing diversity in psychology graduate training programs; it has been noted that publicizing the average GRE scores of the admitted class and overemphasizing a quantitative cutoff for admission rather than employing a holistic review process [74, 75] results in an over-admission of White applicants relative to the general population. Other structural interventions suggested to diversify the REI workforce include providing medical students from minoritized groups with mentors to support their opportunities to conduct research, apply for grants, and present at conferences, and increasing the diversity of the applicant pool invited to interview for REI fellowships [72, 76, 77].

Although the literature on increasing diversity in the REI workforce focuses primarily on racial and ethnic minority providers, truly diversifying infertility care means making training and work opportunities accessible and desirable to applicants whose diverse identities go beyond race and ethnicity. Advocates for diversity in the field should be mindful of the multiple identities that qualified applicants might hold. These include gender identity, sexual orientation, disability status, and neurodivergence. Currently, information about the percentage of REIs, nurses, reproductive mental health clinicians, and affiliated staff who hold these identities is scarce, while proposals for increasing recruitment and retention of multiply diverse individuals are nonexistent. This represents an area for further exploration so best practices can be developed.

Conclusions

Implicit biases are formed through a lifetime of learned associations. Similarly, recognizing and ameliorating them is the work of a lifetime. It involves a willingness to be immersed in unfamiliar settings, form new and meaningful relationships, and become aware of one's tendency to resort to overlearned habits and reactions when tired, stressed, or overworked. Although reducing implicit bias is an aspirational goal, concrete steps at the level of the individual provider, the organization, and the larger system can be put in place to decrease the impact of these biases on the patients they endeavor to serve. Through a combination of individual, organizational, and systemic efforts, the experiences and outcomes of minoritized patients in infertility care can be improved.

References

1. Ethics Committee of the American Society for Reproductive Medicine. Disparities in access to effective treatment for infertility in the United States: an Ethics Committee opinion. Fertil Steril. 2021;116(1):54–63.
2. Weiss MS, Marsh EE. Navigating unequal paths: racial disparities in the infertility journey. Obstet Gynecol. 2022;5:10–97.
3. Sonalkar S, Chavez V, McClusky J, Hunter TA, Mollen CJ. Gynecologic care for women with physical disabilities: a qualitative study of patients and providers. Womens Health Issues. 2020;30(2):136–41.
4. Ha S, Martinez V. Associations between disability and infertility among US reproductive-aged women. Int J Environ Res Public Health. 2021;18(6):3202.

5. Topper PS, Bauermeister JA, Golinkoff J. Fertility health information seeking among sexual minority women. Fertil Steril. 2022;117(2):399–407.
6. Kirubarajan A, Patel P, Leung S, Prethipan T, Sierra S. Barriers to fertility care for racial/ethnic minority groups: a qualitative systematic review. F&S Rev. 2021;2(2):150–9.
7. Lai CK, Skinner AL, Cooley E, Murrar S, Brauer M, Devos T, Calanchini J, Xiao YJ, Pedram C, Marshburn CK, Simon S. Reducing implicit racial preferences: II. Intervention effectiveness across time. J Exp Psychol Gen. 2016;145(8):1001.
8. Traub A. Judy Heumann, who fueled a revolution in disability rights, dies at 75. The New York Times. 2023 Mar 6:D7-L.
9. Aberson CL, Shoemaker C, Tomolillo C. Implicit bias and contact: the role of interethnic friendships. J Soc Psychol. 2004;144(3):335–47.
10. Turner RN, Crisp RJ. Imagining intergroup contact reduces implicit prejudice. Br J Soc Psychol. 2010;49(1):129–42.
11. Lai CK, Marini M, Lehr SA, Cerruti C, Shin JL, Joy-Gaba JA, Nosek BA. A comparative investigation of 17 interventions to reduce implicit racial preferences. J Exp Psychol Gen. 2014;143(4):1765–85.
12. Greenwald AG, Dasgupta N, Dovidio JF, Kang J, Moss-Racusin CA, Teachman BA. Implicit-bias remedies: treating discriminatory bias as a public-health problem. Psychol Sci Public Interest. 2022;23(1):7–40.
13. Sukhera J, Wodzinski M, Teunissen PW, Lingard L, Watling C. Striving while accepting: exploring the relationship between identity and implicit bias recognition and management. Acad Med. 2018;93(11S):S82–8.
14. Chang EH, Milkman KL, Gromet DM, Rebele RW, Massey C, Duckworth AL, Grant AM. The mixed effects of online diversity training. Proc Natl Acad Sci. 2019;116(16):7778–83.
15. Paluck EL, Porat R, Clark CS, Green DP. Prejudice reduction: progress and challenges. Annu Rev Psychol. 2021;72:533–60.
16. Kalev A, Dobbin F, Kelly E. Best practices or best guesses? Assessing the efficacy of corporate affirmative action and diversity policies. Am Sociol Rev. 2006;71(4):589–617.
17. Morewedge CK, Yoon H, Scopelliti I, Symborski CW, Korris JH, Kassam KS. Debiasing decisions: improved decision making with a single training intervention. Policy Insights Behav Brain Sci. 2015;2(1):129–40.
18. Carter ER, Onyeador IN, Lewis NA Jr. Developing & delivering effective anti-bias training: challenges & recommendations. Behav Sci Policy. 2020;6(1):57–70.
19. Brottman MR, Char DM, Hattori RA, Heeb R, Taff SD. Toward cultural competency in health care: a scoping review of the diversity and inclusion education literature. Acad Med. 2020;95(5):803–13.
20. Gutierrez KJ. The performance of "antiracism" curricula. N Engl J Med. 2020;383(11):e75.
21. Kaiser CR, Major B, Jurcevic I, Dover TL, Brady LM, Shapiro JR. Presumed fair: ironic effects of organizational diversity structures. J Pers Soc Psychol. 2013;104(3):504.
22. Stevens F, Shriver E. The shame of implicit racial bias. J Soc Psychol. 2024;164(2):258–72.
23. Boysen GA, Vogel DL. The relationship between level of training, implicit bias, and multicultural competency among counselor trainees. Train Educ Prof Psychol. 2008;2(2):103.
24. Boysen GA, Vogel DL. Bias in the classroom: types, frequencies, and responses. Teach Psychol. 2009;36(1):12–7.
25. Stevens FL, Abernethy AD. Neuroscience and racism: the power of groups for overcoming implicit bias. Int J Group Psychother. 2018;68(4):561–84.
26. DiAngelo R. Nice racism: how progressive white people perpetuate racial harm. Beacon Press; 2021.
27. Shook NJ, Fazio RH. Interracial roommate relationships: an experimental field test of the contact hypothesis. Psychol Sci. 2008;19(7):717–23.
28. Aberson CL. Friendships with blacks relate to lessened implicit preferences for whites over blacks. Collabra Psychol. 2019;5(1):16.

29. Phelan SM, Burke SE, Hardeman RR, White RO, Przedworski J, Dovidio JF, Perry SP, Plankey M, Cunningham B, Finstad D, Yeazel M. Medical school factors associated with changes in implicit and explicit bias against gay and lesbian people among 3492 graduating medical students. J Gen Intern Med. 2017;32:1193–201.
30. Sutton MY, Anachebe NF, Lee R, Skanes H. Racial and ethnic disparities in reproductive health services and outcomes, 2020. Obstet Gynecol. 2021;137(2):225–33.
31. Jackson-Bey T, Morris J, Jasper E, Edwards DR, Thornton K, Richard-Davis G, Plowden TC. Systematic review of racial and ethnic disparities in reproductive endocrinology and infertility: where do we stand today? F&S Rev. 2021;2(3):169–88.
32. Morris JR, Plowden TC, Green LJ, Edwards DR, Jackson-Bey T. Racial and ethnic variation in genetic susceptibility: are disparities in infertility prevalence and outcomes more than Black and White? Reprod Sci. 2022;29(7):2081–3.
33. Komorowski AS, Jain T. A review of disparities in access to infertility care and treatment outcomes among Hispanic women. Reprod Biol Endocrinol. 2022;20:1–7.
34. Byrne A, Tanesini A. Instilling new habits: addressing implicit bias in healthcare professionals. Adv Health Sci Educ. 2015;20:1255–62.
35. Gawronski B. Six lessons for a cogent science of implicit bias and its criticism. Perspect Psychol Sci. 2019;14(4):574–95.
36. Ungar T, Knaak S, Mantler E. Making the implicit explicit: a visual model for lowering the risk of implicit bias of mental/behavioural disorders on safety and quality of care. Healthc Manage Forum. 2021;34(2):72–6.
37. Dyrbye L, Herrin J, West CP, Wittlin NM, Dovidio JF, Hardeman R, Burke SE, Phelan S, Onyeador IN, Cunningham B, Van Ryn M. Association of racial bias with burnout among resident physicians. JAMA Netw Open. 2019;2(7):e197457.
38. Lueke A, Gibson B. Brief mindfulness meditation reduces discrimination. Psychol Consciousness Theory Res Pract. 2016;3(1):34.
39. Ivers NN, Johnson DA, Rogers JL. The association between implicit racial bias and mindfulness in mental health practitioners. J Couns Dev. 2021;99(1):11–23.
40. Braun SE, Mladen S, Crawford M, Edwards S, Kinser P. A constructivist grounded theory exploration of mindfulness for healthcare professional students. Complement Ther Clin Pract. 2023;50:101689.
41. Green AA, Kinchen EV. The effects of mindfulness meditation on stress and burnout in nurses. J Holist Nurs. 2021;39(4):356–68.
42. Suleiman-Martos N, Gomez-Urquiza JL, Aguayo-Estremera R, Cañadas-De La Fuente GA, De La Fuente-Solana EI, Albendín-García L. The effect of mindfulness training on burnout syndrome in nursing: a systematic review and meta-analysis. J Adv Nurs. 2020;76(5):1124–40.
43. Murphy J, Farrell K, Kealy MB, Kristiniak S. Mindfulness as a self-care strategy for healthcare professionals to reduce stress and implicit bias. J Interprof Educ Pract. 2023;30:100598.
44. Hofert SM, Tackett S, Gould N, Sibinga E. Mindfulness instruction for community-hospital physicians for burnout and patient care: a pilot study. J Patient Saf Risk Manage. 2020;25(1):15–21.
45. Galiatsatos P, O'Conor KJ, Wilson C, Myers C, Reeves J, Thomas WJ, Phillips A, Johnson S, Golden SH. A checklist to address implicit bias in healthcare settings during the COVID-19 pandemic: the PLACE strategy. Health Secur. 2022;20(3):261–3.
46. Hagiwara N, Penner LA, Gonzalez R, Eggly S, Dovidio JF, Gaertner SL, West T, Albrecht TL. Racial attitudes, physician–patient talk time ratio, and adherence in racially discordant medical interactions. Soc Sci Med. 2013;87:123–31.
47. Hagiwara N, Lafata JE, Mezuk B, Vrana SR, Fetters MD. Detecting implicit racial bias in provider communication behaviors to reduce disparities in healthcare: challenges, solutions, and future directions for provider communication training. Patient Educ Couns. 2019;102(9):1738–43.

48. Wolsiefer KJ, Mehl M, Moskowitz GB, Cagno CK, Zestcott CA, Tejeda-Padron A, Stone J. Investigating the relationship between resident physician implicit bias and language use during a clinical encounter with hispanic patients. Health Commun. 2023;38(1):124–32.
49. Shandley LM, Hipp HS, Anderson-Bialis J, Anderson-Bialis D, Boulet SL, McKenzie LJ, Kawwass JF. Patient-centered care: factors associated with reporting a positive experience at United States fertility clinics. Fertil Steril. 2020;113(4):797–810.
50. Sun M, Oliwa T, Peek ME, Tung EL. Negative patient descriptors: documenting racial bias in the electronic health record: study examines racial bias in the patient descriptors used in the electronic health record. Health Aff. 2022;41(2):203–11.
51. Goddu AP, O'Conor KJ, Lanzkron S, Saheed MO, Saha S, Peek ME, Haywood C, Beach MC. Do words matter? Stigmatizing language and the transmission of bias in the medical record. J Gen Intern Med. 2018;33:685–91.
52. Cobert J, Mills H, Lee A, Gologorskaya O, Espejo E, Jeon SY, Boscardin J, Heintz TA, Kennedy C, Ashana D, Chapman AC. Measuring implicit bias in intensive care unit notes using word embedding neural network models. Chest. 2024;165(6):1481–90.
53. Gainsburg I, Derricks V, Shields C, Fiscella K, Epstein R, Yu V, Griggs J. Patient activation reduces effects of implicit bias on doctor–patient interactions. Proc Natl Acad Sci. 2022;119(32):e2203915119.
54. Chen AH, Youdelman MK, Brooks J. The legal framework for language access in healthcare settings: title VI and beyond. J Gen Intern Med. 2007;22:362–7.
55. Where Does Title VI Apply? https://www.justice.gov/crt/fcs/T6manual5#:~:text=Where%20Does%20Title%20VI%20Apply%3F&text=3%5D,No%20person%20IN%20THE%20UNITED%20STATES%20shall%2C%20on%20the%20ground,activity%20receiving%20Federal%20financial%20assistance.
56. Ashley W. The angry black woman: the impact of pejorative stereotypes on psychotherapy with black women. Soc Work Public Health. 2014;29(1):27–34.
57. Sfakianoudis K, Maziotis E, Grigoriadis S, Pantou A, Kokkini G, Trypidi A, Giannelou P, Zikopoulos A, Angeli I, Vaxevanoglou T, Pantos K. Reporting on the value of artificial intelligence in predicting the optimal embryo for transfer: a systematic review including data synthesis. Biomedicine. 2022;10(3):697.
58. Kragh MF, Karstoft H. Embryo selection with artificial intelligence: how to evaluate and compare methods? J Assist Reprod Genet. 2021;38(7):1675–89.
59. Fitz VW, Kanakasabapathy MK, Thirumalaraju P, Kandula H, Ramirez LB, Boehnlein L, Swain JE, Curchoe CL, James K, Dimitriadis I, Souter I. Should there be an "AI" in TEAM? Embryologists selection of high implantation potential embryos improves with the aid of an artificial intelligence algorithm. J Assist Reprod Genet. 2021;38:2663–70.
60. Osta K, Vasquez H. Don't talk about implicit bias without talking about structural racism. 2020.
61. https://www.acgme.org/globalassets/pfassets/publicationsbooks/2021-2022_acgme__databook_document.pdf.
62. https://www.aacnnursing.org/news-data/fact-sheets/nursing-workforce-fact-sheet#:~:text=Considering%20racial%20backgrounds%2C%20the%20breakdown,Hawaiian%20or%20other%20Pacific%20Islander.
63. https://www.zippia.com/embryologist-jobs/demographics/.
64. American Psychological Association. Psychology's workforce is becoming more diverse: news on psychologist's education and employment from APA's center for workforce studies. Monitor Psychol. 2020;51(8):19.
65. data.census.gov.
66. Greenwood BN, Hardeman RR, Huang L, Sojourner A. Physician–patient racial concordance and disparities in birthing mortality for newborns. Proc Natl Acad Sci. 2020;117(35):21194–200.
67. Witt RE, Malcolm M, Colvin BN, Gill MR, Ofori J, Roy S, Lenze SN, Rogers CE, Colson ER. Racism and quality of neonatal intensive care: voices of black mothers. Pediatrics. 2022;150(3):e2022056971.

68. Husain F, Razai MS. Ethnic disparities in fertility care: causes and solutions. Obstet Gynaecol Reprod Med. 2022;32(10):240–2.
69. Alspaugh A, Suárez-Baquero DF, Mehra R, Lanshaw N, Joseph J, Combs M, Spiller K, McLemore MR, Franck LS. "Patients want to see people that look like them": aspiring midwives of color as resistance to racism through concordant care in the United States. SSM Qual Res Health. 2023;3:100226.
70. Cheng AW, Nakash O, Cruz-Gonzalez M, Fillbrunn MK, Alegría M. The association between patient–provider racial/ethnic concordance, working alliance, and length of treatment in behavioral health settings. Psychol Serv. 2023;20(S1):145.
71. Domar AD, Smith K, Conboy L, Iannone M, Alper M. A prospective investigation into the reasons why insured United States patients drop out of in vitro fertilization treatment. Fertil Steril. 2010;94(4):1457–9.
72. Richard-Davis G. The pipeline problem: barriers to access of black patients and providers in reproductive medicine. Fertil Steril. 2021;116(2):292–5.
73. Terregino CA, Saguil A, Price-Johnson T, Anachebe NF, Goodell K. The diversity and success of medical school applicants with scores in the middle third of the MCAT score scale. Acad Med. 2020;95(3):344–50.
74. Roberts MC, Ostreko A. GREs, public posting, and holistic admissions for diversity in professional psychology: commentary on Callahan et al. (2018). Train Educ Prof Psychol. 2018;12:286.
75. Callahan JL, Smotherman JM, Dziurzynski KE, Love PK, Kilmer ED, Niemann YF, Ruggero CJ. Diversity in the professional psychology training-to-workforce pipeline: results from doctoral psychology student population data. Train Educ Prof Psychol. 2018;12(4):273.
76. Sullivan LM, Velez AA, Longe N, Larese AM, Galea S. Removing the graduate record examination as an admissions requirement does not impact student success. Public Health Rev. 2022;43:1605023.
77. Taylor S, Iacobelli F, Luedke T, Matthews PA, Monge M, Cooper J, Moreira J, Grippo P, Girotti J, Molina Y, Yanez B. Improving health care career pipeline programs for underrepresented students: program design that makes a difference. Progr Commun Health Partnerships Res Educ Action. 2019;13(5):113.

Index

D. A. Kaplan (ed.), *Cultural Responsiveness in Assisted Reproductive Technology*, https://doi.org/10.1007/978-3-031-76204-8

H

I

J

L

GPSR Compliance

The European Union's (EU) General Product Safety Regulation (GPSR) is a set of rules that requires consumer products to be safe and our obligations to ensure this.

If you have any concerns about our products, you can contact us on ProductSafety@springernature.com

In case Publisher is established outside the EU, the EU authorized representative is:

Springer Nature Customer Service Center GmbH
Europaplatz 3
69115 Heidelberg, Germany

Batch number: 10726135

Printed by Printforce, the Netherlands